Diagnostic Techniques in
Veterinary Dermatology

Diagnostic Techniques in Veterinary Dermatology

Ariane Neuber

DrMedVet CertVD DECVD MRCVS
Director, Derm4Pets
Head of Dermatology, Chiltern Referral Services
Chalfont St Giles, UK

Tim Nuttall

BSc BVSc CertVD PhD CBiol MRSB MRCVS
Head of Dermatology
Royal (Dick) School of Veterinary Studies
University of Edinburgh
Edinburgh, UK

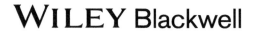

Registered Office(s)
John Wiley & Sons, Inc., 111 River Street, Hoboken, NJ 07030, USA
John Wiley & Sons Ltd, The Atrium, Southern Gate, Chichester, West Sussex, PO19 8SQ, UK

Editorial Office
9600 Garsington Road, Oxford, OX4 2DQ, UK

For details of our global editorial offices, customer services, and more information about Wiley products visit us at www.wiley.com.

Wiley also publishes its books in a variety of electronic formats and by print-on-demand. Some content that appears in standard print versions of this book may not be available in other formats.

Library of Congress Cataloging-in-Publication Data

Names: Neuber, Ariane, 1970- author. | Nuttall, Tim, 1967- author.
Title: Diagnostic techniques in veterinary dermatology : a manual of
   diagnostic techniques / Ariane Neuber, Tim Nuttall.
Description: Hoboken, NJ, USA : Wiley-Blackwell, 2017. | Includes
   bibliographical references and index. |
Identifiers: LCCN 2017005977 (print) | LCCN 2017015845 (ebook) | ISBN
   9781119233046 (Adobe PDF) | ISBN 9781119233060 (ePub) | ISBN 9781405139489
   (paperback)
Subjects: LCSH: Veterinary dermatology. | MESH: Skin Diseases–veterinary |
   Dog Diseases–diagnosis | Cat Diseases–diagnosis
Classification: LCC SF901 (ebook) | LCC SF901 .N48 2017 (print) | NLM SF
   992.S55 | DDC 636.089/65–dc23
LC record available at https://lccn.loc.gov/2017005977

Cover images: courtesy of the authors

Set in 10/12pt Warnock by Thomson Digital, Noida, India

10   9   8   7   6   5   4   3   2   1

Contents

1   Introduction to Dermatological Tests   *1*

2   Looking for Parasites   *21*

3   Hair Plucks and Trichograms   *41*

4   Dermoscopy   *53*

5   Cytology   *57*

6   Fungal and Bacterial Cultures and Identification   *81*

7   Introduction to Histopathology   *105*

8   Allergy Testing   *125*

9   Immune-Mediated Skin Diseases   *159*

10   Endocrine and Metabolic Skin Diseases   *173*

11   Infectious Diseases   *199*

12   Diagnostic Imaging   *215*

13   Otoscopy and Examination of the Ear   *235*

14   Which Test to Choose When   *257*

15   Genetic Tests for Skin Diseases   *277*

     Further Reading   *289*

     Index   *297*

1

Introduction to Dermatological Tests

Recent studies show that skin and ear diseases comprise 25% of all veterinary consultations. They are often complex and ongoing conditions that are a challenge to manage. Very few can be diagnosed on history and appearance alone. The modern approach to dermatology emphasises using the history and clinical signs to construct a logical differential diagnosis list. The diagnosis is then achieved by utilising appropriate tests to eliminate and/or confirm conditions in the differential diagnosis. On the other hand it is all too easy to become over-reliant on tests; it is most important that the clinical pathology is made to fit the history and clinical signs, not *vice versa*.

There is a very wide range of tests that can be used to investigate skin problems, but selecting, performing and interpreting the most appropriate tests in each case requires some experience. Many textbooks and journals, however, concentrate on individual skin conditions and assume that the reader is experienced enough to undertake the relevant diagnostic procedures. In practice, some of the most common reasons for poor management of skin conditions involve the inappropriate use of diagnostic tests, suboptimal execution of test procedures, inadequate sample choice and misinterpretation of results. The aim of this book, therefore, is to provide an illustrated, step-by-step guide to help you select, perform and interpret clinical tests and procedures for a range of dermatological presentations.

What Equipment Will You Need?

A wide range of equipment is necessary for thorough examination of the skin, which may seem daunting. The vast majority, however, are inexpensive, non-specialist items that are common to virtually all veterinary practices and do not need special skills to operate. The few items that are expensive and/or need specific training to use are all optional; they are undoubtedly useful, especially to dermatology specialists, but are not necessary to successfully practise veterinary dermatology.

Essential Equipment

- Good lighting is essential for proper examination of the skin, lesions and collected material. Good fluorescent room lighting is a minimal requirement and a high-intensity spotlight is necessary for any serious examination.

Diagnostic Techniques in Veterinary Dermatology, First Edition. Ariane Neuber and Tim Nuttall.
© 2017 Ariane Neuber and Tim Nuttall. Published 2017 by John Wiley & Sons, Ltd.

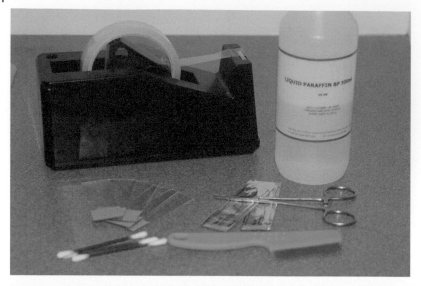

Figure 1.1 Some equipment needed for taking samples for skin parasitology: a flea comb, clear sticky tape, No. 10 scapel blades, cotton buds, liquid paraffin, artery forceps for taking hair pluckings and microscopic slides.

- Flea comb for coat combings (Figure 1.1).
- Hand lens or magnifying glass for close examination of the skin, coat and collected material; the large illuminated lenses sold for reading are most useful (Figure 1.2).
- A good-quality binocular microscope for examining hair plucks, skin scrapes and cytology (Figure 1.3).

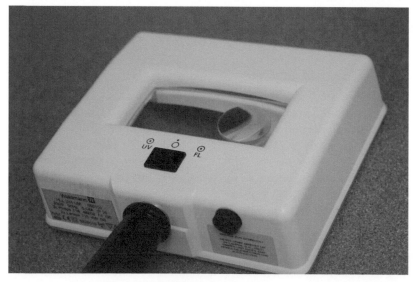

Figure 1.2 A magnifying lens with illumination. In this case the lamp doubles up as a Wood's lamp for dermatophyte detection.

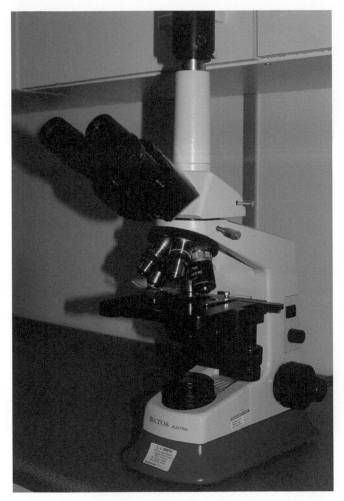

Figure 1.3 A good-quality microscope is essential to be able to correctly identify parasites, cells and microorganisms in the samples examined. The image shows a trinocular microscope with the option to attach a camera to document the findings.

- Glass slides for mounting material; frosted slides are easier to label (Figure 1.1 and Figure 1.4).
- Cover-slips are essential for any microscopic examination (Figure 1.4).
- Immersion oil for using the ×100 oil immersion microscope lens; different types of oil with different viscosities are available. Type A is the least viscous and is often preferred as it is the least messy and the cheapest. Type NVH is the most viscous. For in-house use, type B would also be suitable also but it is messier than type A (Figure 1.4).
- Lens tissue or cloth and cleaning fluid or alcohol for cleaning microscope lenses without damage.
- Otoscope for examining the ears (Figure 1.5).
- Wood's lamp for screening for fluorescent dermatophytes (Figure 1.2).
- Electric clippers for removing hair, allowing access to the skin.

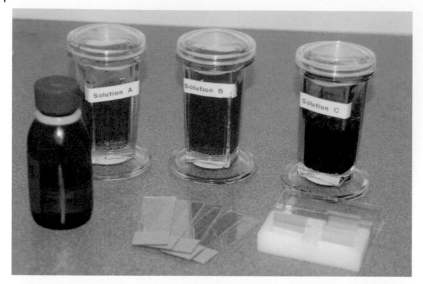

Figure 1.4 Essential microscope equipment: glass slides with a frosted edge for easy labelling, glass cover-slips to improve the optic performance under the microscope, immersion oil and a modified Romanowsky-type rapid staining solution kit.

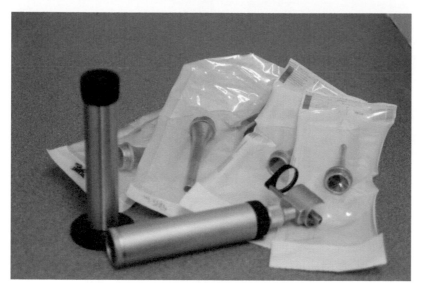

Figure 1.5 Equipment used for otoscopy: a handheld otoscope, various sizes of cones to be attached to the otoscope (all packaged individually after autoclaving to sterilise the cones after each use) and a cone cleaner to remove otic debris after use prior to sterilising.

- Curved scissors for more precise and less traumatic hair removal.
- Fine-tipped curved artery (mosquito) forceps for hair plucks (Figure 1.1).
- Liquid paraffin for skin scrapes (Figure 1.1).
- 20% potassium hydroxide as a clearing agent when looking for parasites or dermatophytes (optional).

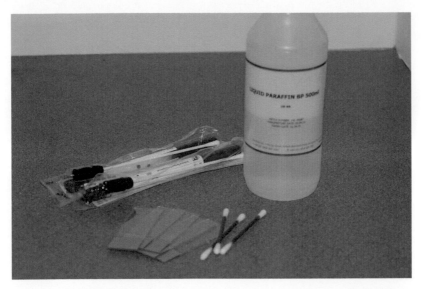

Figure 1.6 Equipment for obtaining samples from the ear canal: cotton buds, bacteriology swabs with transport medium, liquid paraffin and glass slides.

- No. 10 and No. 15 scalpel blades for skin scrapes and biopsies (Figure 1.1).
- Cotton buds for collecting material from the ears (Figure 1.6).
- Adhesive tape (Sellotape®, Scotch Tape® etc.) for skin surface parasites and cytology (Figure 1.1).
- Sterile bacteriology swabs with and without transport media; fine-tipped ENT swabs are useful for taking samples from narrow sites or when using otoscopes etc. (Figure 1.6).
- Sterile universal (30 mL) and bijoux (5 mL) containers for storing and transporting tissue samples (Figure 1.7).
- Diff-Quik® type stain for routine cytology (Figure 1.4).
- Toothbrushes to collect material for dermatophyte culture (Figure 1.8).
- Syringes and needles of various sizes for taking blood samples and aspirates (Figure 1.9).
- Blood collection tubes: plain, EDTA, heparin and gel-clotting tubes.
- Indelible marker pen to mark biopsy and skin test sites.
- 4-, 6- and 8-mm skin biopsy punches (Figure 1.7).
- Basic surgical kit and suture material for performing skin biopsies and closing skin wounds.
- 10% neutral buffered formalin for fixing biopsy specimens (Figure 1.7).

Optional Equipment

- Dermatophyte test medium for in-house dermatophyte culture.
- Lactophenol cotton blue is useful for staining dermatophyte colonies for identification if in-house cultures are performed.

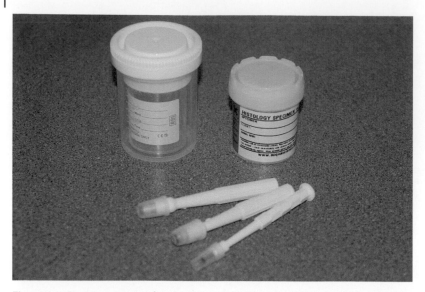

Figure 1.7 Some equipment for obtaining and transporting tissue samples (skin biopsy specimens): single-use biopsy punches in varying sizes and sterile containers with formalin saline for histopathology or empty for tissue culture.

- Special laboratory stains for cytology: Grams, Leishman, Giemsa, Ziehl–Nielsen etc.
- Intradermal allergen test kit for more experienced clinicians with an interest in dermatology to perform allergy testing in atopic dermatitis (Figure 1.10).
- Video-otoscope (Figure 1.11).

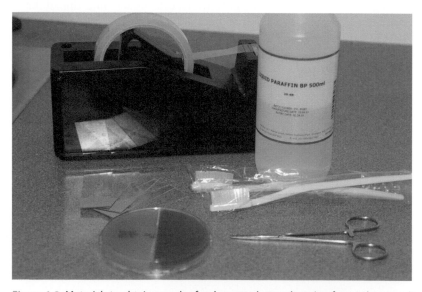

Figure 1.8 Materials to obtain samples for dermatophyte culture/perform in house cultures: clear sticky tape (for direct microscopy), liquid paraffin (for direct microscopy), sterile toothbrushes, artery forceps for hair plucks, glass slides for direct microscopy and a combined dermatophyte test medium (DTM) and Sabouraud agar plate for culture.

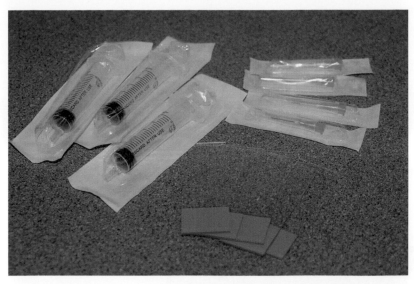

Figure 1.9 Materials for fine-needle aspirates: different gauge sterile single-use needles, 5-ml syringes and glass slides.

Use and Abuse of the Practice Microscope

No piece of equipment is so vital or subject to so much abuse as a microscope. Robust and inexpensive models with binocular lenses and integral light sources are easily mastered and give good results, but need looking after and must be used correctly for the best results.

Which Microscope Should I Buy?

Monocular microscopes or, even worse, those with mirrors for external lights, belong in a museum. The ideal microscope should have binocular eyepieces (with one capable of independent focusing), an integral light source, a focusing condenser, a mechanical stage, coarse and fine focus, and four lenses – ×4, ×10, ×40 and ×100 oil immersion (eyepieces are usually ×10 giving a final magnification of ×40 to ×1000). Dry (non-oil) ×60 lenses with a final magnification of ×600 are sometimes used instead of the oil immersion lens. Wide-field, stand-off eyepieces with rubber cups are best, as they can also be used when wearing glasses by folding the rubber cups down. The light source should provide white light (e.g. by using an LED) or have a daylight filter to convert the yellow–orange tungsten light to daylight (i.e blue–white). More expensive microscopes have a filter mount above the light source so that a variety of other filters can be used, although this is rarely necessary in general practice.

You essentially get what you pay for with microscopes. Despite this, budget models with the above features are perfectly adequate for most routine practice use. Cheaper lenses, however, can result in a curved edge to the field of view, which can be disorientating and/or trigger motion sickness. More expensive, flat-field (or planform)

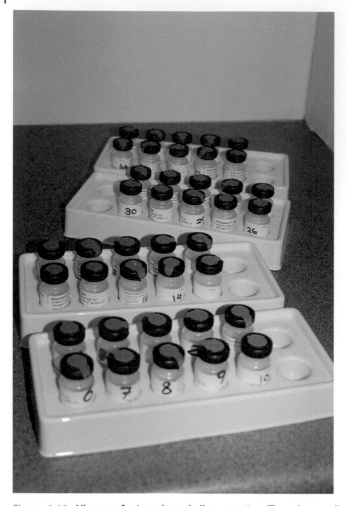

Figure 1.10 Allergens for intradermal allergy testing. The relevant allergens will vary regionally.

lenses achieve an even depth of field across the whole image and avoid edge effects. More regular or intensive users may appreciate the increased robustness, finer movement and improved image that come with more expensive, better-quality models. It is often possible to try various models on loan first to select one that best fits your budget and requirements.

Trinocular mounts or multiple-headed microscopes are more expensive and are generally used where hands-on teaching or archiving of images is important. In general practice, however, cameras can also be useful for real-time video to show other staff and/or clients, and taking still images for clinical records or to send for a second opinion. The best results are from using trinocular mounts connected to digital cameras and monitors. It is also possible attach inexpensive CCD cameras to eyepieces and feed images directly to a computer, although the quality is not usually as good as using a dedicated camera and mount. Some camera-equipped mobile phones and tablets placed against an eyepiece can also take fairly decent images.

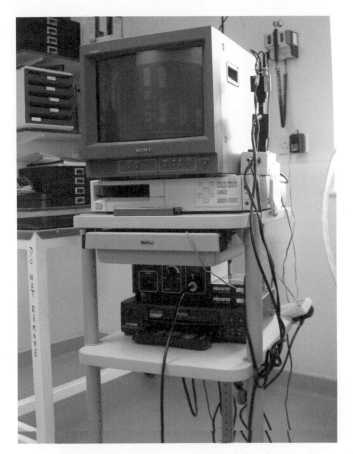

Figure 1.11 A video-otoscope is very helpful for performing deep ear flushes.

Microscope Set-Up: Where Should It Be?

It is important that the microscope is situated where it is comfortable to use. Discomfort will lead to you skimming slides in order to finish them as quickly as possible or, in the worst case, not using the microscope at all. There should be a dedicated site for microscopy with enough working surface and shelving for the microscope, clinical notes, clinical slides and ancillary equipment, such as clean slides, cover slips, immersion oil and cleaning materials. The working surface should be firm and stable. An adjustable seat (ideally with lower back support) will allow different users to maintain a comfortable, upright position. Some users may like to use elbow or forearm pads; placing split foam tubing insulation over the edge of the bench can also help. It is important to examine and adjust the arrangements if using the microscope causes strain.

Microscope Set-Up: Eye-Pieces and Illumination

It is also important to set the microscope up correctly. Incorrect adjustment can result in poor-quality images, eye strain, headaches and motion sickness. If these problems cannot be solved by the fairly simple steps outlined below or cleaning, get the microscope professionally serviced.

- Alter the separation between the eyepieces until you see a single, circular image.
- Focus to get a sharp image with relaxed eyes; don't strain to get the image in focus.
- Adjust the focus between the eyepieces for your eyesight. First focus normally on a slide with one eye looking through the fixed (non-adjustable) eyepiece. Next, close your first eye and then correct the focus for your other eye, if necessary, by adjusting the other eyepiece (using its independent focus). You will now have the two binocular images in perfect focus for each eye. Some microscopes enable you to note down the adjustment, which is useful for multiple users with different eyesight.
- Koehler illumination (Figure 1.12) focuses the light source on the slide, giving the optical illusion that the light comes from the sample. This avoids transillumination and gives you the best light balance and image quality. It is very easy to set up:
  - close the light source lens diaphragm so that you can see the edges in the image field using the ×4 or ×10 objective;
  - focus the condenser until edges of the diaphragm are sharp;
  - adjust the condenser centring screws until the light source is centred in the field of view;
  - open the diaphragm so that it is no longer visible and there is even illumination of the field of view;
  - some older microscopes do not have a light source lens diaphragm – if this is the case, hold a thin piece of card, paper, a paper-clip, or the tip of a pen or pencil against the light source and focus the condenser until you see a sharp image outline in the image field.

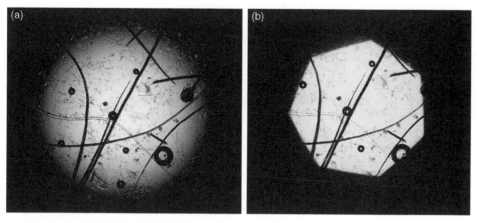

Figure 1.12 Koehler (Köhler) Illumination provides optimum contrast and image quality by focusing and spreading the light source evenly over the field of view. In these figures the light source diaphragm has been closed to set up Koehler illumination (in the absence of a light source diaphragm this can be approximated by holding a paperclip, piece of card or pencil point against the light source). a) The edge of the diaphragm is not in focus with the sample, which will result in poorer-quality images. b) Adjusting the condenser focus wheel (which moves the condenser lens independently of the slide stage) will bring the edge into focus and optimise the image.

- You can now adjust the iris diaphragm to give the clearest image for each lens:
  - for parasites and dermatophytes it is useful to close the iris diaphragm – the image is poorer but the increased contrast makes the parasites or fungi stand out better on unstained samples;
  - for cytology of stained preparations under high power, open the diaphragm to reduce contrast and improve the detail of the nucleus, cytoplasm, granules and microorganisms.

Dark Field Microscopy

Dark field microscopy is rarely used in clinical practice and few practice microscopes have dark field capability. However, it can be useful in liquid phase non-stained preparations (e.g. urine sediments, *Leptospira*, *Treponema paraluiscuniculi*, some endoparasites, insects in bedding, forage mites in foods etc.). It is also fairly easily to quickly modify most microscopes to do this.

The principle is that the centre of the light source is occluded, leaving the specimen illuminated only by scattered light from the margin. This gives a bright view of the specimen surrounded by a dark background. Dark field microscopes have occluding discs built in to the condenser. However, a similar effect can be achieved using discs of black card or insulation tape fixed to glass slides or discs and held against the light source, fitted to the light source filter holder or held against the base of the condenser. Ideally the edge of the disc should be just wider than the field of view for each lens. The condenser diaphragm and light intensity should be adjusted to give the best contrast for each view.

Scanning the Field

You should always use a cover-slip (or cover glass). The only exceptions are tape-strip preparations where the tape is, in effect, its own cover-slip. Microscope lenses are designed to 'look' through a cover-slip and fluid layer, which provides a flat optical surface, puts material in a similar focal field, avoids air–fluid interfaces and reduces contrast. Curved surfaces (including oil on top of the cover-slip) act as mini-lenses and cause serious distortion. Cover-slips can also protect the lenses from scratches and the mounting fluid, and provide a defined search area for skin scrapes etc. Mounting fluids include immersion oil and liquid paraffin or potassium hydroxide, if these were used for skin scrapes or for clearing hairs prior to examination for dermatophytes etc. Cover-slips can be permanently sealed to slides using mounting solutions such as DPX (or, if necessary, clear nail varnish), but this is only really needed if the slides are to be archived. It is important to use enough mounting fluid to seal the cover-slip to the slide without gaps or air bubbles, but not so much that it gets onto the microscope lenses or stage. Be very careful not to get any DPX or similar mountant onto the microscope lenses or stage.

Initially, visually examine the slide to orientate it, and appreciate the depth of material, degree of staining and possible areas of interest. It is useful to check the quality of staining visually or under low power before placing a cover-slip, as the slide can be re-stained at this stage if necessary. You should then study the slide at progressively higher magnification. Low-power lenses (×4–×10) are useful to scan large areas; with scrapes, plucks etc., start at one corner of the cover slip, proceeding down to the opposite edge, across one visual field and back up again to methodically search all the collected material. Use the high-power lens (×40) to close in on areas of interest. Use the oil-immersion lens (×100) last of all to avoid getting oil on the other lenses.

It is important that microscopic preparations are thin enough to allow proper examination without having to continually change focus. This is time consuming, tiring and diagnostic findings are easily missed. It is also time consuming to examine preparations that are too thin and spread out. It further follows that any material outside the area of the cover-slip will not be examined at all.

Cleaning

Cleaning is really, really important. In the first instance, make every effort to avoid contaminating the rest of the microscope with oil and debris. Many non-oil immersion lenses are not oil-proof, and will need replacing if oil gets in. Dried oil and skin debris can also clog up and jam stages and focus wheels. Clean the lenses and stage with lens cleaner and lint-free, fine tissue or lens cloths immediately after use. Commercial lens cleaner is best, but methylated spirits or similar alcohols are also effective. Do not use anything that will leave a residue, or coarse paper or cloths that could damage the lenses or leave fine particles of lint etc. Dried on immersion oil and debris can be removed by carefully rubbing the lens on polystyrene soaked in lens cleaner.

Stains

Diff-Quik* Type Stains

There are several Diff-Quik® type stains available. These are modified Romanowsky or Wright–Giemsa stains used to identify cells and microorganisms. They are the most commonly used stains in practice by virtue of their ease of use and interpretation. There are three pots: fixer (usually methanol or methylated alcohol, which is pale blue to green), stain 1 (eosinophilic – red) and stain 2 (basophilic – deep blue to purple). Staining efficiency declines over time and the pots can also accumulate skin debris, *Malassezia* and bacteria that can contaminate slides. In a busy laboratory, dispose of old solutions, rinse the pots and replenish from the stock solutions every 1–2 weeks.

There is a variety of ways to dry, fix and stain cytology samples. These have their advantages and disadvantages, and to some extent the method depends on personal preference. However, it is helpful to think about the sample and the method that might be best in each situation.

Two-Stain Method
Dip air-dried smears or tape-strips in each pot five to ten times for 1 second each time. The staining time will need to be longer for thicker, oily or waxy preparations. Rinse under a tap or with distilled water (directing the flow against the back of the slide stops

you flushing your preparation down the sink) and gently blot dry using textured paper towel without damaging the stained preparation. Wait for the rest of the water to evaporate or use a hand- or hair-dryer to completely dry the slide before applying a mounting agent and cover slip.

One-Stain Method

With this method simply put a drop of the basophilic stain directly onto the cytology preparation, place a cover-slip and examine. Alternatively, the stain can be rinsed off and the preparation dried as above. With tape-strips, place one drop of the stain on the slide, stick the tape down over the stain, blot away the excess and examine. This approach is very quick and easy, and particularly suitable for tape-strips or waxy preparations that are hard to dry and stain. This method, however, leads to a more monochromatic stain. This is perfectly adequate for identifying microorganisms, such as bacteria and *Malassezia*, but distinguishing different cell types is harder.

Checking Staining

Once the slide is ready, check the staining under low power; if it is adequate add a drop of oil and a cover slip; if not, re-stain. If necessary oil can be removed from slides for re-staining: place a piece of lens tissue on the slide, add one to two drops of xylene, acetone or methanol, allow the oil to pass into the lens tissue, and then carefully move it across the slide to remove the oil without damaging the smear. De-staining may be necessary if the slide is over-stained (the basophilic stain in particular can colour over cellular detail) or if using an alternative stain (e.g. Gram or Ziehl–Nielsen) is appropriate. Slides can be immersed in acetone, ethanol or methanol (you can also use the Diff-Quik® fixer in pot one) until sufficiently decolourised.

Heat Fixing

Waxy or oily preparations can be difficult to air dry and, as they are soluble in alcohol, may be lost during fixing and using the two-stain method described earlier. Heat fixing, by passing the slide through a Bunsen or spirit burner or hand- or hair-dryer until it is just hand hot, and then staining with the eosinophilic and basophilic stains, can avoid this. Heat fixing can easily damage cytology preparations if it overdone, however, and remember to let the slides cool before staining to avoid cracking them. Careful and thorough air drying using a hand- or hair-dryer and then staining in the usual fashion gives good results with most oily or waxy samples.

Staining Tape-Strips

Tape-strips can be stained by directly immersing the tape in the solutions. This is most easily done by attaching the two ends of the tape to a microscope slide to form a loop on the surface or over the end of the slide. After rinsing, detach one end of the loop and stick the tape flat against the slide, blot out the excess water and examine. The tape traps a thin layer of water next to the slide, so it is not usually necessary to use a cover-slip. Most fixatives dissolve adhesive tape and are best avoided – if using the two-stain method (see earlier) just dip the tape in the eosinophilic and then the basophilic stain. The stains will also turn some tapes opaque, and it may be necessary to experiment to find a locally available, compatible combination.

Other Romanowsky-Type Stains

Several other similar but distinct Romanowsky-type stains exist, but their use is mainly restricted to specialist laboratories as they are less straightforward and take longer than Diff-Quik® stains. **Wright's** (also known as Wright's–Giemsa) and **May–Grünwald** stains are particularly good at distinguishing fine cellular detail and are most frequently used for examining peripheral blood smears and bone marrow preparations. **Leishman's** (which is very similar to Wright's stain) and **Giemsa** are highly effective differential stains used to identify malaria, trypanosomes, other parasites and bacteria in peripheral blood smears, bone marrow specimens and other tissues. The stains are difficult and tedious to make up, and are best obtained from commercial sources.

Gram Staining

Gram staining is a relatively simple technique, but with the advent of Diff-Quik® type stains its use in practice has become less common. The technique is widely used in bacteriology to differentiate Gram-negative (which stain pale red–pink) and Gram-positive (which stain purple–blue) bacteria. Cell wall damage, aging or death may cause Gram-positive bacteria to appear Gram-negative. Gram stains can be performed on smears prepared from tissue samples or cultured colonies. There are various methods, which vary in slight details. One technique is as follows.

1) Air dry and gently heat fix the smear by passing the slide briefly through a Bunsen flame until just hot to the touch.
2) Cover the slide with crystal violet solution for 1 minute. Briefly wash in tap water and drain.
3) Cover with Gram's iodine solution for 1 minute. Wash off with tap water, drain and then blot up remaining water.
4) To decolourise the preparation, cover with 95% alcohol for 10 seconds, wash off with tap water and drain. Thick smears may need longer, but be careful not to overdo it.
5) Cover the slide with safranin solution (the counterstain) for 30 seconds, wash off with tap water, and then drain and blot dry prior to microscope examination.

Lactophenol Cotton Blue

Lactophenol cotton blue is widely used to stain fungal hyphae, microconidia and macroconidia for identification. It is commercially available and easy to use with preparations taken from fungal cultures in practice.

1) Place one to two drops of lactophenol cotton blue onto a microscope slide.
2) Tease a small amount of hyphae from the surface of a fungal culture into the stain.
3) Carefully place a cover-slip on the preparation for microscopic examination.

Clear adhesive tape is particularly good for collecting material for transfer to microscope slides and preserving the natural orientation of fungal elements.

1) Place one to two drops of lactophenol cotton blue onto a microscope slide.
2) Cut off a small piece of tape (approximately $0.5\,\text{cm}^2$), taking care not touch the adhesive surface.
3) Using forceps, gently touch the adhesive side to a fungal colony.

4) Lower the tape fungal (i.e. adhesive) side down onto the drops of stain and place a cover-slip for microscopic examination.
5) Alternatively, place the tape fungal side up, add one to two drops of stain onto the tape and then place the cover-slip.

Ziehl–Nielsen Stain

Ziehl–Nielsen (ZN) staining is used to identify mycobacteria that stain poorly or not at all with Gram or Romanowsky stains because of the mycolic acid waxes in their cell wall. Heating allows the carbol fuchsin stain to penetrate the cell wall, where it forms a complex with the mycolic acids. This fails to decolourise with mild acid treatment – hence the term acid fast. ZN stains can be used on cytology smears, histopathology sections and culture material, but are rarely performed outside of histopathology or cytology laboratories.

1) Cover the sample preparation with carbol fuchsin stain.
2) Heat the stain so that it gently steams for at least 5 minutes. Add more stain if necessary to prevent the preparation drying out and do not let the sample boil.
3) Remove from the flame and allow to cool slightly to prevent the glass slide cracking in the next step.
4) Cover with acid–alcohol for 20 seconds then rinse in tap water to stop the decolourisation.
5) Counterstain with methylene blue for 60 seconds, then rinse in tap water and blot dry.

Other Stains

There are various other stains that, again for reasons of time, expense and ease of use, are rarely performed outside of histopathology or cytology laboratories. Some stains that may be used include:

- **Haematoxylin and eosin (H&E)** is the most common tissue stain used in histopathology. Haematoxylin stains cell nuclei blue, while eosin stains cytoplasm, connective tissue and erythrocytes pink or red;
- **Periodic acid-Schiff (PAS)** stains carbohydrates such as glycogen, glycoprotein and proteoglycans. It is used to distinguish glycogen storage diseases and identify fungi in tissue sections;
- **Sudan stains** (such as Sudan III, Sudan IV, Oil Red O, and Sudan Black B) are used to detect lipids;
- **Methylene blue** is occasionally used to highlight nuclei in cytology specimens. It can also be used to stain hyphae, microconidia and macroconidia from cultured fungi.

Different staining methods are suitable for different types of samples and to examine the specimen for different types of cells and microorganisms. Table 1.1 summarises the uses of the various types of stain.

Using Internal and External Laboratories

Using your in-house laboratory is quicker, but may not be any cheaper once the full running costs are taken into account, and may not be any easier or more accurate

Table 1.1   Indications for the most common stains used on cytology samples and histopathology sections.

Stains	Uses
Modified Romanowsky or Wright-Giemsa (e.g. Diff-Quik®, Rapi-Diff®)	Routine rapid in-clinic staining of cytology samples and blood smears Differentiates cells, nucleus, cytoplasm, cytoplasmic granules, bacteria and fungi All organisms that stain with these stains will appear dark blue and the stains do not differentiate Gram-negative and Gram-positive bacteria
Haematoxylin and eosin (H&E)	Routine first-line histopathology stain May be combined with other stains to highlight specific organisms and substances
Gram	To identify bacteria in cytology samples and histopathology sections Differentiates Gram-negative and Gram-positive bacteria
Ziehl–Nielsen	To identify acid-fast bacteria, mainly mycobacteria but also *Nocardia* and *Rhodococcus*, and some protozoa (e.g. *Cryptosporidium*)
Grocott–Gomori's methenamine silver	Stains both living and dead fungal organisms
Periodic acid–Schiff (PAS)	Detects polysaccharides (e.g. glycogen), glycoproteins, glycolipids and mucins in histopathology sections Will stain living but not dead fungi
Giemsa	Accurate identification and differentiation of cells in cytology samples, bone marrow aspirates and blood smears To identify certain microorganisms (e.g. trypanosomes, spirochaetes, *Histoplasma*, *Chlamydia* and *Chlamydophila*, and protozoa)
Wright	Accurate identification and differentiation of cells in blood smears Combination Wright–Giemsa staining is widely used
Leishman	To identify leucocytes, blood-borne parasites and trypanosomes in blood smears
Sudan (Sudan II, Sudan III, Sudan IV, Oil Red O, and Sudan Black B)	To identify fat in cytology samples, histopathology sections and faeces
Congo red	To detect amyloid in histopathology sections
Toluidine blue	Detects mast cell granules in cytology samples and histopathology sections
Calcofluor-white	Fluorescent stain that identifies fungi, algae and related organisms on hairs, cytology samples and histopathology sections Most commonly used with fluorescent microscopes but stained hair samples on a standard microscope can be illuminated with a Wood's lamp to detect dermatophytes

depending on your experience and the equipment available. It is also important that all equipment is maintained properly and that quality control is conducted where appropriate (e.g. haematology and biochemistry analysers).

There are some tests – including serology, endocrine assays, microbial culture and sensitivity, and histopathology – that can only be performed in specialised laboratories. Most reputable laboratories perform these tests to a high standard and are open about their quality assurance measures. It is useful to develop a relationship with your laboratory; you will come to be familiar with their format and results and they will know what to expect from you. It also makes it easier to call in for advice – many laboratories now also have a network of clinical specialists that can give you advice on particular cases and results. It is also perfectly appropriate to use different laboratories for different tests, depending on their field of expertise, e.g. haematology and biochemistry, serological assays, endocrine assays, histopathology etc.

Dermatohistopathology, in particular, is becoming an increasingly specialised field and it is crucial that biopsy specimens go to a pathologist with a particular interest in skin diseases and who is clinically up to date. Many skin conditions can only be confirmed on histopathology and a number of new conditions are described each year. Some of these may be quite rare, leaving the pathologist in the ideal position to collate and disseminate information from their clinical colleagues.

How to Get the Best From an External Laboratory

- Take the appropriate samples. The bulk of this book is concerned with this, but check with the laboratory first if you are unsure. Some samples, for instance, may need special treatment or storage before despatch.
- Fill the submission forms in correctly, concisely and accurately. The amount of information will vary depending on the sample, but identification, age, sex and breed should be a minimum. Objective tests (e.g. blood tests) will require little else, but more clinical information can help the laboratory staff interpret the results.
- Skin biopsy specimens should be sent with a complete history, description of the clinical signs and differential diagnosis list. It can also be very helpful to attach photographs (it is very easy now to submit digital images by email) of the lesions. Each specimen should be submitted in a separate pot, clearly labelled with the biopsy site, to help match the histopathology to the clinical lesions.
- Package and label the samples correctly. You must ensure that legal requirements for posting pathological specimens are adhered to. Most laboratories now provide appropriate packaging and mailing containers, often with prepaid postage or a courier service. Guidelines for regulations in the UK can be found on: http://www .royalmail.com/sites/default/files/Guidance-Document-Infectious-Substances-171012 .pdf.
- Always consider test results in light of the history and clinical signs. If they do not fit, then discuss them with the laboratory. It may be necessary to re-evaluate the clinical data, test results or re-submit samples, but an incorrect diagnosis can lead to inappropriate and potentially life-threatening treatment. Very few diagnoses come out of the blue – virtually all rely on clinicopathological correlation of all the available data. Remember to use your clinical skills, and make the diagnosis fit the data – do not twist the findings to justify a diagnosis.

Sensitivity, Specificity, and Positive and Negative Predictive Value

Many journal articles and textbooks will refer to these statistical terms when referring to diagnostic tests. They can be qualified in absolute terms if figures are known (e.g. a test may have a sensitivity of 83%) or estimated in more relative terms (e.g. a test is highly sensitive but poorly specific). They describe the reliability with which tests can be used to confirm or rule out particular conditions. It is therefore important that clinicians have some understanding of these concepts when considering test results or trying to interpret published papers etc.

Sensitivity refers to the probability that a test will be positive if an animal has the condition tested for – in other words, how likely are false-negative results? **Specificity** refers to the probability that if animal does not have the disease, the test will be negative – in other words, how likely are false-positive results? An ideal test would have 100% sensitivity and specificity, but in practice virtually all tests will have some false-negative and false-positive results. An example of this would be using skin scrapes to detect *Sarcoptes* mites: if you find mites, then you can be nearly 100% sure that the animal has scabies, i.e. skin scrapes are highly specific for *Sarcoptes* infestation – there are no false-positives. Negative skin scrapes on the other hand do not rule out the possibility of scabies as you will not find mites in a large proportion of affected animals; i.e. skin scrapes are poorly sensitive for *Sarcoptes* infestations – there are many false-negatives.

The predictive values refer to the proportion of individuals for whom the test result is true. The **positive predictive value** (PPV) is the proportion of animals with a positive test that actually have the condition – i.e. that are correctly diagnosed. Conversely, the **negative predictive value** (NPV) is the proportion of animals with a negative test that do not have the condition.

The difference between these two sets of figures is that the sensitivity and specificity refer to inherent properties or accuracy of the test, whereas the PPV and the NPV give you some idea of the clinical usefulness of the test in a defined population that is tested. This is only useful, however, if the prevalence of the condition in the population is known as this has an effect on predictive values. For this reason, the sensitivity and specificity are more commonly quoted.

		Presence of the condition		
		Positive	Negative	
Test result	Positive	**True positive**	**False positive**	PPV
	Negative	**False negative**	**True negative**	NPV
		Sensitivity	Specificity	

Sensitivity = true positive/(true positive + false negative)
Specificity = true negative/(true negative + false positive)
PPV = true positive/(true positive + false positive)
NPV = true negative/(true negative + false negative)

Worked Example

Let us say that 100 dogs with pruritus have a serology test for *Sarcoptes* performed. Of these, 10 dogs have *Sarcoptes*: nine are positive on an enzyme-linked immunosorbent assay (ELISA) and one is negative. Of the remaining 90 dogs with another diagnosis, five are also positive on the ELISA.

		Presence of the condition		
		Positive	Negative	
Test result	Positive	**9**	**5**	PPV
	Negative	**1**	**85**	NPV
		Sensitivity	Specificity	

Sensitivity $= 9/(9 + 1) = 90\%$
Specificity $= 85/(85 + 5) = 94\%$
PPV $= 9/(9 + 5) = 64\%$
NPV $= 85/(85 + 1) = 99\%$

The test has a high sensitivity detecting 90% of *Sarcoptes* cases, and is highly specific, as 94% of animals with other dermatoses had a negative test. **In this population** of 100 tested animals the PPV is 64%, meaning that approximately two thirds of animals with a positive test have *Sarcoptes*, and the NPV is 99%, virtually excluding *Sarcoptes* in animals with a negative ELISA. In this example, the prevalence of *Sarcoptes* in the population is 10%. See how changing the prevalence (but keeping the sensitivity and specificity) affects the PPV and NPV. The PPV, in particular, can be poor for conditions with low prevalences, and, where possible, positive results for rare diseases should be confirmed with an alternative test.

When considering sensitivity and specificity it is also important to understand why the test has been used, the clinical presentation and what the expected outcome is. For example, urinary cortisol:creatinine ratios (UCCR) are quick, cheap and easy tests that can be used to diagnose canine hyperadrenocorticism (HAC). They are highly sensitive, as virtually all dogs with HAC have an elevated UCCR, but poorly specific, as UCCRs are also elevated in many other conditions. The diagnostic value in sick, polydipsic/polyuric animals can therefore be low; the UCCR is often elevated, but this can be of little clinical significance. It can, however, be a useful test in an otherwise healthy animal with alopecia, as a negative test will effectively eliminate HAC.

Before considering which test to perform, it is, therefore, important to think carefully about which differential diseases need to be investigated and which questions the clinician would like to have answered. Without careful consideration of these factors, the tests cannot give useful answers and this can effectively cost a lot of the client's money without reaching a diagnosis, which is most frustrating both for the attending vet and client. Although packages offered by commercial laboratories can be useful in some cases, using them without reflection is probably not the most effective use of the resources available to manage any given case.

2

Looking for Parasites

Introduction

Ectoparasites are a major cause of skin problems, particularly in patients with pruritus, alopecia (Figure 2.1) and scaling (Figure 2.2). Parasitic infestations are important differentials that should be confirmed or eliminated early in the investigation of virtually all animals presenting with skin problems. Techniques used to detect ectoparasites and/or immunological reactions to them include: visual inspection, coat combing (Figure 2.3), tape-strips, skin scrapes (Figure 2.4), faecal examination, intradermal tests and/or serology, and trial therapy. All of these approaches have their advantages and disadvantages. The sensitivity and specificity, furthermore, vary both between tests and the ectoparasites they are used to detect. Interpretation can therefore be difficult for the inexperienced.

Visual Inspection

A careful visual inspection of the skin and coat is mandatory in all cases of skin disease. This should cover the whole body, including the underside, feet and ears.

Technique

1) Manually groom the coat, carefully palpating and parting the hairs to reveal the underlying skin. Long hair should be parted, examined and lifted out of the way to allow further inspection.
2) Look at both surfaces of the feet, gently splaying the digits to expose the interdigital skin and, in cats, protrude the claws to reveal the claw sheath.
3) Evert skin folds as much as possible, including the cutaneous marginal pouch (Henry's pocket) (Figure 2.5) on the caudal margin of the pinna.
4) Searching the entire body with a hand lens is impractical, unless you have the time and patience, but it is useful to examine suspicious areas and predilection sites in more detail.
5) A full otoscopic examination can and should be done in all but very fractious animals.

Ectoparasites that you should be able to find with or without a hand lens/otoscope include the following.

Diagnostic Techniques in Veterinary Dermatology, First Edition. Ariane Neuber and Tim Nuttall.
© 2017 Ariane Neuber and Tim Nuttall. Published 2017 by John Wiley & Sons, Ltd.

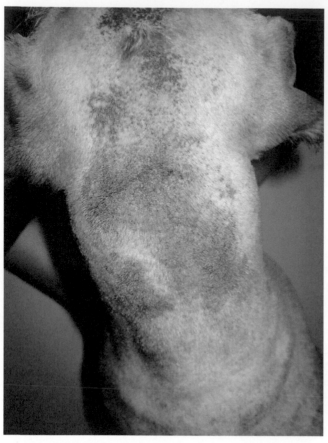

Figure 2.1 Alopecia and comedones in a dog with demodicosis. This is a good place to perform a deep skin scraping, looking for *Demodex* spp. mites.

- **Chiggers** (*Eutrombicula* spp.) or **harvest mites** (*Trombicula* [previously *Neotrombicula*] spp.; also called berry bugs in Scotland). The engorged larvae form characteristic aggregations of bright orange dots, although these are easy to miss on a cursory examination. Typical sites include interdigital skin (Figure 2.6), claw sheath in cats, distal limbs, axillae, ventral body, tail (often the very tip in cats), chin, facial folds and ears, particularly the cutaneous marginal pouch (Henry's pocket).
- **Ticks** – these are large, grey and distended (0.5–1.0 cm) after a blood meal; however, they are brown–black and much smaller (particularly immature forms) before a blood meal, and harder to find in haired skin. *Otobius* (the soft spinose ear tick) are found in the ear canals.
- **Lice** – large (2–3 mm), slow-moving, white–brown insects attached to hairs.
- **Fleas** – large (2–3 mm), red–brown and fast-moving or their faecal material (stationary) (Figure 2.7).
- **Otodectes** – these moderately large (0.4–0.5 mm), white–brown, readily mobile mites (Figure 2.8) can often be seen among debris in the ear canal, especially with a video-otoscope.

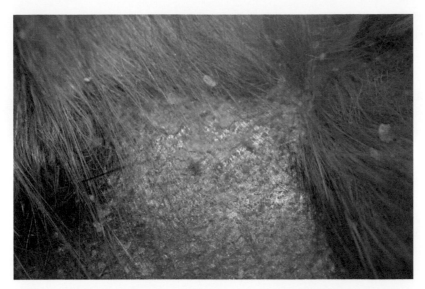

Figure 2.2 Scaling in a rabbit with cheyletiellosis. This is a good type of lesion to use some sticky tape to collect material for microscopy.

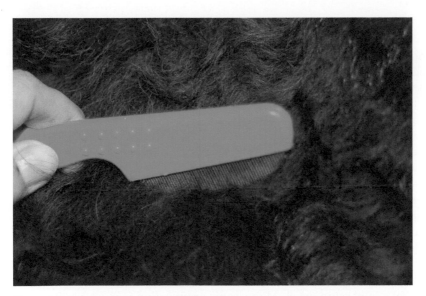

Figure 2.3 A flea comb is very useful to perform a coat combing. Comb the whole coat, collect the material on a piece of paper, remove hair and transfer debris to Petri dish or glass slide for examination. Alternatively, suspicious material can be used for a wet paper test.

- Other **surface parasites** such as *Cheyletiella* (0.3–0.4 mm) (Figure 2.9), *Chorioptes* and *Psoroptes* (0.5–0.8 mm) may also be seen. These are again moderately large mites that live among surface debris, and it is usually the movement of the debris caused by the mites' activity that is seen rather than the actual mites. This has given rise to the colloquialism 'walking dandruff' for cheyletiellosis.

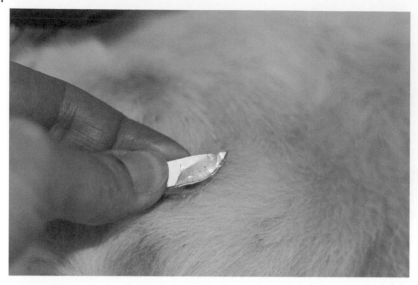

Figure 2.4 Skin scraping on the lateral elbow in a yellow Labrador Retriever with suspected sarcoptic mange.

Coat Brushings

Surface debris can be collected by a flea comb or stiff brushes. Vigorously brush the coat for 30–60 seconds trying to collect as much as possible from the skin surface. Heavy coats can prevent effective brushing and large amounts of hair can be difficult to sift through and examine. Try to remove excessive amounts of hair before examining the skin surface debris.

The material can be brushed onto dark card or a petri dish for examination with a hand lens. Most surface ectoparasites, such as lice, *Cheyletiella*, *Chorioptes*, *Psoroptes* etc., show up best against a dark background. It may be possible to find flea eggs (Figure 2.10), although these are rapidly lost into the environment. Flea faeces, conversely, are more obvious on a light background although the 'wet-paper' test is even more effective (see later in this section). Adult fleas will not hang around for examination, but should be obvious if encountered.

You can add the debris to liquid paraffin or potassium hydroxide on a microscope, apply a cover slip and examine using the ×4 lens. Adhesive tape can also be used to mount the collected debris on a microscope slide, although this does create bubbles and air interfaces that can obscure detail. Microscopic examination is more sensitive, but more time consuming. Trapping adult fleas with adhesive tape or drowning them in alcohol or formalin can nevertheless aid speciation, which may be useful when investigating the epidemiology of a flea infestation.

Flea faeces, which are largely partly digested blood, leave a reddish brown stain on moistened white paper or cotton wool – the so-called 'wet-paper' test (Figure 2.11). Adhesive tape-strips (see next section) may be a more sensitive way to detect small fragments, however. Dirt and other debris are easily distinguished by their grey–black–brown stains.

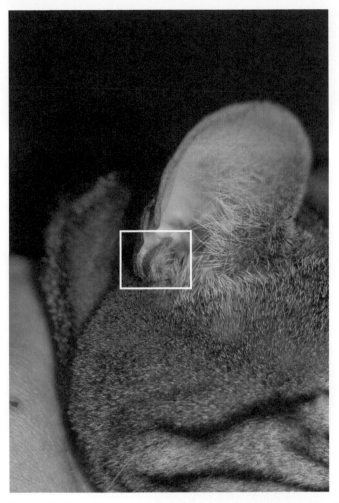

Figure 2.5 Henry's pocket in a cat. This is a body site that harvest mites can often be found in.

Otic cytology is particularly used to look for *Otodectes*, although other parasites such as *Demodex* (Figure 2.12) can also be seen in material from the ear canal. Debris from the external ear canal can be collected using cotton buds, ear loops or curettes, fine spatulas or forceps. Firmer foam buds with a triangular or spiral shape are also effective. Pushing cotton buds too far into the ear canal can impact debris deep into the horizontal canal, as the ear canal narrows towards the tympanic membrane. Flexible, red rubber or plastic instruments are best; metal spatulas, curettes and forceps must be used with care in unsedated animals as sudden movements could result in injury to the ear canal. Break up the collected debris into liquid paraffin or potassium hydroxide (see later in this chapter) on a microscope slide, place a cover-slip and examine under low power (×4 lens or ×10 lens to check suspicious objects).

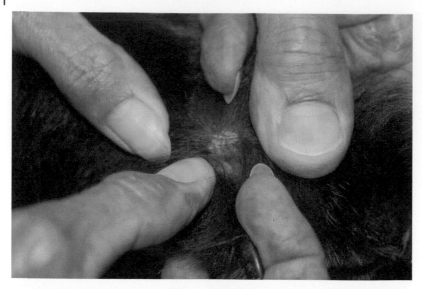

Figure 2.6 Harvest mites showing as orange to red dots in the interdigital areas of a dog. The mite infestation was associated with erythema and pruritus in this case.

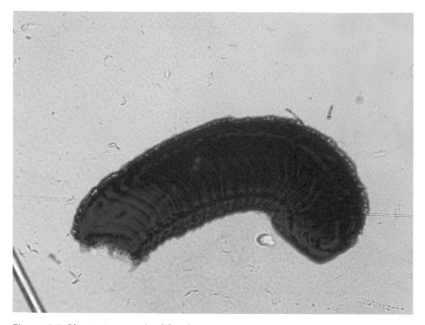

Figure 2.7 Photomicrograph of flea faeces. *Source:* Courtesy of Luisa Cornegliani.

Tape-Strips

Adhesive tape can be used to remove the outer layers of the stratum corneum with attached ectoparasites or microorganisms. Apply clear adhesive tape repeatedly to the

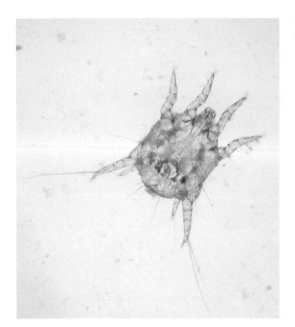

Figure 2.8 Photomicrograph of an adult *Otodectes* mite from a dog with otitis.

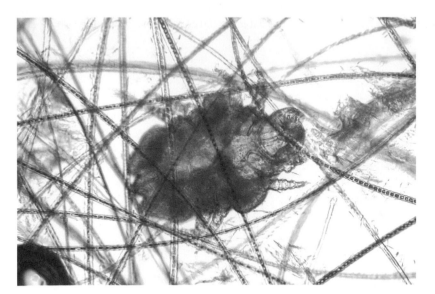

Figure 2.9 Photomicrograph of a *Cheyletiella* spp. mite from a rabbit with dorsal scaling.

skin until skin debris is clearly stuck to it and the tape is no longer sticky. Part the hairs to ensure that samples are from the skin and proximal hair shaft rather than the relatively sterile distal hair shaft. You can also gently shorten long hair, but be careful not to disturb the skin surface. Stick the tape to a microscope slide (no cover-slip is necessary) and

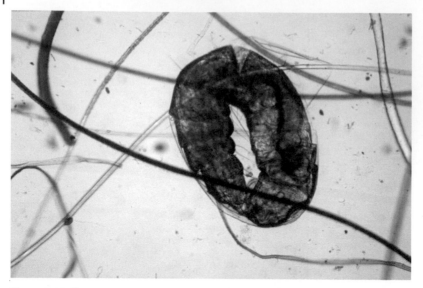

Figure 2.10 Flea eggs can rarely be seen on the animal. *Source:* Courtesy of Luisa Cornegliani.

examine with the ×4 lens, using the ×10 lens to check any suspicious material in greater detail. Flea faeces, lice, *Cheyletiella*, *Otodectes* and their eggs are all easily seen. Flea faeces, which are partly digested blood, are bright red. Crusts from fresh haemorrhage are also red, but other inflammatory exudates are largely serous and yellow–brown.

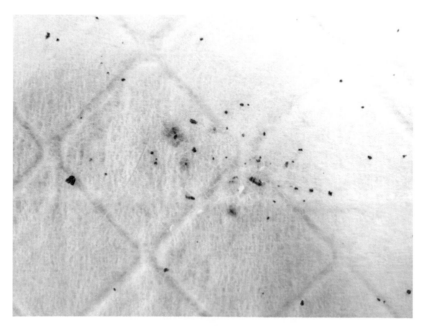

Figure 2.11 Flea faeces dissolving on a wet white paper to reveal brown–red hue indicative of the blood digested by the flea. *Source:* Courtesy of Meng Siak.

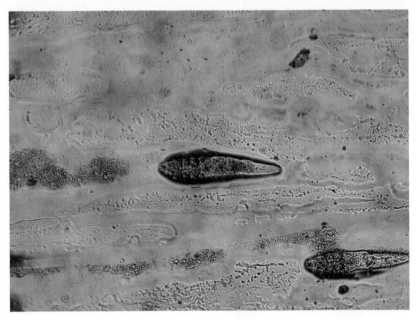

Figure 2.12 Photomicrograph of *Demodex* spp. mites in ear wax. *Source:* Courtesy of Luisa Cornegliani.

Short-tailed *Demodex*, which are more superficial, can sometimes be found. *Demodex* can usually be found by firmly squeezing the skin before applying adhesive tape to the surface. This may be as effective as hair plucks and skin scrapes (see later in this chapter) provided that the skin is squeezed firmly enough to expel the mites from the hair follicles. Degreasing and follicle-clearing strips (e.g. Nivea Clear-Up Strips®) can also be used to collect *Demodex* mites. The area of skin is wetted before applying the strips, which are then left to dry for 10–15 minutes before removing them for microscopic examination.

Hair Plucks

Hair plucks are usually taken to look for evidence of demodicosis (Figure 2.13) and dermatophytosis, or to examine the hair shaft to determine the stage of the growth cycle and identify any abnormalities (this is also referred to as a trichogram). Regardless of the reason, the technique is much the same (see Chapter 3). Hair plucks for ectoparasite examinations can be mounted on a microscope slide in liquid paraffin (Figure 2.14) or in potassium hydroxide to clear the hairs and associated keratinaceous debris. The sample is then covered with a cover-slip and methodically examined with the ×4 lens, using the ×10 lens to study particular areas in more detail. Plucked hairs can also be mounted on adhesive tape and stuck to a microscope slide, but this leaves lots of bubbles and air interfaces that obscure the finer detail and make interpretation difficult.

Hair plucks are very useful in situations where skin scrapes may be difficult to perform. This could include fractious animals or sensitive sites where sedation is necessary, and/ or scarred and thickened skin where it is difficult to achieve sufficiently deep scrapes.

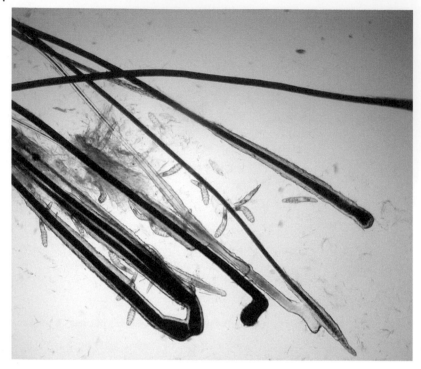

Figure 2.13 Hair plucking showing numerous *Demodex* spp. mites. *Source:* Courtesy of Federico Leone.

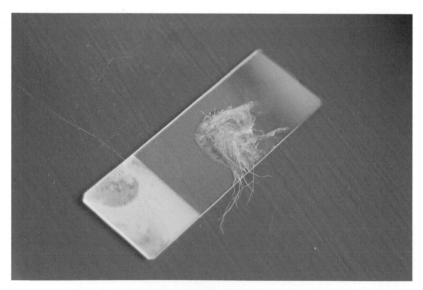

Figure 2.14 Hair mounted on glass slide. A cover-slip needs to be applied prior to microscopic examination to avoid air interfaces creating distortion.

Hair plucks from areas of follicular casts, comedones and/or from around areas of lichenified skin with discharging sinus tracts usually yield good results. They are nevertheless generally less sensitive than skin scrapes.

Skin Scrapes

Skin scrapes are usually performed to find ectoparasites. Multiple scrapes should be taken, but it is important to avoid being indiscriminate. It is best to target your scrapes to primary lesions (Figure 2.15) at the predilection sites and avoid excoriated skin. This does entail using the history and clinical signs to rank the likelihood of different parasites in the differential diagnosis. Do not be too rigid in deciding which parasites may or may not be present though. Different parasites live at different levels within the skin and it is important to collect material from each layer. It is good practice to do a full sequence of surface, superficial and deep scrapes at each site. It is, in reality, difficult to precisely differentiate each level and attempts to do so may result in missing the parasites.

Technique

1) Carefully clip any hair with scissors or electric clippers, but do not disrupt the skin surface and superficial debris, if present.
2) Apply liquid paraffin (or potassium hydroxide – see later in this chapter) to the skin. Wipe off the excess to leave a thin film. Some dermatologists instead put a drop of oil or potassium hydroxide on the scalpel blade just before scraping the skin (see later in this chapter).

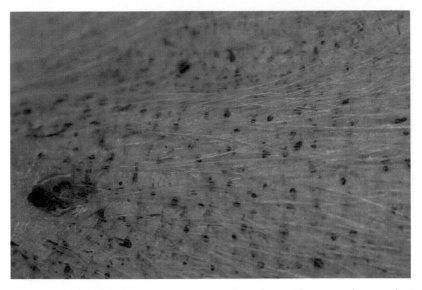

Figure 2.15 Comedones are a primary lesion in demodicosis. This is a good area to obtain a skin scraping from.

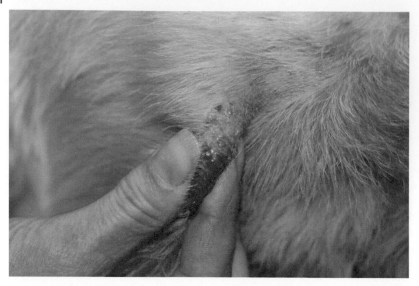

Figure 2.16 For a deep skin scraping in cases where *Demodex* spp. mites are suspected, pinching the skin to apply pressure helps extrude mites further to the surface and increases the chances of finding the mites.

3) Pinch the skin to help force *Demodex* mites towards the surface (Figure 2.16). Let the skin relax and then hold it taut to provide a flat area for scraping and to avoid bunching.

4) Scrape with a No. 10 or No. 20 blade. Their curved shape allows you to scrape large areas and minimises the risk of cutting or tearing the skin. No. 15 blades have a similar shape but are much smaller and therefore scrape smaller areas. They can, however, be useful for difficult sites, such as the feet and ears.

5) Scrape by moving the blade across the skin perpendicular to the direction of the cutting edge. Using this technique you can apply a fair amount of pressure with little risk of cutting the skin. Some dermatologists prefer to blunt blades before use to reduce the risk of cutting the skin. You can also use skin scrape spatulas, which are much blunter than scalpel blades.

6) Rotate the blade up and away from the skin at the end of each scrape to collect material and avoid pushing it into the surrounding hairs. Keep transferring material to a microscope slide to avoid losing anything from the more superficial layers.

7) Scrape until capillary oozing appears (showing that you have at least reached the superficial dermal capillary plexus), but do not collect too much blood (Figure 2.17); it obscures the view making parasites very difficult to see.

8) Too much hair and debris also makes it difficult to find anything so divide the collected material if necessary.

9) Evenly mix the material into enough liquid paraffin or potassium hydroxide to form a thin, homogeneous layer under a cover-slip. Too little fluid results in air bubbles and interfaces. Using too much can result in loss of material as it flows out from under the cover-slip, where it can also get on the microscope and lenses.

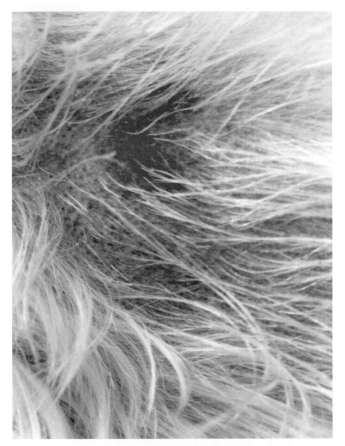

Figure 2.17 **For a deep skin scraping, mild capillary bleeding needs to be visible after the procedure, to ensure that the scraping was deep enough to find** *Demodex* spp. mites.

10) All ectoparasites are visible with the ×4 lens, which makes for quick scanning. Look for movement and check with the ×10 lens if unsure. Scan the whole slide in a methodical fashion, so every bit of the material is examined.

Pustules and Draining Sinus Tracts

Examination of material from pustules, furuncles and draining sinus tracts is an effective way to detect *Demodex* mites associated with secondary bacterial infection, especially deep pyoderma and furunculosis. Find a relatively fresh lesion and then either squeeze the skin to express purulent material or rupture an intact pustule with a needle. Collect the material directly onto a microscope slide, or transfer using a spatula or scalpel blade. Mix the material evenly in some liquid paraffin, apply a cover-slip and examine as described for skin scrapes. You can also make a thin smear of the material, let it dry, add a drop of liquid paraffin and then place the cover-slip.

Potassium Hydroxide *Versus* Liquid Paraffin

Potassium hydroxide (KOH) is an alternative to liquid paraffin. It clears hairs and keratinaceous debris, making parasites easier to see, but it is caustic to the animal, you and the microscope, and should be used with care. Nothing stronger than a 5% solution should be used on the skin but a drop of 10% or 20% KOH can be placed on the slide and gently warmed for 30–60 seconds to enhance clearing. This is lethal to mites, however, and the lack of movement can be a drawback. Mites will be alive and moving in a 5% solution but this takes up to 30 minutes to clear debris.

A 20% KOH solution can be mixed with material collected in liquid paraffin and left for 20–30 minutes to dissolve keratinaceous debris and the liquid paraffin. Using 20% KOH in 40% dimethyl sulphoxide or after treatment with alcohol solvents can aid removal of the oil. Centrifuge the solution, discard the supernatant and transfer the pellet to a microscope slide. This method is time consuming but has the advantage of concentrating material (especially useful if multiple scrapes are taken) and avoids using KOH on the skin.

KOH should never be used near mucous membranes or delicate structures and the skin should be rinsed with water immediately after use.

Vacuuming

Vacuuming the skin is an unusual technique that nevertheless has been shown to be effective in recovering fleas, lice, *Cheyletiella*, *Otodectes*, *Psoroptes*, *Sarcoptes* and *Demodex*, as well as house dust and forage mites. In one report this was more sensitive than skin scrapes for detecting surface-living mites. Debris from the coat and skin surface is collected using a filter attached to a handheld unit or hose of a conventional vacuum cleaner. The collected material can then be mixed with potassium hydroxide (see previous section) or a flotation solution (see next section) before microscopic examination. Some animals, however, find the noise and sensation of the vacuum disturbing.

Faecal Examination

Faecal examination is not commonly performed in skin cases. It is useful for endoparasites, although these are more frequently associated with pruritus and other problems in horses, small mammals and exotic species. It can be helpful in cases with concurrent diarrhoea. It may reveal fleas, lice, *Demodex* spp. and *Cheyletiella* in over-grooming animals (where tape-strips, skin scrapes etc. are less sensitive), hookworms in hookworm pododermatitis, and forage mites if contaminated foodstuffs are ingested. It is particularly useful for finding *Demodex gatoi* and fleas in cats with self-induced alopecia. Identifying pollen grains in faeces may be useful in determining pollen exposure.

Technique

1) Place 2–5 g of fresh faeces in a universal container or other suitable pot.
2) Add 30–60 mL of a saturated salt (NaCl) solution (saturated zinc sulphate or sugar solutions are also used).

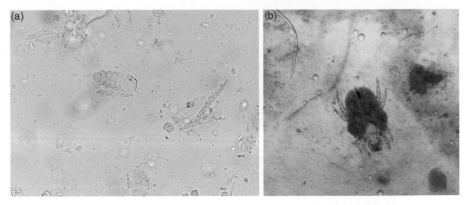

Figure 2.18 Ectoparasites found in faecal flotations from affected cats. a) *Demodex gatoi*. *Source:* Courtesy of Catherine Milley. b) *Cheyletiella*. *Source:* Courtesy of Ana Rios.

3) Add some 0.5 mm glass beads and vigorously mix or vortex to break up the sample.
4) Sieve the mixture to remove large clumps of faecal matter and debris.
5) Fill a suitable flat-topped tube with the sieved solution until the meniscus protrudes beyond the neck of the tube.
6) Place a cover-slip over the meniscus and leave for 15 minutes.
7) Lift off the cover-slip with the associated fluid and place it, fluid side down, onto a microscope slide.
8) Examine the slide for parasites (Figure 2.18), eggs and pollen grains with the ×4 lens, using the ×10 lens to examine any suspicious material in more detail.

Parasites in the Environment

Environmental parasites are a special case, as their presence on the animal is transitory and easily missed, and they are best sought in the animal's surroundings, bedding or food. These include mosquitoes, *Culicoides* midges, *Simulium* blackflies, *Phlebotomus* sandflies, *Tabanus* and other horseflies, *Stomoxys*, *Haematobia*, *Hydrotaea irritans*, *Hippobosca* and other biting flies, *Dermanyssus gallinae*, the red poultry mite, and forage mites. *Hydrotaea* are normally found on the affected animals, and other species are often obvious in and around the animal's environment. However, insect or mite traps can be useful, although expert identification of the insects or mites may be necessary to differentiate potential parasites from harmless environment arthropods. Trombiculid mites (harvest mites or chiggers) are free-living environmental mites as adults, but the parasitic larvae are usually found on the affected host.

Specificity and Sensitivity

The specificity of these techniques is very high. Any physical evidence is near 100% specific for an infestation; the one exception is *Demodex* mites which may be commensal (see later in this chapter). It is less likely, but still possible, that other parasites, such as lice, *Otodectes* and *Cheyletiella*, are incidental findings. The sensitivity of these techniques, however, is more variable. In general tape-strips and impression smears are least sensitive, hair-plucks mid-way, and skin scrapes most sensitive. This is, however, complicated by your skill and experience in technique and lesion selection. Sensitivity is also directly related to the number of samples that you take and particularly to choosing the best sites to obtain samples from.

Finding *Cheyletiella* and *Otodectes*

Finding these parasites is usually straightforward, but can vary with presentation. Adult and immature mites, eggs and faecal pellets can be found in 80–100% of the typical cases of mild to moderate pruritus and profuse scaling or otic discharge. The sensitivity can fall to 50% or less, however, in cases with more pruritus and fewer specific clinical signs. This may be related to increased self-trauma and/or mite-specific hypersensitivity reducing the number of parasites.

Finding *Demodex*

Finding *Demodex* is usually straightforward provided that you scrape down to the dermis (i.e. capillary bleeding occurs). Chronically inflamed, thickened skin can be difficult to scrape, and hair plucks, material expressed from furuncles or even punch biopsies are more rewarding. It is particularly difficult to scrape the thickened, mucinotic skin typical of Shar-Peis. Specific body sites may also present difficulties, with the feet being more difficult to scrape to the level of the dermis as it is very deep in this location. In some cases, scarring complicates matters further.

In clinical demodicosis there are usually large numbers of mites representing all stages of the life cycle. Because they are commensal, however, one or two adults occasionally turn up as incidental findings in other cases. Your clinical judgement is important (i.e. did you suspect demodicosis, how likely is it, are the history and clinical signs compatible etc.), but if necessary treat for demodicosis, repeat the skin scrapes and carefully evaluate any clinical improvement. Dead *Demodex* quickly disintegrate, appearing as translucent 'ghosts' on skin scrapes and cytology. Finding *Demodex* mites on patients routinely treated with moxidectin may occasionally be more challenging.

Repeated scrapes will help you to assess the response to therapy. There should be an increasing ratio of dead and adult mites to live and immature mites. If not, re-evaluate your treatment regime and look for an underlying cause, particularly in adult-onset demodicosis and cases complicated by a secondary pyoderma.

A *Demodex*-specific polymerase chain reaction (PCR) test (see Chapter 10 for more about PCR tests) is now available, following the work of Ivan Ravera. However, he concluded that *Demodex* can be found in all healthy dogs. This test is rapid and highly sensitive using material from hair plucks and scrapes, but it has not been validated in the diagnosis of demodicosis. It is likely to have a very high false-positive rate and currently cannot be recommended.

Finding *Sarcoptes*

Sarcoptes are not commensal so any mites, eggs or faecal pellets are significant. Finding *Sarcoptes* can be very difficult though. Look for non-excoriated primary lesions (crusted erythematous papules) at the predilection sites (pinnal margins, elbows, hocks and ventral chest). Take multiple scrapes and consider concentrating the collected material as described earlier.

An enzyme-linked immunosorbent assay (ELISA) for serum-specific *Sarcoptes* IgG is a good alternative. In the original study, sensitivity and specificity were 92% and 96% respectively, although this has been a little lower in more recent studies. Sera from dogs infested with *Cheyletiella*, *Demodex*, *Linognathus*, *Otodectes* and fleas are generally negative. False-negative serology can occur in the first month following infestation before an adequate IgG titre is generated. False-positive reactions can occur in dogs that have been previously exposed; titres usually fall to normal over several weeks but this can take up to 6 months. False-positive reactions are also seen in some atopic dogs strongly reactive to *Dermatophagoides* house dust mites as these species share cross-reacting antigens with *Sarcoptes*. This can be relevant as *Sarcoptes* is an important differential diagnosis in canine atopic dermatitis.

The pinnal pedal scratch reflex (eliciting ipsilateral hind limb movements by rubbing the pinna against itself) has been shown to have good sensitivity and specificity compared to detection of mites, eggs or faeces, and/or clinical resolution following a therapeutic trial. Other dermatologists, however, believe that this reflex indicates otic pruritus and is not specific for *Sarcoptes* infestations.

Therapeutic trials are warranted in cases where mites cannot be demonstrated but where there is a suggestive history and clinical signs, and/or a positive pinnal scratch reflex and/or positive serology. Amitraz, selamectin, moxidectin, doramectin, ivermectin, sarolaner, fluralaner and afoxolaner should be effective in the majority of cases, with some of these drugs not currently licensed to be used for this indication. However, isolated reports of treatment failures underline the importance of looking at all the available evidence before ruling *Sarcoptes* in or out.

Fleas and Flea Allergic Dermatitis

Evidence of fleas is reportedly found in less than 50% of animals with flea allergic dermatitis (FAD), probably because of a combination of the immune response and increased grooming. Heavier infestations are easier to detect but may be less pathogenic in the absence of FAD and be incidental to the main dermatosis (e.g. secondary flea infestation in an atopic dog). Strictly speaking, FAD cannot be diagnosed in the absence of positive flea-specific serology and/or intradermal tests (IDTs) consistent with type 1 and/or type 4 hypersensitivity responses.

Reports of positive IDTs to flea extracts vary from 2% to 77%. This probably reflects the proportion of atopic dermatitis (AD), FAD and concurrent AD/FAD cases seen at different centres as well as the reagents used. Many flea-specific tests use crude whole-body extracts, although the major flea allergens appear to be salivary proteins. An 18 kD major allergen has been cloned, sequenced and termed Cte f 1. Reactivity to Cte f 1 is seen in approximately 80% of animals naturally or experimentally sensitised to fleas, but this low sensitivity makes purified Cte f 1 unsuitable for diagnostic use. In studies of animals with confirmed FAD, whole-body extracts were less sensitive in IDTs compared to purified flea salivary antigens. In other studies of dogs with AD and FAD, FcεRIα (the high-affinity IgE receptor) based ELISAs, using purified flea salivary antigens, were more sensitive than IDTs with whole-body extract. The sensitivity, specificity, and positive and negative predictive values of both the whole-body and purified salivary antigens in IDTs were, however, superior to those for an FcεRIα-based ELISA using the purified flea salivary antigen in a population of dogs with confirmed FAD. IDTs and serum IgE levels have been correlated with clinical FAD in dogs, although other studies suggested that anti-flea IgE and IgG were present in healthy and affected dogs, and levels did not correlate with clinical severity. Positive IDT reactions to whole-body extracts have been reported in 24–67% of healthy animals. These did not, furthermore, appear to be predictive of developing FAD in the future. Controlled live flea challenge is highly specific and sensitive for FAD, but is not available outside certain specialist centres.

Common Mistakes and Pitfalls

- Poor lesion selection – learn to recognise and understand the significance of different skin lesions. It is especially important to avoid secondary lesions.
- Not taking enough scrapes or other samples – four scrapes should be the minimum, particularly for cases where sarcoptic mange is suspected (you can never take too many though).
- Tape-strips are taken from the outer layer of the coat (i.e. the distal hair shaft) – part the coat and take samples from the skin and proximal hair shaft.
- Scrapes are too shallow – do not try to anticipate which parasites are present and where they are, and make sure that each scrape goes down to the dermis.
- Scrapes are too deep – collect material during the scrape to avoid losing more superficial material.
- Relying on one test – apply them in a logical sequence, using the least invasive (usually the least sensitive, unfortunately) first. If necessary, look at all of the history, clinical signs, test results and response to therapy to make a diagnosis.
- Misinterpreting parasite-specific serological and intradermal test results. It is important to understand that these assess the immunological response to the parasites and you have to work out how relevant this is.

Parasite Identification Guide

The parasite identification guide (Figure 2.19) is arranged to help you identify common parasites in a clinical setting, working through a series of easily visualised characteristics. It does not follow precise anatomical classification or taxonomy. The features used for individual speciation, furthermore, are beyond the resolution of most practice microscopes and are not necessary in most clinical situations. They are therefore beyond the scope of this book, but can be found in specialist parasitology textbooks if necessary.

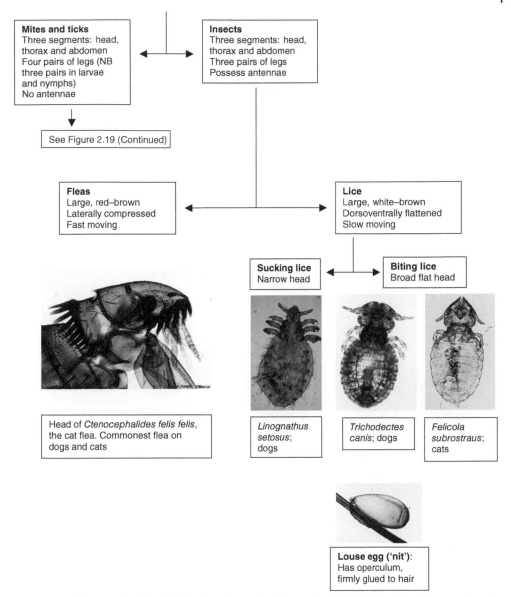

Mites and ticks
Three segments: head, thorax and abdomen
Four pairs of legs (NB three pairs in larvae and nymphs)
No antennae

Insects
Three segments: head, thorax and abdomen
Three pairs of legs
Possess antennae

See Figure 2.19 (Continued)

Fleas
Large, red–brown
Laterally compressed
Fast moving

Lice
Large, white–brown
Dorsoventrally flattened
Slow moving

Sucking lice
Narrow head

Biting lice
Broad flat head

Head of *Ctenocephalides felis felis*, the cat flea. Commonest flea on dogs and cats

Linognathus setosus; dogs

Trichodectes canis; dogs

Felicola subrostraus; cats

Louse egg ('nit'):
Has operculum, firmly glued to hair

Figure 2.19 Ectoparasite identification key. *Source:* Boehringer Ingelheim Animal Health, reproduced with permission.

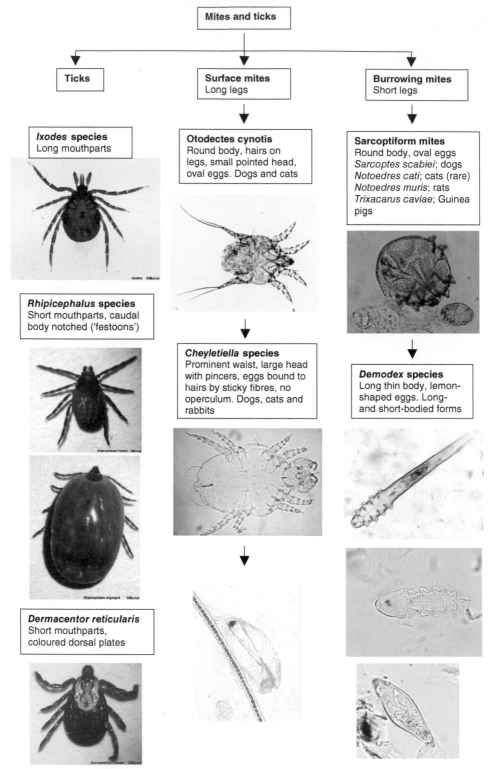

Figure 2.19 (*Continued*)

3

Hair Plucks and Trichograms

Introduction

Hair plucks are straightforward, minimally invasive procedures that are useful in many situations. These include:

- confirming self-trauma, especially in cases of feline alopecia;
- detecting *Demodex* mites;
- detecting dermatophytosis;
- determining hair growth cycles;
- investigating hair follicle and shaft disorders.

Hair plucks for the latter two indications are often referred to as trichograms.

Technique

1) Grasp the hairs with a pair of fine (mosquito-type) forceps close to the skin (Figure 3.1). Curved ones are easier to use and the tips are less likely to pinch the skin, especially in difficult areas such as the interdigital skin. Placing rubber or plastic sleeves (e.g. from cut down intravenous infusion tubing) over the tips of the forceps gives a better, more even grip of the hairs and will reduce crush artefacts (which is important for trichograms). Grasping the hairs with your fingertips more or less eliminates crushing, but the less secure grip may result in collecting fewer of the more tightly attached anagen hairs.
2) Pull in the direction of hair growth with a firm even pressure. Too little pressure will yield fewer hairs and increase the proportion of the looser telogen hairs. Too much pressure crushes the hair shaft. Jerking the hairs can break them, leaving the proximal end of the shaft in the follicle. Do not be discouraged by your early attempts; it takes practice to apply just the right amount of pressure.
3) Place the hairs in some liquid paraffin on a microscope slide and apply a cover slip. You can also mount the hairs in potassium hydroxide to clear them prior to examination particularly if looking for parasites (see Chapter 2).
4) Alternatively, you can mount the hairs on the slide using adhesive tape. This can, however, leave a lot of bubbles and air interfaces that obscure fine detail.
5) Aligning the hairs (i.e. root to root, tip to tip) makes interpretation easier.

Diagnostic Techniques in Veterinary Dermatology, First Edition. Ariane Neuber and Tim Nuttall.
© 2017 Ariane Neuber and Tim Nuttall. Published 2017 by John Wiley & Sons, Ltd.

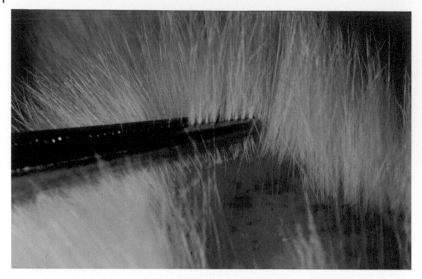

Figure 3.1 Technique for hair plucks: grasp the hairs with a pair of fine (mosquito-type) forceps close to the skin.

6) Scan under low power (×40) initially. Assess the number, length and diameter, relative abundance of primary and secondary hairs, adherent parasites and eggs, as well as any abnormalities that require further inspection. It is important to gauge how many hairs are affected, as infrequent minor abnormities, such as broken hairs, may not be significant.

7) Use high power (×400–×1000) to examine individual hairs and areas of interest in more detail. Start at the hair bulb and move distally along the shaft. Identify the stage of the hair growth cycle; bulb abnormalities; peribulbar *Demodex*; follicular casts; smooth shaft with a defined cuticle, cortex and medulla; adherent scale, eggs or spores; shaft defects and fractures; pigmentation, and size and distribution of melanosomes; and, finally, the presence of a tapered tip.

Hair Pluck Findings and their Significance

Hair Follicle Growth Phase

Growing, **anagen** hairs have large active bulbs with non-keratinised proliferating tissues (Figure 3.2). They are fairly tightly attached to the surrounding skin. Grossly these are larger than the diameter of the hair shaft, are smooth, may appear moist or sticky and are flexible. On the microscope slide they may appear squashed or bent over.

Resting, **telogen** hairs are more loosely attached to the skin and epilate more easily. The hair bulbs are largely keratinised and therefore appear dry and align with the hair shaft. They form leaf-shaped tapered points with slightly roughened edges that have been likened to a fine artists' or make-up brush (Figure 3.3). The lower portion of the hair shaft

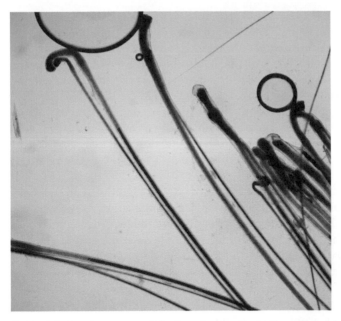

Figure 3.2 Growing, anagen hairs have large active bulbs with non-keratinised proliferating tissues. *Source:* Courtesy of J. Declercq.

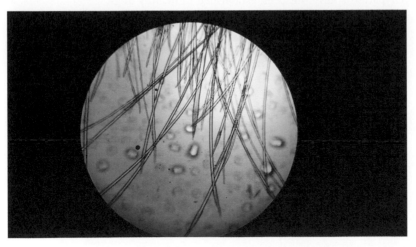

Figure 3.3 Hair pluck showing predominantly telogen hairs. *Source:* Courtesy of D. Sanmiguel.

typically lacks pigment, where it has been reabsorbed during the transition from anagen (catagen).

The lower part of the hair shaft may be covered in shed epidermal cells and sheets from the follicle, which probably arise from the outer root sheath and follicular epidermis. Be careful not to mistake these for dermatophyte spores (see later in this chapter).

Dogs and cats normally shed old hairs and grow new coats in a mosaic pattern in the spring and autumn. This is governed by day length and can be disrupted in artificially lit household environments. Some degree of shedding and new hair growth throughout the year is therefore normal. Hair growth can also be influenced by clipping and grooming. In most animals, hair plucks will usually reveal a mixture of anagen and telogen hairs, with the latter predominating. Exceptions are the Arctic breeds, which can have long resting phases with predominantly telogen coats, and breeds such as Poodles, that require haircuts and have predominantly anagen coats. This is the reason why the latter breeds, like humans, suffer anagen defluxion and hair loss during chemotherapy and other treatment with cytotoxic drugs. This is otherwise relatively uncommon in animals.

An excess of telogen hairs or a completely telogenised coat is suggestive of an endocrine or metabolic disorder, although telogen hairs can also predominate in Arctic-type and other plush-coated breeds. Telogen effluvium follows severe illness, pyrexia, metabolic conditions, pregnancy and lactation or malnutrition etc. that causes the coat to synchronously enter telogen. The coat is lost following normal wear and tear, trauma, grooming or in exogen (the expulsion of the old telogen hairs before replacement with a new anagen cycle). Telogen hairs are also seen in dermatoses characterised by follicular arrest, such as cyclical (also recurrent or seasonal) flank alopecia (Figure 3.4), some follicular dysplasias and the alopecia of follicular arrest seen in Pomeranians, Chows and related breeds ('alopecia X') (Figure 3.5). Interpreting anagen–telogen ratios can be helpful, but should not be regarded as definitive as there is marked breed and seasonal variation, and precise hair growth cycle patterns have not been established in healthy dogs.

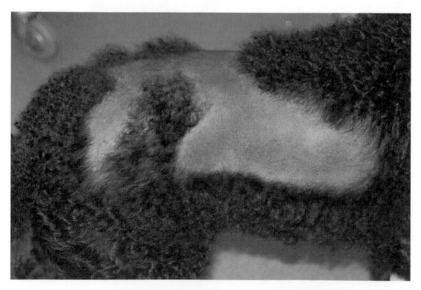

Figure 3.4 Patient affected with cyclical (also recurrent or seasonal) flank alopecia.

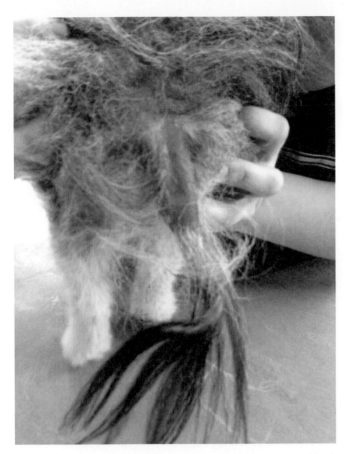

Figure 3.5 Alopecia of follicular arrest seen in Pomeranians with alopecia X.

Hair Bulb Abnormalities

Stretched and broken hair bulbs (so-called 'pinged' hairs after an elastic band analogy) result from excessive pulling or jerking of hairs, or pulling them against the lie of the hair follicle. The hair shaft within the hair follicle stretches and then breaks, leaving an irregular, tapered end with no discernable hair bulb. This can also be a feature in anagen defluxion or hair shaft abnormalities that weaken the hair shaft (see later in this chapter), but the fracture site is usually more abrupt.

Anagen deluxion is associated with severe metabolic or toxic insults that damage the actively dividing cells in the hair bulb and interrupt anagen. This results in abnormal irregular, pinched and distorted hair bulbs and proximal shafts. Hairs commonly fracture at these weak points.

So-called 'exclamation point' hairs are associated with **alopecia areata** (Figure 3.6). These hairs have a normal diameter in the distal shaft but a narrow proximal shaft and club-shaped hair bulb giving the appearance of an exclamation mark (!).

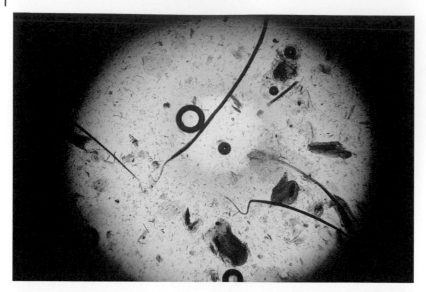

Figure 3.6 Photomicrograph of a trichogram from an Eringer cow with alopecia areata. The hair bulbs resemble the so-called 'exclamation point' hairs associated with alopecia areata in humans affected by the disease. *Source:* Courtesy of Silvia Rueferacht.

Follicular Casts

Follicular casts are tightly adherent collars of keratinaceous debris seen around the proximal shaft (Figure 3.7). They are associated with follicular hyperkeratosis, and can be seen in demodicosis, dermatophytosis, endocrine dermatoses, follicular dysplasias, sebaceous adenitis and primary keratinisation defects.

Hair Shaft Defects

Healthy hairs should taper evenly to a fine tip. A normal trichogram will usually exhibit a range of larger primary (guard) and finer secondary (undercoat) hairs, although this depends on the breed and type of coat. In reality, there is no hard and fast demarcation, and a range of hair shaft diameters will be seen. Normal hairs have three layers (Figure 3.8): a thin outer cuticle of overlapping scales; the keratinised cortex; and the inner medulla made up of glycogen granules and occasional air bubbles. This may be hard to discern in pigmented hairs. Hairs are straight in most breeds, but may gently curl in breeds such as Poodles, Rex cats etc.

Fractured hairs (Figure 3.9) exhibit blunt, split or frayed ends. Fractures, especially of the distal ends, commonly result from **self-trauma**, and the remaining hair shaft and bulb should appear normal. Fractures can also be associated with any **bulb and/or shaft defects**. This can occur at any level of the hair shaft, but is often seen in the proximal or mid shaft. Various other hair shaft defects are usually present. **Trichorrhexis nodosa** is an uncommon condition that macroscopically appears as a mid-shaft swelling. Higher

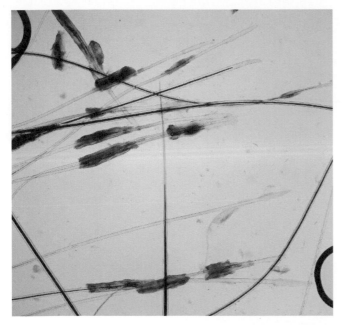

Figure 3.7 Follicular casts attached to the proximal hair shaft in a dog with demodicosis. *Source:* Courtesy of J. Declercq.

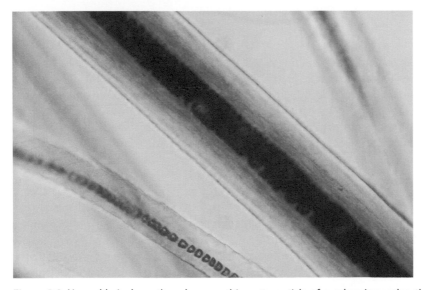

Figure 3.8 Normal hairs have three layers: a thin outer cuticle of overlapping scales; the keratinised cortex; and the inner medulla made up of glycogen granules and occasional air bubbles.

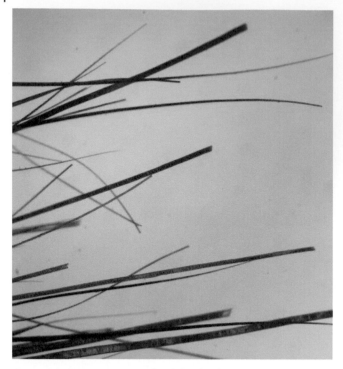

Figure 3.9 Fractures, especially of the distal ends, commonly result from self-trauma. This finding is particularly helpful in feline patients if the owner is unaware of self-trauma. *Source:* Courtesy of J. Declercq.

magnification reveals that the swelling consists of a frayed point, which looks like two paintbrushes pushed together. The hairs usually fracture at this weak point. The cause is unclear, but it appears to be associated with trauma (self-trauma, grooming, bathing etc.) to inherently weak hairs.

Various **hair shaft abnormalities** are recognised. These include twisted hairs, swellings, nodules and splits and are usually associated with familial or hereditary hair shaft abnormalities and, less commonly, with chemical or physical trauma.

Pigmentation and Macromelanosomes

The degree of pigmentation of the hair will vary with the coat colour. Non-pigmented hairs are almost transparent viewed with a microscope, whereas black hairs are heavily pigmented, obscuring most of the internal detail of the shaft. In pigmented hairs, melanin is normally evenly distributed throughout the cortex in small granules (micromelanosomes) (Figure 3.10). Abnormally large and irregularly dispersed melanin aggregates (macromelanosomes) are seen in colour-dilute coats (Figure 3.11), and

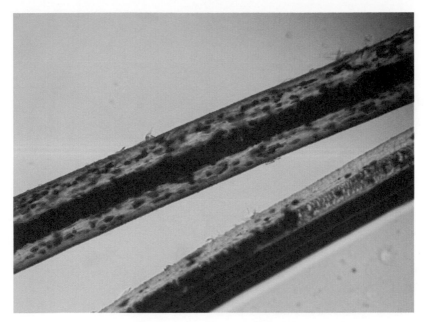

Figure 3.10 Black hairs with the melanin evenly distributed throughout the cortex in small granules (micromelanosomes).

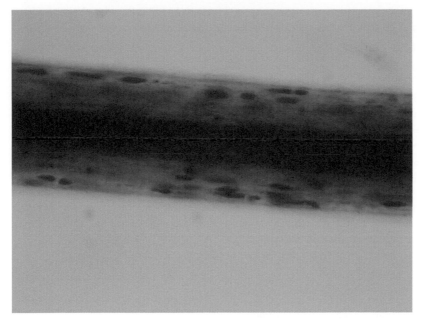

Figure 3.11 Abnormally large and irregularly dispersed melanin aggregates (macromelanosomes). These give the optical illusion of turning black coats grey or blue, and brown coats fawn or red. In some animals (e.g. Weimeraners and blue cats) the macromelanosomes do not cause any problems. However, in many colour-dilute dog breeds they are large enough to disrupt hair growth and distort the hair shaft, resulting in follicular dysplasia and alopecia.

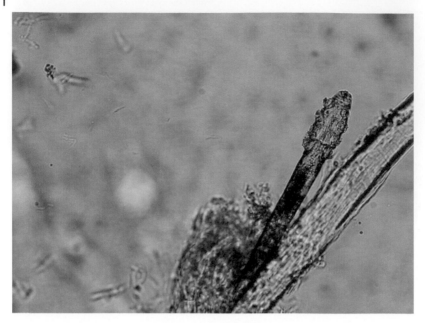

Figure 3.12 Hair pluck with long-bodied *Demodex* (*D. injai*). *Source:* Courtesy of Luisa Cornegliani.

are a feature of colour-dilution alopecia and black-hair follicular dysplasia. Macro-melansomes can distort and weaken the hair shaft resulting in fracture.

Parasites

Long-bodied *Demodex* adults, larvae, nymphs and eggs are intimately associated with the hair follicle and can be frequently found around the hair bulb and proximal shaft in cases of demodicosis (Figure 3.12). Hair plucks are less sensitive than skin scrapes, but are particularly useful in pedal demodicosis, especially if heavy scarring makes scrapes difficult, or as an initial test in fractious animals that would otherwise require sedation for skin scrapes (see Chapter 2). Hair plucks are less sensitive at detecting short-bodied *Demodex* species, which are more superficial and are associated with follicular openings and epidermal pits, and *Demodex injai* in dogs, which can be associated with sebaceous glands rather than hair shafts.

Eggs attached to the hair shaft are diagnostic of louse or *Cheyletiella* infestations. *Cheyletiella* eggs are small, operculated and loosely attached at their base by silken fibres (Figure 3.13). Louse eggs are large, macroscopically visible, and prominently cemented to the hair along most of their length (Figure 3.14).

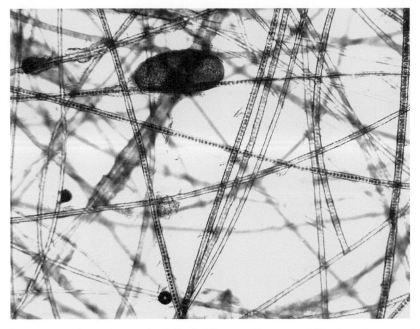

Figure 3.13 Photomicrograph of *Cheyletiella* eggs. They are smaller than nits, operculated and more loosely attached at their base by silken fibres. *Source:* Courtesy of Luisa Cornegliani.

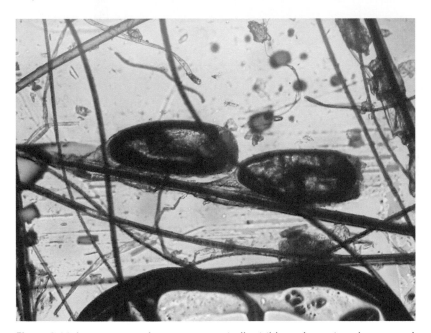

Figure 3.14 Louse eggs are large, macroscopically visible, and prominently cemented to the hair along most of their length. *Source:* Courtesy of Luisa Cornegliani.

Dermatophytosis

Dermatophyte-infested hairs are disrupted and often fractured. The normal architecture of the hair shaft is destroyed and hyphae may be visible, especially in hairs cleared with potassium hydroxide. Rafts of tiny, bubble-like ectothrix spores can be seen surrounding affected hair shafts (Figure 3.15). These findings are highly specific for dermatophytosis, but hair plucks are less sensitive than Wood's lamp examination or fungal culture. This can, nevertheless, be a useful technique for confirming the diagnosis by examining fluorescing hairs.

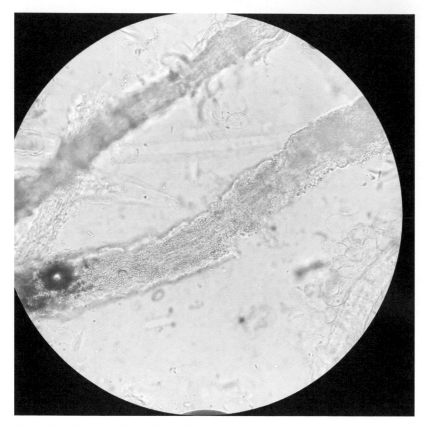

Figure 3.15 Dermatophyte-infected hair with ectothrix spores on the hair shaft. *Source:* Courtesy of J. Ngo.

4

Dermoscopy

Dermoscopy (also known as dermatoscopy or epiluminescence microscopy) describes examination of the skin, hair and skin lesions with a dermoscope (or dermatoscope) (Figure 4.1, Figure 4.2). At its most basic level this can be accomplished using a handheld illuminated magnifier. However, higher-quality equipment will yield much better magnified images. These are commonly used to assess skin lesions in humans, and are starting to become more widely in used in animals.

Dermoscopes

Dermoscopes generally use 10–20× magnification, but much higher optical magnification is now available in some high-end units. Digital magnification is also available, albeit with some loss of fidelity of the image at high magnification. Dermoscopes can be non-polarised immersion, polarised immersion or hybrid types. Both types are available in optical and digital (wired or wireless) formats, and digital cameras, smartphones or tablets can be connected to optical units. Most dermoscopes now use LED light sources. The number of LED units varies, but generally the more there are, the better the image quality.

Immersion dermoscopes have a non-polarised light source and a transparent lens plate. Mineral oil or alcohol is applied to the skin and the dermascope lens applied to the area of interest. This gives a high-quality image, avoids reflections and can be better for scale and uneven surfaces. However, immersion dermascopes are messy and less convenient, and applying the lens may affect cutaneous blood vessels and blanch the lesion.

Polarised non-immersion lenses do not need to contact the surface and therefore do not require a fluid layer. The polarised light will cancel out reflections from the skin surface. They are more convenient and can be quickly scanned over several lesions. The image quality is usually very good, especially for blood vessels. Linear-polarised light is best for the skin surface, and cross-polarised light is better for deeper structures. If necessary, the impact of surface scale can be minimised by wiping oil over the surface or tape-stripping.

Diagnostic Techniques in Veterinary Dermatology, First Edition. Ariane Neuber and Tim Nuttall.
© 2017 Ariane Neuber and Tim Nuttall. Published 2017 by John Wiley & Sons, Ltd.

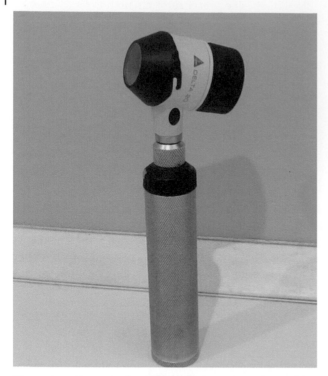

Figure 4.1 A dermoscope used to closely examine the skin surface. *Source:* Courtesy of Fabia Scarampella.

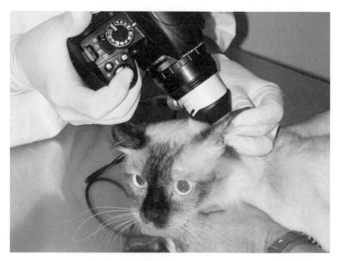

Figure 4.2 Using the dermoscope on a feline patient with suspected dermatophytosis. *Source:* Courtesy of Fabia Scarampella.

Table 4.1   Uses of dermoscopy in humans.

Condition/lesion	Example
Nodules and plaques	Melanoma Basal cell carcinomas Squamous cell carcinomas Cylindroma Dermatofibromas Haemagiomas and haemangiosarcomas Seborrhoeic keratosis Pigmented and other naevi Viral papillomas
Parasites	Lice *Demodex* *Sarcoptes* (India ink can be used to highlight the epidermal burrows)
Infections	Fungal infections
Alopecia	Alopecia areata Female androgenic alopecia Monilethrix Netherton syndrome Woolly hair syndrome
Others	Nail lesions Corns Calluses Foreign bodies

Uses of Dermoscopy

In humans, dermoscopy is mainly used to assess pigmented lesions to distinguish benign conditions from melanoma and other malignant neoplasia (Table 4.1). The sensitivity and specificity are better than for standard examination, leading to both earlier diagnosis and a reduction in unnecessary surgical excision. Dermoscopes can also be used to more precisely delineate ill-defined lesions and more accurately plan surgical margins reducing the need for overly large or repeat excisions. Digital dermoscopy can enhance image size and quality, and allows recording of images to show a patient or owner, for further analysis (including remote viewing and second opinions), to plan procedures and to monitor lesions for changes with time.

Dermoscopy is starting to be used for a range of similar indications in animals. One study comparing dogs with histopathogically confirmed pattern baldness to healthy dogs showed significant reductions in hair follicle unit thickness, number of secondary hairs and hair shaft diameter. Detection of comma-like hairs is consistent with dermatophytosis (Figure 4.3), and dermoscopy has been shown to have 94% specificity and 64% sensitivity relative to fungal culture (compared to 88% and 76% for Wood's lamp examination, and 97% and 31% for hair pluck examination). In healthy horses,

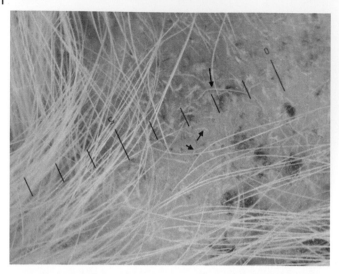

Figure 4.3 Close-up through the dermoscope of a feline patient with dermatophytosis. *Source:* Courtesy of Fabia Scarampella.

dermoscopy could be used to asses hair density, hair shaft thickness and pigment patterns, but could not identify cutaneous blood vessels.

The ease, low cost and non-traumatic nature of dermoscopy are very attractive. It is likely that further studies of hair and skin in both healthy and diseased animals will help establish normal and disease-associated patterns that will help in the diagnosis of various skin conditions.

5

Cytology

Introduction

Cytology is the study of cells. Specifically, it refers to the microscopic examination of stained smears from the skin surface, ulcers, scales, exudate, cerumen and of material collected from deeper tissues by needle aspirates. These may include lymph nodes, nodules or internal organs.

The techniques are relatively simple to perform, and vary, in most cases, from the non- to minimally invasive. Most can be performed on fully conscious animals with minimum risk and no lasting harm. Sedation may be necessary in some fractious animals and when aspirating deep tissues and internal organs. Damage to organs, tissues, contamination by infectious organisms and tumour seeding are possible adverse effects, but these are rare provided some care is exercised. Cytology involves acquiring a sample with one of the techniques described below, processing the cells by drying the specimen, fixing the cells, staining the slide and interpreting the sample under the microscope.

Interpretation of cytological preparations can be difficult, requiring some knowledge and experience. It is, however, important to remember that you do not need to make a diagnosis in every case. A partial interpretation, for instance differentiating an inflam- matory from a neoplastic lesion, can still be valuable. Many veterinary laboratories now offer a cytology service for staining, examining and interpreting fixed specimens. Making a duplicate smear, examining it yourself and comparing your interpretation to the cytologist's report is an excellent way to learn.

The specificity and sensitivity of the findings vary from low to high depending on the condition and the skill of the clinician in obtaining and interpreting the sample. It is important to realise that most cytology techniques only sample a very small proportion of the available cells and may therefore be non-diagnostic simply by being non- representative. Cytology, unlike histopathology, does not yield any information about tissue architecture or invasiveness of lesions. Clinicians should therefore be careful not to over-interpret negative findings.

Indications for Cytology

Cytology is a relatively cheap, quick and easy technique that can yield results rapidly and allow decisions to be taken without the need for costly and invasive procedures. Due to the relatively cheap running costs and overheads, it is a good practice builder, giving a

Diagnostic Techniques in Veterinary Dermatology, First Edition. Ariane Neuber and Tim Nuttall.
© 2017 Ariane Neuber and Tim Nuttall. Published 2017 by John Wiley & Sons, Ltd.

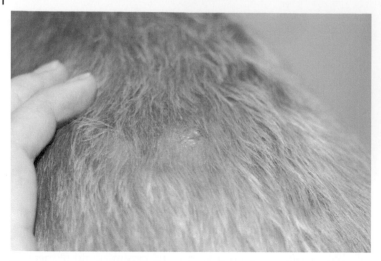

Figure 5.1 Large dorsal pustule in a dog with pyoderma. The pustule can be ruptured with a small injection needle and the purulent material collected with a glass slide touched several times onto the surface.

competitive advantage over practices that do not offer this in-house technique. The instant and yet very effective help this technique offers the clinician is very good for the decision-making process for the case it is used for, and improves the quality of medicine practised. It is also a valuable client education tool. It should be routinely considered in almost all dermatology cases.

Indications for cytology include:

- erythematous areas;
- papular and pustular eruptions (Figure 5.1);
- scaling and crusting diseases;
- areas that are greasy to the touch;
- all suspected neoplasms and other nodules;
- lymphadenopathy;
- papules and plaques;
- vesicles, bullae, pustules, abscesses, cysts and sinus tracts;
- extensive and persistent ulcers (Figure 5.2);
- atypical and/or unusual lesions;
- lesions not responding to treatment as expected;
- conditions where a precise, rapid diagnosis is essential – treatment is expensive, has serious side effects or euthanasia may have to be considered;
- for a rapid assessment of excised material.

In other words, most patients with cutaneous diseases will benefit from cytology. Cytology can be diagnostic or very helpful in a number of conditions:

- *Malassezia* otitis or dermatitis;
- staphylococcal otitis or dermatitis;
- bacterial overgrowth syndrome;
- other bacterial infections;

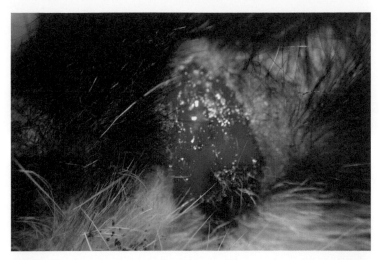

Figure 5.2 An large ulcer in a feline patient with eosinophilic granuloma due to flea allergic dermatitis. Sampling of this lesion can be achieved by simply pressing a glass slide lightly onto the surface to collect some material.

- dermatophytosis;
- deep fungal infections;
- pemphigus foliaceus;
- sterile pyogranuloma syndrome and histiocytosis;
- neoplasia, particularly to differentiate epithelial, mesenchymal and round cell tumours, and to assess the degree of malignancy. Some round cell neoplasms, such as histiocytomas or mast cell tumours, can be identified on cytology (Figure 5.3). However, histopathology is

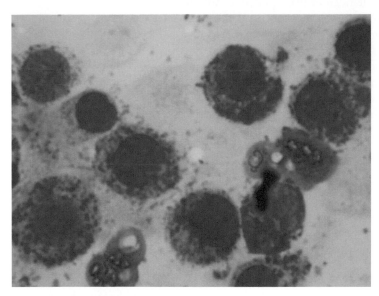

Figure 5.3 Photomicrograph of a fine-needle aspirate from a dog with a discreet cutaneous mass. There are numerous mast cells with eosinophilic granules. The cells show anisocaryosis and anisocytosis.

essential to confirm the grade for mast cell tumours. Knowing in advance which type of neoplasm is present, enables the clinician to plan the surgery effectively.

Cytological Techniques

There are several different methods to obtain samples, some of which are better suited to certain conditions and situations than others. Techniques include:

- adhesive tape-strips;
- direct impression smears;
- indirect impression smears;
- otic cytology;
- needle cores;
- fine-needle aspirates.

Adhesive Tape-Strip Cytology

Adhesive tape can be used to remove the outer layers of the stratum corneum and adherent microorganisms. A very wide range of brands of adhesive tape are available, which vary markedly in their adhesive properties, clarity and ability to survive immersion in Diff-Quik® type stains. Useful brands include Cellux™, and 3M Scotch™, Pressure Sensitive™ and Diamond Clear™ tapes. You may need to experiment with locally available tape and stains, as not all are compatible.

1) Use a strip of tape just slightly longer than a microscope slide.
2) Apply the middle portion of the tape repeatedly to the skin until keratinocytes and superficial debris are clearly stuck to it and it is no longer adhesive (usually six times). You can use a one-handed or two-handed technique to hold and apply the tape, but the most important points are to only handle the tape at the ends and apply sufficient pressure in the middle to collect surface material.
3) Once the sample has been collected, attach the two ends of the tape to a microscope slide to form a loop on one surface or over one end and stain with Diff-Quik® (see Chapter 1). Alternatively, place a drop of the purple, basophilic stain (third pot) on a slide and stick the tape down over it.
4) Blot the excess water or stain away, and then scan the slide with the ×4 or ×10 lens before examining areas of interest with the ×40 or ×100 oil immersion lens. No cover-slip is necessary.

Adhesive tape-strip cytology is an excellent method to sample dry, greasy, scaling or eroded lesions in order to identify *Malassezia*, bacteria, inflammatory cells and exfoliated neoplastic cells. It is especially useful for irregular surfaces or restricted sites such as the interdigital skin. Tape-strips are less useful with moist lesions, such as pustules, exudates, erosions or ulcers, as material frequently fails to adhere to the tape.

Direct Impression Smears

Impression smears are especially useful for moist or seborrhoeic lesions that will not stick to adhesive tape. Direct impression smears are made by applying the microscope slide directly to the lesion. It may be necessary to gently debride the surface to reveal representative cells. In this case, you should also take an impression smear from the original surface or underside of the crust to ensure that all possible representative surfaces have been sampled. Direct impression smears can also be made from the cut surfaces of excised lesions for quick identification of suspected tumours or inflammatory lesions.

1) Rupture intact pustules and papules with a sterile needle if necessary.
2) Firmly press a microscope slide once directly onto the lesion.
3) Avoid multiple impression smears at the same site as the smear can rapidly become too thick to properly stain and examine.
4) To repeatedly sample the same lesion, move the slide along each time so that you end up with a series of impressions of the lesion, each slightly deeper than the last.
5) Air dry and stain with Diff-Quik® or an alternative stain (see Chapter 1).

Indirect Impression Smears

Indirect impression smears are appropriate when the slide cannot be apposed to the skin and adhesive tape-strips are unsuitable. Indications include sampling pustules, the interdigital skin and other inaccessible sites such as the ears.

1) Gently debride the surface to representative tissue if necessary.
2) Rupture intact papules or pustules with a sterile needle if necessary.
3) For deep dermatoses with draining sinus tracts, find an intact furuncle and gently squeeze the skin to express fresh material onto the surface. Remember that this may be painful.
4) Collect and transfer the material to a microscope slide with a cotton bud, curette or spatula.
5) Make a thin smear on the microscope slide, taking great care to avoid rupturing the cells. Material collected using a cotton bud can be gently rolled onto the slide, which is less damaging to the cells and can give better-quality impression smears. Cotton buds can, however, deposit cotton fibres, which could be mistaken for fungal hyphae.
6) Air dry and stain.

Wet-Prep Impression Smears for *Dermatophilus*

Dermatophilus is most commonly seen in farm animals and horses, but occasional cases are reported in dogs, cats and small mammals. Impression smears can be used to demonstrate the characteristic cocci arranged in parallel branching chains ('railroad tracks'). A narrow clear capsule may be visible around the cocci.

Simple impression smears can be made from fresh pus in acute active cases. This can be difficult in chronic drier cases, and a 'wet-prep' impression smear is more rewarding. For this, crusts should be vigorously emulsified with a few drops of sterile saline on a slide using a scalpel blade. A drop of the basophilic (pot 3) Diff-Quik® or Rapi-Diff® stain is added before placing a cover-slip over the sample for a quick examination and diagnosis (useful on farms and in stables). Alternatively, the sample can be air dried and stained with Diff-Quik®/Rapi-Diff® or a Gram stain.

Kunkers, Tissue Grains or Sulphur Granules

Kunkers, tissue grains or sulphur granules are various terms used to describe more or less solid, gritty, yellow to red or pigmented material within purulent discharges. They consist of concretions of organisms surrounded by inflammatory exudates and necrotic tissue. They are very distinctive and are most commonly seen with unusual infections associated with filamentous bacteria, fungi, oomycetes (*Pythium* or *Lagendium* spp.) and parasites (e.g. *Habronema*). The causative organisms may be seen on impression smears made from crushed material.

Otic Cytology

Otic smears are used to look for *Otodectes* and *Demodex* (Figure 5.4) (see Chapter 2), as well as identifying microorganisms and cells in cases of otitis.

1) Debris is best collected from the external ear canal after initial examination but before cleaning.
2) Material can be collected using cotton buds, ear loops or curettes, fine spatulas or forceps. Firmer foam buds with a triangular or spiral shape can also be effective. Pushing cotton buds too far into the ear canal can impact debris deep into the horizontal canal, as the ear canal narrows towards the tympanic membrane. Flexible, red rubber or plastic instruments are best; metal spatulas, curettes and forceps must be used with care in unsedated animals as sudden movements could result in injury to the ear canal.
3) Insert the cotton bud or curette down to the junction of the vertical and horizontal ear canals, and gently rotate to collect material. This can be done under direct

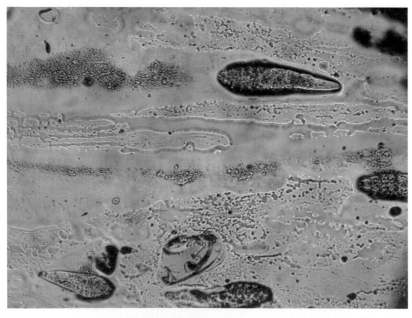

Figure 5.4 Unstained cytological preparation of ear wax showing numerous *Demodex* spp. mites within the cerumen. *Source:* Courtesy of Luisa Cornegliani.

visualisation through an operating otoscope. Material can also be directly collected using very fine ENT swabs or aspirated (see Middle Ear Cytology) through the operating channel of a video-otoscope. However, this more precise sampling may require sedation to keep the patient still during the procedure.

4) Gently roll or smear the material onto a microscope slide, air dry and stain as above. It may be more difficult to dry and stain very waxy or oily preparations, but air drying, fixing and staining with longer immersion in Diff-Quik® or other appropriate stains (see Chapter 1) gives good results with most samples, and is preferable to heat fixing.

In uncooperative patients, a gloved finger can be inserted into the ear canal and the material obtained dabbed onto a slide instead of using a cotton bud. However, the technique does not allow access to debris that is deeper in the ear canal.

Middle Ear Cytology

Cytology samples can be taken from the middle ear using an operating or, more accurately, a video-otoscope, while the patient is under general anaesthesia.

1) After cleaning the external ear canals, perform a myringotomy if the tympanic membrane is intact, but appears opaque, discoloured or bulging, or when middle ear disease is strongly suspected or has been confirmed by computed tomography (CT) or magnetic resonance imaging (MRI) scanning. Under direct visualisation use an ear curette, fine wood- or wire-mounted ENT swab or urinary catheter to rupture the tympanic membrane aiming for the caudal-ventral quadrant to enter the tympanic bulla and avoid structures associated with hearing and balance. Special myringotomy needles and knives are also available for this purpose.

2) Insert the swab through a ruptured tympanic membrane or myringotomy incision into the middle cavity to obtain samples for culture and cytology. The swab can be housed in a wide-bore tube until adjacent to the tympanic membrane to help prevent contamination from the ear canals (the microbial population and antibiotic resistance patterns can vary between the external ear canal and the middle ear).

3) Alternatively, you can pass a fine tube into the middle ear, instil 0.5–1.0 mL of sterile saline and then aspirate the fluid back. This is a particularly useful technique when using a video-otoscope. The aspirated fluid can be cultured and/or spun down for cytology. Place the fluid sample in an Eppendorff or similar microcentrifuge tube, centrifuge, decant the supernatant and then re-suspend the cell pellet in the small volume of remaining fluid. Place the drop of fluid on a microscope slide, place another slide up against the drop held at a 45° angle and then draw back to spread the sample (as for a haematology smear). Cytospin® cytology centrifuges will make a cytology impression direct from the fluid sample, but are not widely available in general practice.

4) Air dry and stain.

Needle Cores

Needle cores are a quick, cheap and minimally invasive way of investigating cutaneous masses and enlarged lymph nodes. Their disadvantage is that they only obtain a few cells, which may not be representative, and give no information about tissue architecture and invasiveness. Cytology is nevertheless a useful screening technique that can yield much information, although it should not be regarded as a replacement for biopsy and histopathology. Needle cores and fine-needle aspirates (see next section) can be used to sample deeper or internal lesions under endoscopic or ultrasonographic guidance.

1) Clip the hair over the site and swab with alcohol.
2) Fix the mass against the skin and insert a 21–23-gauge needle. Larger needles recover more cells but cause more trauma and haemorrhage, which may dilute the sample and maker it harder to interpret.
3) Reposition the needle several times and withdraw.
4) Fill a 2- or 5-mL syringe with air, attach to the needle and express the material in the needle hub onto a microscope slide. It is helpful to hold the end of the needle over the microscope slide while you do this, as the pressure of attaching the syringe can express the material collected in the needle.
5) Use the air in the syringe to express the material in the needle onto one end of a microscope slide.
6) Use a second slide to make a smear. While the cytology preparation is still moist, place a second slide over the first and allow it to attach by surface tension. Draw the two slides apart to form a smear. You are aiming to make a cell monolayer without damaging the cells; it takes some practice to achieve the right balance of pressure, so do not be discouraged by your first attempts.
7) Air dry and stain.

Fine-Needle Aspirates

It may be difficult to obtain material by simple needle cores from very firm or fluid-filled lesions. These may need aspirating using a syringe, which can harvest more material and cells, but also causes more trauma, damaged cells and haemorrhage. The technique is largely similar to that for a needle core (see previous section).

1) Attach a 2–5-mL syringe to the needle.
2) Insert the needle into the lesion and pull back the plunger a few millimetres. The more pressure, the more material and cells, but also the more risk of trauma and haemorrhage.
3) Reposition both the needle and syringe several times, maintaining the negative pressure. Be careful to keep the needle tip within the lesion at all times to avoid sampling the surrounding tissues.
4) Release the plunger while the needle tip is still in the lesion to avoid aspirating air and forcing the sample into the syringe barrel.
5) Withdraw the needle and detach it from the syringe. Draw up a few millilitres of air into the syringe and re-attach to the needle, taking care not to lose the sample.
6) Express the sample onto a microscope slide, make a smear, air dry and stain.

Cytological Findings

Red Blood Cells (Erythrocytes)

These are small, round anucleate, red–orange cells (Figure 5.5). Their biconcave shape may or may not be obvious depending on how fresh the sample is, infection, trauma etc.

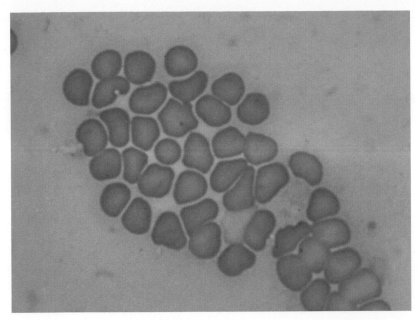

Figure 5.5 Photomicrograph of a group of erythrocytes found in an impression smear.

Red blood cells are frequent findings in cytology samples and are often the most numerous cell type present. They are associated with haemorrhage, infection, inflammation, trauma and ulceration, but their presence is non-specific. Heavy blood contamination and dilution of samples can make it difficult to detect and identify representative cells. It may therefore be better to re-sample from another site. Fresh haemorrhage will also result in the non-specific presence of circulating leucocytes.

Keratinocytes

These are large, flat and angular, and are translucent or stain pale blue to pale purple (Figure 5.6). They may have melanin or keratohyaline granules. These are tiny, smaller than most bacteria, and stain yellow–brown–black with Diff-Quik®, in contrast to microorganisms, which stain blue–purple (see later in this chapter). You may see occasional nucleated keratinocytes. Some appear to be rolled, forming large trapezoid to cigar shapes, which often stain deep purple to blue and may represent keratincotyes originating from hair follicles.

Angular and rolled keratinocytes are a normal, non-specific finding in almost all cutaneous cytology. Numerous nucleated cells can be seen in lesions that have eroded into the deeper, living layers of the epidermis and in dermatoses characterised by parakeratosis, such as zinc-responsive dermatosis, *Malassezia* dermatitis and necrolytic migratory erythema (superficial necrolytic dermatitis or hepatocutaneous syndrome).

Acantholytic Cells

Acantholytic cells are similarly large, flat cells, although they usually more rounded and less angular than keratinocytes and are invariably nucleated (Figure 5.7). They

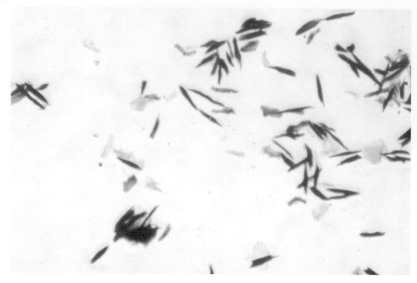

Figure 5.6 Photomicrograph of numerous keratinocytes. Some lie flat and are very pale blue and angular, while the majority of keratinocytes in this field are rolled up and show up well with dark purple staining.

usually stain purple to blue, but some may exhibit ballooning degeneration with a pale, almost unstained cytoplasm. They may exfoliate as individual cells or form rafts, and are frequently associated with numerous neutrophils and, in some cases, eosinophils.

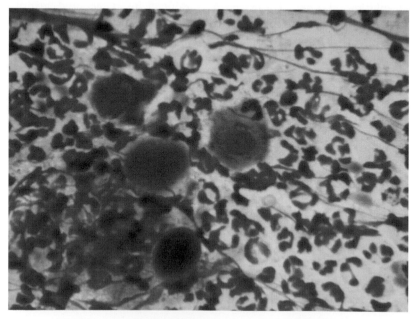

Figure 5.7 Photomicrograph of an impression smear of a patient with pemphigus foliaceous. Numerous acantholytic cells as well as neutrophils, which are mostly non-degenerate, are found. Some nuclear streaming is also seen.

Acantholytic cells are typical and highly suggestive of pemphigus foliaceus, but they can also be seen in severe bacterial or dermatophyte infections. It is important, therefore, to check the neutrophils for signs of degeneration (see later in this chapter) and evidence of intracellular bacteria. If bacteria are seen in a cytological preparation containing acantholytic cells, ideally a course of antibiotics should be administered prior to taking samples for histopathological examination to avoid confusion over pyoderma versus pemphigus foliaceus as the primary disease. Careful review of the clinical presentation can also help differentiate pemphigus foliaceus from staphylococcal pyoderma (see Table 14.5). A sample for dermatophyte culture should always be taken when pemphigus foliaceus is suspected, as certain species of dermatophytes can cause lesions that both macroscopically and histopathologically strongly resemble this autoimmune condition but treatment of the two diseases is obviously markedly different.

Acanthocytes (or spur cells), on the other hand, are red blood cells with a spiked cell membrane due to abnormal thorny cytoplasmatic projections and this term should not be confused with acantholytic epidermal cells.

Fibroblasts and Other Mesenchymal Cells

The dermis normally contains a sparse population of fibroblasts, myofibroblasts and other mesenchymal cells, so small numbers are normal in most cytology smears. It is impossible to precisely identify the cells without special cytochemical staining, as they all appear small and elongated to spindle-shaped with a small, oval to spindle-shaped nucleus. The cytoplasm usually stains a homogeneous pale blue. Increased numbers of activated cells can be seen in inflammatory lesions. They are larger, occasionally oval to round, and may have deeper-staining, vacuolated cytoplasm and active nuclei with a more open chromatin pattern. It is possible to mistake these for neoplastic cells.

Inflammatory Cells

Neutrophils

Neutrophils are polymorph leucocytes with a non-staining cytoplasm (Figure 5.8). The cytoplasm is frequently invisible on microscopy, but you may be able to see the slightly refractive margin and pick out cells highlighted against stained debris in the background.

Neutrophils are associated with infection, inflammation and ulceration. **Degenerate** or **toxic neutrophils** are a good indication of infection. They appear swollen and have indistinct nuclei with an open and disrupted chromatin pattern (karyorrhexis). Nuclear streaming is common, as the cells are fragile and vulnerable to trauma. Nuclear streaming may be mistaken for fungi or filamentous bacteria, but has a red–pink stain (microorganisms stain dark blue–purple with Diff-Quik®), is irregular and non-parallel (stretched chewing gum is a good analogy) and can usually be traced back to a ruptured nucleus. Intracytoplasmic bacteria may also be seen in infections (see later in this chapter). **Non-degenerate** neutrophils appear to be smaller, with dark, shrunken nuclei (pycnosis) and nuclear streaming is less common. They are more usually associated with sterile inflammation, but there is no exact differentiation between degenerate and non-degenerate neutrophils – both may be seen in the same smear and their presence or absence should not be relied on to exclude the possibility of an infection.

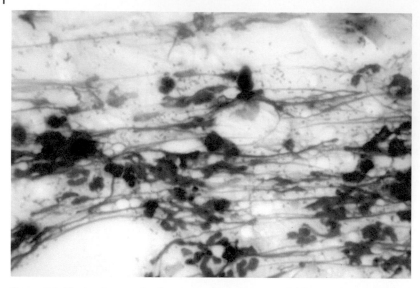

Figure 5.8 Photomicrograph of a smear of purulent material from a dog with *Pseudomonas* otitis. Numerous neutrophils, mostly degenerate, rod shaped bacteria and nuclear streaming can be seen.

Eosinophils

Eosinophils are also polymorph leucocytes, but their cytoplasm contains numerous, prominent eosinophilic granules (Figure 5.9). These are easily visible using Diff-Quik® type stains and light microscopy. Feline eosinophilic granules appear to be larger and more

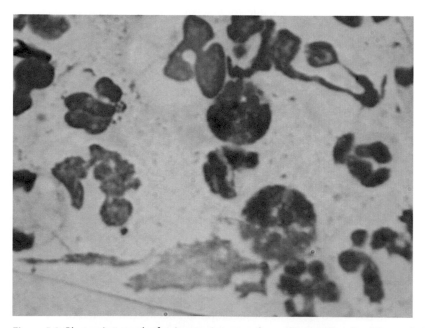

Figure 5.9 Photomicrograph of an impression smear from a German Shepherd Dog with GSD pyoderma. There are neutrophils, occasionally with intracellular cocci, as well as eosinophils with prominent eosinophilic granules.

rod-like than those in dogs. Free granules released from degranulated or ruptured cells are commonly seen. Eosinophils are frequently associated with parasites, hypersensitivity and apparently idiopathic eosinophilic dermatoses, but can also been with mast cell tumours (mast cells produce eosinophilic chemotactic factors) and, less commonly, with fungal infections and foreign body reactions (including hair granulomas).

Basophils

Basophils are another type of polymorph leucocyte with intensely basophilic staining granules. These can obscure the nucleus, making it difficult to distinguish basophils from mast cells. Basophils are rarely seen in cytology preparations, but can be associated with hypersensitivity.

Monocytes and Macrophages

Cells of the monocyte–macrophage lineage are large, round to oval mononuclear cells. **Monocytes** (also termed histiocytes in tissues) have a prominent round to oval or bean-shaped nucleus surrounded by a pale blue–grey cytoplasm. They resemble large lymphocytes or lymphoblasts, but tend to have more cytoplasm with an eccentrically placed nucleus. Histiocytic cells can be found in fine-needle aspirates from histiocytomas (Figure 5.10).

Macrophages are activated monocytes/histiocytes. They are large, round to oval cells with a large oval to bean-shaped eccentric nucleus that typically has an open chromatin pattern. The abundant cytoplasm is usually pale blue–grey with numerous vacuoles. These may be quite large, containing phagocytosed microorganisms, degenerate cells and other debris.

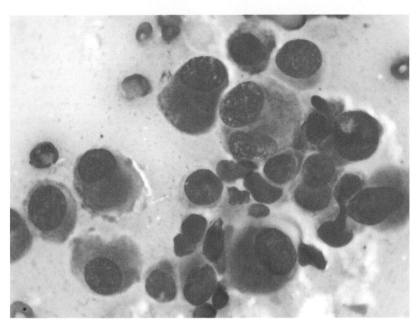

Figure 5.10 Fine-needle aspirate from a dog with a cutaneous mass. Numerous histiocytes are seen showing marked anisocytosis and anisocaryosis, typical for this condition. A small number of erythrocytes is also present.

Multinucleate giant cells are a particular form of activated macrophage. They are very large, much larger than other cell types seen on cytology, with multiple nuclei, ranging from two or three to ten or more in very large cells. These are typically eccentric, arranged around the margin at one pole of the cell. The cytoplasm is similar to that in macrophages.

Monocytes and macrophages are commonly seen in variable numbers in infections and inflammation, particularly chronic inflammation. They are typically associated with mycobacterial, filamentous bacterial and deep fungal infections, idiopathic sterile pyogranuloma syndrome and histiocytic lesions. Multinucleate giant cells are highly suggestive of foreign body reactions and fungal infections.

Lymphoid Cells

Lymphoid cells seen on cytology include small lymphocytes, large lymphocytes (lymphoblasts) and plasma cells. Lymphocytes are small, round cells with a dense, dark-staining nucleus that occupies almost all the cell, leaving just a thin rim of homogeneous, pale blue–grey cytoplasm. Lymphoblasts are similar, but two to three times larger, and usually have a less dense nucleus with a more open chromatin pattern and more cytoplasm. Plasma cells are small, oval cells with a dark blue-staining cytoplasm. The nucleus is usually located at one pole of the cell and has a coarse pattern with dense clumps of chromatin (often said to resemble a clock face). There is typically a narrow, pale-staining band adjacent to the nucleus (often referred to as a halo), which is the Golgi body.

A few lymphocytes and plasma cells are found in any inflammatory dermatosis, especially chronic lesions. Large numbers suggest neoplasia, lymphocytic/plasmacytic pododermatitis or, rarely, reactive lymphoid hyperplasia syndromes (lymphocytosis). Lymphoblasts are rarely seen, except in lymphoid neoplasia.

Mast Cells

Mast cells are medium-sized, round to oval cells with numerous, small, prominent dark blue–purple (metachromatic) granules that frequently obscure the nucleus. Extracellular granules, released from degranulated and ruptured cells, are commonly seen. Low numbers of mast cells are a normal feature, so they can occasionally be seen in almost all cytology specimens. Increased numbers can be a feature of allergic and parasitic dermatoses, but very large numbers are usually associated with mast cell neoplasia (see later in this chapter).

Inflammatory Lesions

Inflammatory lesions are characterised by mixed populations of otherwise normal cells, such as neutrophils, eosinophils, lymphoid cells, monocytes/macrophages, mast cells, epithelial cells and fibroblasts. The relative numbers of these cell types can be indicative of certain patterns of inflammation.

- 75% or more granulocytes are suggestive of acute inflammation and 50% or more monocytes suggest chronic inflammation, although these are rough guides only.
- Degenerate neutrophils are commonly seen with infections.
- Pyogranulomatous inflammation (mixed degenerate neutrophils, monocytes and activated macrophages) can be associated with less common bacterial, mycobacterial and fungal infections, or idiopathic sterile pyogranuloma syndrome.

- Eosinophils suggest parasites, allergy, eosinophilic granuloma complex or foreign bodies (including free keratin and hair shafts in furunculosis). Certain species (horses and cats) and breeds of dogs (Arctic breeds) are more prone to sending eosinophils into inflammatory lesions that would be neutrophilic in other dog breeds.
- Multinucleate giant cells are suggestive of fungal infections and foreign body reactions.
- Look carefully for microorganisms (see later in this chapter). Intracellular organisms phagocytosed by neutrophils or macrophages confirm infection. Extracellular organisms, in contrast, may simply be contaminants. As ever, it is important to correlate the clinical appearance with the cytological findings. Mycobacteria do not stain with Diff-Quik® type stains and do not always stain well with Ziehl–Nielsen, but their presence can sometimes be inferred by observing tiny, rod-shaped vacuoles in macrophages and occasionally in surrounding tissue debris.

Lymph Node Cytology

Lymph nodes predominantly consist of lymphocytes, which dominate all lymph node cytology. Reactive lymph nodes are characterised by increased numbers of both small lymphocytes and lymphoblasts, but the former are more numerous, making up at least 50% of the cell population. Depending on the type of associated inflammation or infection, other inflammatory cells and/or microorganisms may be present in variable numbers. An excess of lymphoblastic cells is suggestive of lymphoma, although this should always be confirmed by histopathology. Metastasis to local lymph nodes typically manifests as a reactive pattern (i.e. mostly small lymphocytes) with the presence of other cells consistent with the primary neoplasm.

Microorganisms

Malassezia

Malassezia appear as small oval to peanut or snowman shapes, often forming rafts on the surface of keratinocytes. They most frequently stain blue–purple, but can appear red–pink or pale blue (Figure 5.11). Using the ×100 oil immersion lens is the most accurate way to find *Malassezia*, but with practice they can be easily identified using the ×40 dry lens. Some *Malassezia* fail to stain, but their refractile cell wall can be picked out, especially with a closed condenser iris (see Chapter 1) to increase contrast. This failure to stain may be due to lipids or biofilms produced by certain strains under certain circumstances. *M. pachydermatis* is most commonly isolated from dogs, although other lipid-dependent species have also been isolated from cats and other species. *Malassezia* species can be differentiated on morphology as some have more cylindrical or spherical shapes, although full identification also needs culture and genetic analysis, and it is debatable whether this is of much clinical benefit.

There is no standard accepted cut-off value to diagnose *Malassezia* dermatitis. Estimates of *Malassezia* populations on healthy skin range from less than eight yeasts/cm^2 to less than one yeast per high power field (×400). Estimates of clinically significant *Malassezia* numbers range from more than two yeasts per high power field to more than ten yeasts per oil immersion field (×1000). It is likely that these figures reflect differences in technique, breed and body sites. Furthermore, *Malassezia* are often found

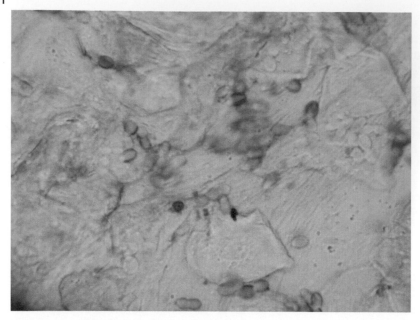

Figure 5.11 Impression smear from an erythematous lesion in a dog with atopic dermatitis and secondary *Malassezia* dermatitis. The photomicrograph shows numerous translucent angular kerati-nocytes and numerous pale-stained and unstained ('ghost') yeast organisms. Only the outline can be seen if the stain is not taken up and sometimes changing the focus can help identify these yeasts.

in rafts associated with squames and may not be uniformly distributed across a slide. Hence an individual's clinical experience and acumen is as important as relying on numbers. Most dermatologists use a benchmark of five or more yeasts per high power field. In practice, it is unusual to find more than one to two *Malassezia* yeasts/field on healthy skin, although they are more common in the ear canals. *Malassezia* are mostly associated with surface overgrowth and inflammatory cells are therefore rare. Scattered neutrophils and macrophages may, however, be present in seborrhoeic dermatitis and the rare cases of *Malassezia* folliculitis or suppurative *Malassezia* otitis. Some animals suffer from *Malassezia* hypersensitivity: in patients with compatible clinical signs and some yeast present, it may be prudent to perform trial therapy to establish how much of an influence the yeast population has on the patient's condition.

Dermatophytes

Dermatophytes are not commonly seen on cytology preparations, although hyphae and ectothrix spores can be seen on hair plucks (see Chapter 3). Spores and hyphae may, however, be seen on impression smears from some cases. Fungal elements typically stain pale blue to purple with Diff-Quik®. Hyphae form branching networks; these may stain uniformly, but more commonly there is a stained cell wall with a clear central cytoplasm and outer halo. These can be differentiated from nuclear streaming (see Neutrophils, earlier in this chapter) as they tend to be blue rather than red–pink, form parallel lines with cross-links and are independent of cell nuclei.

Ectothrix spores (microconidia) form aggregates of small, blue-staining round, oval or flask-shaped bodies. Macroconidia are commonly seen on cytology, but are

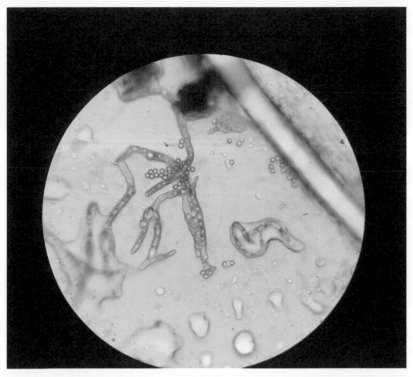

Figure 5.12 Photomicrograph of fungal spores and hyphae from a patient with *Trichophyton terrestre* infection. *Source:* Courtesy of Jacquelyn Diamond.

environmental contaminants as dermatophyte macroconidia are only seen in culture. Macroconidia are large, variably segmented bodies with a thick wall. They may stain blue–purple, but are frequently pigmented gold, green, brown or black depending on the species involved (Figure 5.12).

Other Fungi

A wide variety of fungi are associated with skin infections, usually following direct inoculation. Typical clinical signs include nodules, draining sinus tracts, ulcers and non-healing wounds. Fungal elements may therefore be seen on direct impression smears, indirect impression smears from exudates or aspirates from nodular lesions.

Hyphae, microconidia and occasionally macroconidia from a range of saprophytic, environmental fungi can be seen (Figure 5.13). With Diff-Quik® they normally stain blue, but pigmented species may appear to be gold, green, brown or black. *Cryptococcus* are large, round basophilic (i.e. staining blue–purple) yeast-like organisms with a thick, clear capsule. The capsule is particularly obvious when highlighted against stained debris. *Blastomyces* are also large, round and basophilic, but lack the thick non-staining capsule. *Sporothrix* are small, cigar-shaped basophilic organisms with a thin, non-staining cell wall. *Histoplasma* are similarly small and basophilic, with a clear wall, but are spherical rather than elongated. *Coccidioides* form characteristic spherules full of endospores in affected tissues. *Lagendium* and *Pythium* are oomycetes that can cause severe cutaneous lesions in horses and dogs. They are confined to certain geographical

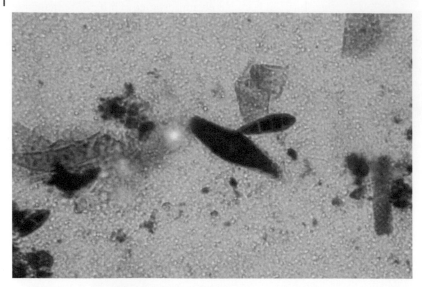

Figure 5.13 Macroconidia from environmental fungi can sometimes be seen on cytology. These are not involved in the aetiology of the dermatitis and are an incidental finding.

locations. On cytology, pyogranulomatous, suppurative or eosinophilic inflammation with occasional hyphae can be seen.

Algae

In some geographic locations there are ubiquitous algae with a low pathogenic potential that rarely cause cutaneous disease (feline) or disseminated disease. These *Prototheca* species (*Prototheca zophii* and *Prototheca wickerhami*) show up as round to oval organisms with a clear cell wall and granular basophilic cytoplasm on Romanowsky-type staining; they are 1–14 μm × 1–16 μm in size. They are usually found extracellularly but can also be within neutrophils or macrophages. Mature forms have a pink to deep purple nucleus.

Bacteria

Virtually all bacteria are basophilic on Diff-Quik® preparations, i.e. they stain blue–purple. This does not reflect whether they are Gram-positive or Gram-negative. Their identity can therefore only be inferred from morphology and knowledge of likely organisms on most cytology preparations. Full identification will require further tests and culture.

Bacterial overgrowth syndrome is characterised by large numbers of bacteria, often of several different forms, with no or only minimal numbers of inflammatory cells. Bacteria are also readily seen with other surface and superficial infections. They may, in contrast, be difficult to detect in deep pyodermas, particularly if there is a lot of fibrosis and scarring. You should therefore make a thorough search of the smear to locate any intracellular organisms and be prepared to send material for bacterial, mycobacterial and/or fungal culture before deciding that a pyogranulomatous lesion is sterile.

The presence of intracytoplasmic bacteria is a definite indicator of infection. Extracellular bacteria, particularly in low numbers, may simply be contaminants from the surface of the skin. This information can be useful in mixed infections, allowing you to identify the most important species when reviewing bacterial culture and antibiotic sensitivity results.

Staphylococci are relatively large cocci that often form diploid or irregular arrangements of four to eight organisms (their name is derived from the Greek for a bunch of grapes). **Streptococci** are smaller and often appear to form chains. **Micrococci** and **enterococci** are also small, but form irregular groups. Rod bacteria (bacilli) are easily differentiated from cocci; common species recovered from the skin include *Pseudomonas*, *Proteus* and **coliforms** (remember that Gram-negative organisms will be basophilic and stain blue–purple with Diff-Quik®). **Corynebacteria** are Gram-positive rod-shaped bacteria.

Mycobacteria do not take up Diff-Quik®, but pyogranulomatous inflammation and the presence of small, clear, rod-shaped vacuoles in macrophages are suggestive. You may also see clear rod-like shapes highlighted against stained background debris. Many, but not all, mycobacteria stain red with Ziehl–Nielsen, but this is rarely performed in practice laboratories. Cytology smears, swabs and biopsy material should be therefore sent to an external laboratory for further staining and culture if you suspect a mycobacterial infection.

Less commonly, a variety of other bacterial organisms including filamentous forms, short rods, curved rods etc. may be seen on cytology. Their identity should be confirmed by culture if you think they are relevant to the skin condition. *Simonsiella* can sometimes be found on cytology (Figure 5.14). These are non-pathogenic bacteria and are most likely transferred onto the skin surface by licking. They are therefore an indication that pruritus is present.

Bacteria mimics include:

- melanin (micromelanosomes) – small yellow–brown–black granules within keratinocytes; variable size and shape;

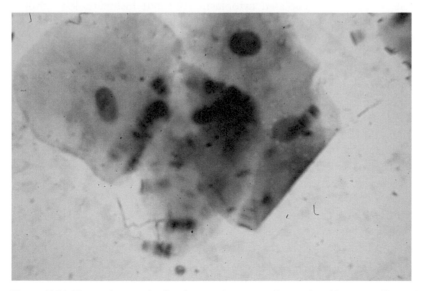

Figure 5.14 Photomicrograph of an impression smear from a dog. Numerous *Simonsiella* groups are seen attached to parakeratotic keratinocytes as groups of tightly aligned short filaments (giving the impression of a larger striated structure).

- keratohyalin – small pink to purple irregular granules within keratinocytes;
- stain precipitate – amorphous granular pink to purple background debris.

Leishmania and Other Protozoa

Leishmania (see Chapter 11, Diagnosis of Infectious Diseases) can be seen on cytology preparations from affected skin, lymph nodes, spleen or bone marrow. They are most commonly seen in the cytoplasm of macrophages, although free organisms can also be present. There are usually moderate to large numbers of amastigotes present, forming small, basophilic rod-like structures, each associated with a tiny adjacent kinetoplast and surrounded by a clear cell wall.

Cutaneous *Toxoplasma* and *Neospora* are very rare and it is therefore very unusual to see them in cytology preparations. If found, they present as crescent- or spindle-shaped tachyzoites with a red to purple nucleus and light blue cytoplasm. Both species look identical on cytology and polymerase chain reaction (PCR) is needed to distinguish them.

Neoplasia

Neoplastic lesions are characterised by relative uniformity of cell type. The majority of cells conform to a single type, although there is usually a subpopulation of red blood cells, neutrophils and other inflammatory cells.

Neoplastic Cell Types

Neoplastic cells can be characterised into three cytological types: epithelial, mesenchymal (or spindle cell) and round cell.

- **Epithelial cell tumours** have large well-defined cells with prominent cell adhesions and organisation. They aspirate well, forming sheets or gland-like arrangements. Glandular cells often have vacuolated cytoplasm. Without histopathology and/or further immunohistochemistry it is usually impossible to identify these cells beyond describing them as an epithelial cell tumour or adenoma (if they appear to be glandular) or, if more malignant, a carcinoma or adenocarcinoma.
- **Mesenchymal (spindle) cells** are medium to large cells that aspirate poorly in unorganised clumps with no cell adhesions. They are spindle-shaped or irregular with poorly defined margins, which may be seen as irregular tufts or wisps of cytoplasm. Without histopathology and/or further immunohistochemistry it is usually impossible to identify these cells beyond describing them as a mesenchymal tumour or, if more malignant, a sarcoma.
- **Round cell tumours** exfoliate well, but as individual cells with no adhesions or organisation (although it large numbers they may appear to be clumped together). They often have a distinct identity (see later in this chapter).
- **Lipomas** are difficult to stain. The aspirate appears as oily drops on the slide, which is usually sufficient for diagnosis. If necessary, you can heat fix (see Chapter 1) or leave the smear to thoroughly dry overnight. Lipocytes form large, regular sheets of cells with prominent vacuoles and small, dark nuclei at the cell margin. It is possible to mistake a different tumour for a lipoma if the aspirate misses the target nodule or lymph node and samples the surrounding fat.

More malignant tumours show less differentiation and may therefore be progressively difficult to place in these categories.

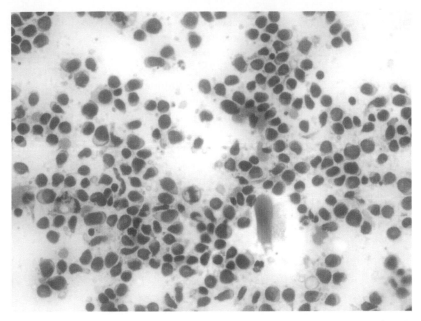

Figure 5.15 Impression smear cytology from a dog with epitheliotropic T-cell lymphoma. There are numerous pleomorphic and dysplastic lymphocytes with a mitotic figure in the centre of the image.

Round Cell Tumours

Mast cell tumours consist of more or less well-differentiated mast cells (see earlier in this chapter). Eosinophils are commonly seen, as mast cells produce eosinophil chemotactic factors. More malignant mast cell tumours are progressively less well differentiated, losing the characteristic metachromatic granules. Very malignant, anaplastic mast cell tumours may appear to be non-granular malignant round cells tumours that will require special staining techniques for identification.

Lymphomas (Figure 5.15) consist of abnormal lymphocytes (see earlier in this chapter). There is usually a uniform population of an excess of large lymphoblasts, although small cell lymphomas can also be seen. The latter may be difficult to differentiate from benign, reactive lymphoid hyperplasia with careful examination for malignant features (see later in this chapter) or immunohistochemistry or PCR techniques to identify the clonal origin of the cells (neoplasia is usually monocloncal, whereas reactive, inflammatory lesions are usually polyclonal).

Benign cutaneous histiocytomas consist of typical histiocytes (see earlier in this chapter) with abundant pale blue–grey cytoplasm, large eccentric round to oval, indented, vesicular nuclei and frequent mitoses.

Localised or disseminated histiocytic sarcomas (malignant histiocytosis) consist of a mixed population of spindle cells and pleomorphic round cells with a histiocyte-like appearance, marked cellular atypia and multiple, frequently bizarre, mitoses. Multinucleate giant cells may also be seen.

Cutaneous **plasmacytomas** usually consist of dense populations of more or less well-differentiated plasma cells with occasional mitoses. Plasma cells are characterised by a round nucleus in a round to oval cell. The nuclei contain coarsely clumped chromatin and small, solitary nucleoli. The cells contain variable amounts of amorphophilic to pale basophilic cytoplasm. Binucleate and multinucleate cells can be found.

Transmissable veneral tumour cells exfoliate easily on aspiration. They are round cells that are contagious and sexually transmitted. The cells have a round nucleus with a fine chromatin pattern and usually single nucleolus. The abundant cytoplasm is pale blue and contains characteristic, clear, cytoplasmatic vacuoles. Mitotic figures are commonly observed.

Melanomas consist of variously differentiated melanocytes. Well-differentiated melanocytes are easily identified, as there are numerous brown–black granules in the cytoplasm (c.f. the blue–purple metachromatic granules in mast cells). Progressively more malignant and less well-differentiated melamomas have fewer granules, so may be harder to identify. Poorly differentiated, anaplastic cells may have no granules and will be impossible to identify without specific immunohistochemical staining.

Malignancy

Malignancy should be considered as a sliding scale from highly aggressive anaplastic tumours to benign, localised neoplasia that borders on hyperplasia. Features of malignancy include:

- large, pale nuclei;
- variation in nuclear and cytoplasmic shape, size or staining;
- multiple or large nucleoli;
- basophilic, granular cytoplasm;
- multiple or abnormal mitotic figures;
- multinucleated and/or giant cells;
- anaplasia (i.e. lack of differentiation).

By convention, at least three features should be consistently present across the slide.

Algorithmic Approach

It can be difficult, even for experienced clinicians, to make a precise diagnosis from a cytology preparation as the histological context is missing. It is, nevertheless, possible to gain a great deal of useful information from most samples that can help in eliminating certain conditions, narrowing the list of differential diagnoses, indicate the direction of further investigation and help you give a more accurate prognosis. For instance, cytology can used to differentiate neoplastic from inflammatory lesions, prompt the collection of biopsy material for microbial culture as well as histopathology, show that metastatic or recurrent lesions have the same cell type or indicate the likely degree of malignancy of a tumour. For this, it is important to avoid empirical decision making, and instead follow a logical, algorithmic, 'decision tree' type approach (Figure 5.16).

Common Pitfalls and Mistakes

- Errors in lesion selection, especially sampling chronic or secondary non-representative lesions.

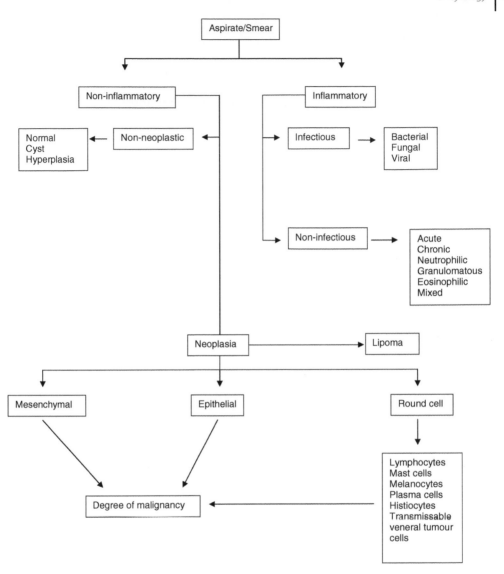

Figure 5.16 Algorithm for cutaneous cytology.

- Mistakes in sample collection, particularly making smears and staining – keep practising, you will get better.
- Over-reliance on a single finding – look for diagnostic changes and patterns that are consistent over the whole preparation.
- Over-reliance on a single lesion – sample several lesions and look for consistent findings.
- Over-interpretation of a negative finding – be very careful not to assume that something is not there just because you cannot see it.

- Failure to recognise significant cell types and organisms – learn the normal and abnormal appearance, checking with textbooks if you are unsure.
- Taking a quick look or an empirical approach to diagnosis – look over the smear methodically and use a logical algorithmic decision-making process.
- Over-reliance on cytology – be aware of the limitations of these techniques and use cytology as a support and adjunct, not a replacement, for histopathology and microbial culture.

6

Fungal and Bacterial Cultures and Identification

Introduction

Suspected fungal and bacterial infections are very common reasons for taking samples. Cytology (see Chapter 5) can be a very useful tool to confirm the presence of infection in animals with compatible clinical signs suggestive of an infection. However, full confirmation and identification of the causative organisms often requires further sampling for culture.

Commensal and Transient Organisms

Normal skin is colonised by a variety of **resident** bacteria and fungi; they colonise mucocutaneous junctions, the skin surface, superficial epidermis and distal hair follicles. The sum of all microorganisms found on the skin makes up the skin microbiome (Figure 6.1). Changes in the skin microbiome are found in conditions such as atopic dermatitis (Figure 6.2) or pyoderma. It is unclear if these changes occur as a cause or effect of the underlying condition.

The commensal organisms are usually acquired in early life by maternal transfer from the vagina, through nursing and through grooming. They are not pathogenic under normal circumstances and may help prevent colonisation by pathogenic species through competition for nutrients etc. Resident microorganisms include *Malassezia*, coagulase-negative staphylococci, streptococci, micrococci, *Acinetobacter* and others, especially in the ears and mucocutaneous junctions.

Transient species, such as coagulase-positive staphylococci, *Escherichia coli*, *Proteus* and *Pseudomonas*, can also contaminate the skin, but usually fail to colonise and cause infections in healthy skin. Transient bacteria can be acquired from the environment or by faecal and/or oral contamination. Transient contamination of the skin and hair coat by spores from a variety of environmental fungi is also common. Dermatophytes can also be cultured from clinically normal animals, and it is thought likely that this also represents environmental contamination rather than carrier status. Persian cats (and possibly Yorkshire Terriers) may be an exception, as their long hair may make normal grooming and removal of spores impossible (although it is also possible that they have specific immune defects and/or an altered skin microenvironment that favours colonisation and infection).

Diagnostic Techniques in Veterinary Dermatology, First Edition. Ariane Neuber and Tim Nuttall.
© 2017 Ariane Neuber and Tim Nuttall. Published 2017 by John Wiley & Sons, Ltd.

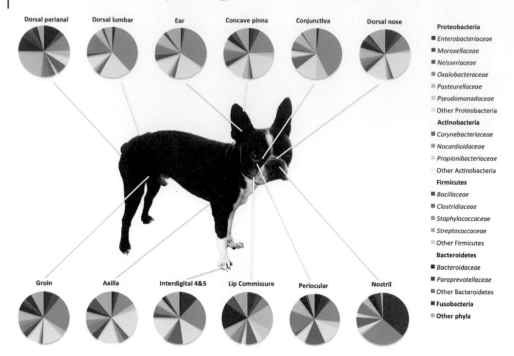

Figure 6.1 Bacterial phyla and families in healthy dogs. Average of most common bacterial phyla and families identified in different sites in the skin of healthy dogs. *Source:* Hoffmann et al. 2014. Reproduced with permission of PLoS.

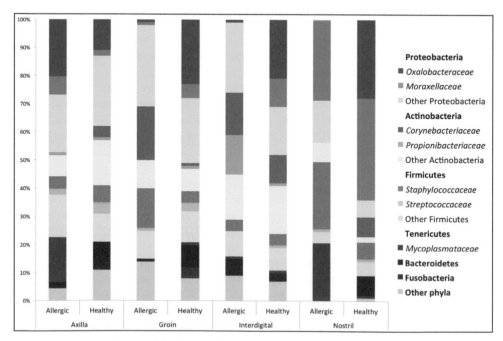

Figure 6.2 Bacterial phyla and families in allergic versus healthy dogs. Average of most common bacterial phyla and families identified in axilla, groin, interdigital skin and nostril in allergic and healthy dogs. *Source:* Hoffmann et al. 2014. Reproduced with permission of PLoS.

Both resident and transient species cause skin infections. Potential pathogens, especially coagulase-positive staphylococci and *Malassezia*, are often found at muco-cutaneous junctions from where they are seeded to the skin by licking and grooming. Mucosal reservoirs are therefore an important source of transient contamination and potential infection. Infection with Gram-negative species can result from oro-faecal contamination.

When to Perform Cultures

Culture, with or without antimicrobial sensitivity testing, is not necessary in all situations. Cytology can be a quick, easy and cost-effective way to detect the presence of infection and identify the likely microorganisms. Some microbes, such as staphylococci, *Malassezia* and dermatophytes, have a relatively predictable pattern of antimicrobial susceptibility and empirical selection of treatment is often successful. Culture is, however, advisable in a number of situations:

- when cytology reveals rod bacteria, as their identity and antibiotic susceptibility are less predictable and often limited (Figure 6.3);
- empirical antimicrobial therapy does not resolve the infection as expected (Figure 6.4);
- after multiple antibiotic courses, particularly with broad-spectrum drugs;
- with life-threatening infections, where the choice of drug must be right first time;

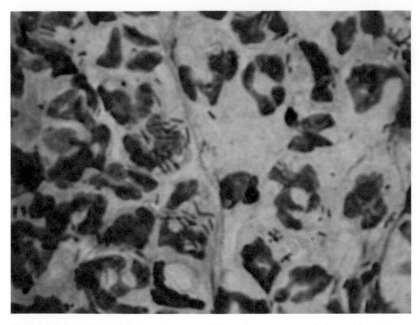

Figure 6.3 Numerous degenerate neutrophils and numerous rod-shaped bacteria, some of which are intracellular, in a dog with *Pseudomonas* otitis.

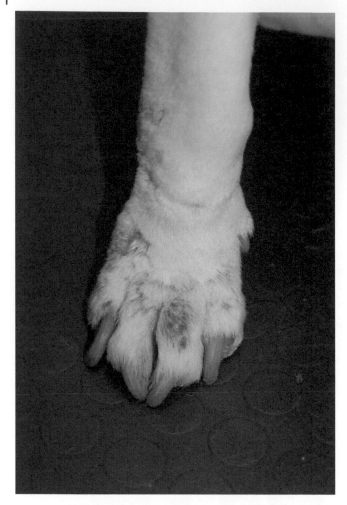

Figure 6.4 Persistent deep pyoderma in a dog on antibiotic therapy.

- where the microorganism must be identified to allow proper selection of treatment and to give an accurate prognosis;
- to confirm the diagnosis where the treatment is expensive and/or may have serious adverse effects;
- where you suspect antimicrobial resistance (e.g. postoperative meticillin-resistant staphylococci) – antimicrobial resistance should be suspected in:
  - non-healing wounds;
  - postoperative infections;
  - nosocomial (i.e. healthcare-acquired) infections;
  - cases not responding to empirical therapy, where there are bacteria present despite ongoing antibiotic therapy;
  - antibiotic treatment within the last 3 months, especially if there have been multiple courses of broad-spectrum drugs.

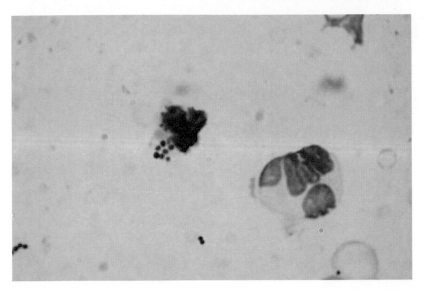

Figure 6.5 Photomicrograph of an impression smear from a dog with pyoderma. Note the degenerative neutrophils and the cocci and diplococci of different sizes.

It is helpful, where possible, to perform cytology as well as taking material for culture. Most cultures are qualitative rather than quantitative (it is possible to perform quantitative cultures, but the techniques are complicated and time consuming, and not suitable for routine clinical use). Cultured organisms may or may not be involved in the infection, particularly if they are normal commensal or resident mucosal organisms. Cytology, in contrast, yields semi-quantitative data, including the number of organisms involved, whether they have been phagocytosed (Figure 6.5), and their relationship to cutaneous cells and structures. The relative abundance and likely importance of different organisms revealed by cytology can be useful when culture detects multiple species with differing antimicrobial susceptibility patterns.

Prior Antibiotic Therapy

Ideally, antibiotic therapy should be discontinued before taking samples for culture. Antibiotic concentrations will usually fall to trivial levels unlikely to affect cultures within five half-lives of the last dose; in practical terms this is usually 24–48 hours for most oral antibiotics but may be longer for long-acting injectable formulations. However, this may not be feasible. In practice, microbiology laboratories should be able grow bacteria in the face of antibiotic treatment if you see them on cytology, although they may need to use enrichment techniques or extend the cultures. It is therefore very important to note any prior or ongoing antibiotic therapy on the submission form.

Obtaining Material for Culture

Material for culture can be obtained by a variety of means depending on the lesions involved. It is important to obtain representative samples and avoid surface

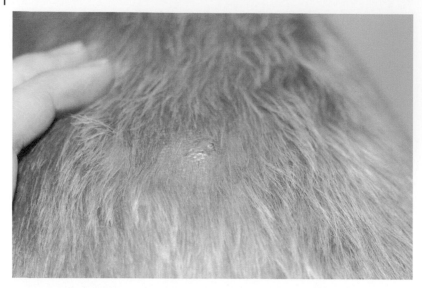

Figure 6.6 Photograph of a pustule in a dog with pyoderma. Opening the intact pustule with a small sterile needle will reveal fresh material suitable for sampling.

contamination that may not be relevant. You should select primary lesions, such as intact pustules (Figure 6.6), furuncles and nodules, and the leading edge of epidermal collarettes and ulcers, trying to avoid chronic, ulcerated and/or excoriated lesions. If rods have been identified on cytology, otic discharge can also be submitted for culture (Figure 6.7). If, in the face of multiple lesions, you are not sure, take several samples.

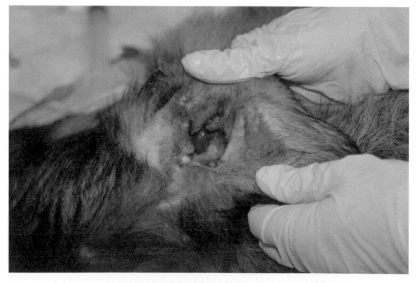

Figure 6.7 Haemorrhagic and purulent material in the ear canal of a dog with *Pseudomonas* otitis. After rods were found on cytology, a swab was taken of the purulent material for culture and sensitivity testing.

You may need to carefully debride crusts to expose deeper lesions and/or disinfect the surface with alcohol. Remember to let the alcohol evaporate before sampling, as residual traces can inhibit subsequent microbial growth. It is also important to avoid exposure to formalin and formalin fumes. Inhibition of microbial growth by formalin can be a problem when biopsy specimens are also taken for culture and histopathology.

Coat Brushings

Coat brushings are usually taken for fungal rather than bacterial cultures. Vigorously brushing or combing the coat with a toothbrush, small grooming brush (Figure 6.8) or carpet square will collect loose hair, scale and dermatophyte spores. When rubbed through the coat, these develop a static charge that attracts fungal spores. The spores can be transferred to dermatophyte test medium (DTM) or Sabouraud agar (Figure 6.9) by lightly touching the surface to deposit loose scale, hair and spores. Gently tapping the neck of the toothbrush against the side of the plate can help dislodge material if necessary. Brushes and carpet squares can be sent to external laboratories for culture, but it is important to use non-airtight containers (e.g. loosening the top of a universal tube or using an envelope) to avoid bacterial overgrowth during transit.

Coat brushings have the advantage of sampling almost the entire coat and are therefore more sensitive than hair plucks (see next section in this chapter). They are preferred for detecting carriage in non-lesional animals, but their disadvantage is that the culture is not directly linked to a lesion. It is possible, though uncommon, to get false-positive cultures from animals whose coats are transiently contaminated from an

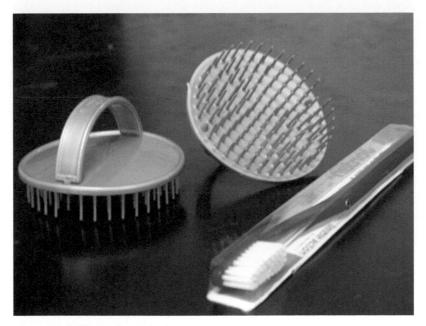

Figure 6.8 Toothbrush and hand brush suitable for obtaining a sample for dermatophyte culture with the McKenzie brush technique.

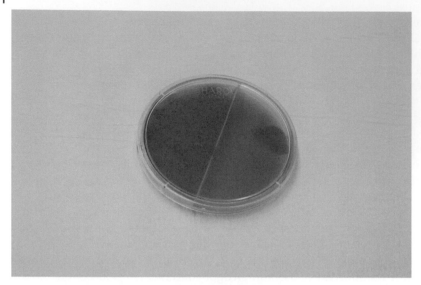

Figure 6.9 Dermatophyte test medium (DTM) and Sabouraud agar in one plate (DermDuet™).

environmental source but who do not have dermatophytosis. Coat brushings are not recommended for bacterial cultures for the same reason; they are likely to isolate a range of species from the skin and hair that may or may not be relevant to the presenting skin disease. Horses, farm animals and small mammals, such as rodents and rabbits, have large number numbers of saprophytic fungi on the skin and coat, which can interfere with dermatophyte cultures. Gently cleansing the skin with a detergent or wiping with alcohol before sample collection may help reduce contamination but could also result in a false-negative culture if not left to dry thoroughly prior to sampling.

Hair Plucks

Hair plucks are widely used for dermatophyte cultures. Plucked hairs can be directly placed on culture media or sent to an external laboratory as above. Hair plucks have the advantage of localising the culture to the clinical lesion and are therefore unlikely to result in any false-positives. Because only a few hairs are sampled though, viable fungi may be missed and this technique can be less sensitive than coat brushing. The best results are obtained from taking fluorescing and/or broken hairs from the edge of active lesions. Dermoscopy (see Chapter 4) can be useful to detect potentially infected hairs for culture.

Swabs

Bacteriology swabs are used to collect material from the surface of the skin. A variety of swabs is available but standard cotton-tipped swabs in transport medium for aerobic and anaerobic culture are best for routine clinical use. Swabs without transport medium are only really suitable for on-site laboratories where the sample will be rapidly processed or placed in culture medium. Special swabs for anaerobic or other fastidious organisms can be used if these species are suspected.

Swabs can be taken directly from the skin surface, although there is a risk that this may simply reveal commensals or secondary, opportunistic invaders. This can be avoided by cleaning the skin with alcohol (see earlier in this chapter), although be careful with superficial pustules as the alcohol can penetrate the thin overlying stratum corneum. Intact pustules can be ruptured with a sterile needle to expose fresh pus that can then be collected using a swab. It can be difficult to find intact pustules in dogs and cats, so you may need to sample the edge of an epidermal collarette or carefully lift the crust off a recently ruptured pustule. In cases of erythematous papulopustular dermatitis, good samples can be obtained swabbing material from a papule debrided with a sterile needle. Fresh material can be expressed from draining sinus tracts and intact furuncles by digital pressure.

Ear Swabs

Material for culture can be collected from the external ear canals using a bacteriology swab in much the same way as material is taken for cytology (see Chapter 4). Samples for culture should ideally be taken before those for cytology and before cleaning the ear to avoid any potential contamination or false-negative cultures. If a conscious sample is taken and the patient is not amenable to having the ears examined, it can be helpful to insert a finger gloved in a sterile glove to obtain some material. The debris can subsequently be transferred onto a bacteriology swab and submitted as usual. It is important, where appropriate, to culture material from both the external ear canals and middle ear, as the bacteria and their antimicrobial susceptibility patterns can differ between these sites. Samples from the middle ear are taken after cleaning the external ear canals to avoid contamination.

Biopsy

Biopsies are preferred for deeper lesions and the skin surface should be prepared with alcohol to reduce contamination for this purpose. Similar to preparing the skin when intact pustules are sampled, the alcohol needs to evaporate off before obtaining the sample to avoid false-negative cultures. Using local anaesthetic at the biopsy site could also inhibit bacterial growth, so it may be better to use a ring block, local nerve block or general anaesthesia. Instead of preserving the tissue sample in formalin, a section of tissue that has been harvested using sterile techniques is placed on a sterile swab saturated in sterile saline solution to avoid drying and placed in a sterile sample container, such as a urine pot, and submitted for culture. If necessary, the epidermis can be trimmed off using a sterile scalpel blade to reduce contamination and restrict culture to the dermis and subcutis. It is best to collect samples for culture before samples for histopathology to avoid formalin splashes or fumes accidentally sterilising the sample.

How to Interpret Bacterial Culture and Sensitivity Results

Culture and sensitivity testing will speciate the bacteria involved in the infection as well as giving an indication as to which antibiotic to choose. However, culture and sensitivity test results need to be interpreted in the light of the body site sampled, ideally in

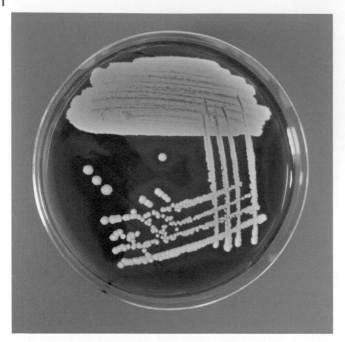

Figure 6.10 Blood agar plate with growth of *Staphylococcus pseudintermedius* and *Staphylococcus aureus*. *Source:* Courtesy of Annette Loeffler.

conjunction with cytology results and the patient history. It is important to treat the patient, not the laboratory result. For example if, on cytology, a mixed infection of yeast, cocci and rods is seen, and the culture shows *Staphylococcus pseudintermedius* (Figure 6.10) and *Streptococcus* spp. but no other organisms were cultured, it is important to call the laboratory to ask them to subculture again as the rod-shaped organisms must have been missed.

The results will be reported either as Kirby-Bauer (Figure 6.11) disc data (which present the results as resistant, susceptible or intermediate) or the minimum inhibitory concentration (MIC) (Figure 6.12); if available, the MIC is preferred as this gives some indication of the degree of resistance and whether this can be overcome by altering the antibiotic dose. However, commercial MIC tests use a restricted range of concentrations and may report the results as resistant, susceptible or intermediate rather than giving the exact MIC.

Kirby-Bauer Disc Diffusion Versus Minimum Inhibitory Concentration

Most *in vitro* susceptibility testing has traditionally been performed utilising the Kirby-Bauer method, whereby discs saturated in an antibiotic solution on a culture plate were used to determine a growth-free zone achieved by diffusion of the antibiotic into the culture medium. The larger size of the growth-free zone (zone of inhibition [ZI]) is, the more susceptible the bacteria are to that antimicrobial. The ZIs are compared to agreed breakpoints to determine whether the infection will be susceptible, intermediate or resistant to the antibiotics tested.

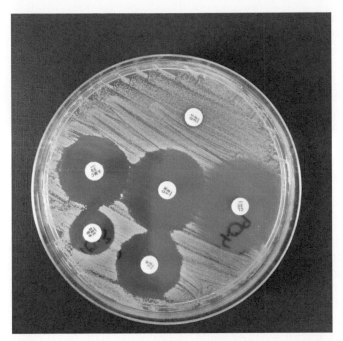

Figure 6.11 Kirby-Bauer disc diffusion test plate showing antibiotic plates on surface of test medium resulting in varying inhibitory rings in the bacterial growth on the plate. *Source:* Courtesy of Annette Loeffler.

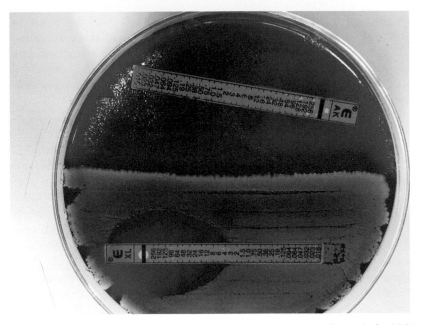

Figure 6.12 Minimum inhibitory concentration (MIC) testing using E-strips®; the MIC is the concentration where the edge of the zone of inhibition touches the strip. *Source:* Courtesy of Stephen Steen.

Kirby-Bauer tests have their limitations. In particular, they do not give the clinician information about the exact concentration needed to suppress bacterial growth. The minimum inhibitory concentration (MIC) is the lowest concentration of an antibiotic (usually reported in µg/mL) that completely inhibits growth of the bacteria. Broth dilution methods culture the bacteria with doubling dilutions of each antibiotic. E-strips® and Oxoid's MIC evaluator® use paper strips impregnated with antibiotics at differing concentrations along the strip. These produce an elliptical zone of inhibition, with the MIC read as the concentration where the edge of the zone of inhibition touches the strip. The lower the MIC, the more susceptible the bacteria are to that antibiotic and the MICs are compared to agreed breakpoints to determine whether the infection will be resistant, intermediate or susceptible to the antibiotic.

Using Breakpoints to Determine Whether an Infection will be Susceptible or Resistant

In vitro bacterial culture and antimicrobial susceptibility testing are performed using µg/mL antimicrobial concentrations assuming that you will administer systemic treatment. The tested concentrations are relevant to those that can be achieved at the target tissues following systemic administration of the drug. Breakpoints are used to determine whether the infection is likely to be susceptible or resistant to each antimicrobial. Briefly, if the ZI exceeds the breakpoint or the MIC is less than the breakpoint then it is likely that the antimicrobial will achieve a therapeutic concentration in the target tissue and the infection should respond to systemic treatment (i.e. the infection is susceptible). However, if the ZI is less than the breakpoint or the MIC exceeds the breakpoint then it is unlikely that the antimicrobial will achieve an effective concentration in the target tissue and the infection is not likely to respond to systemic treatment (i.e. the infection is resistant).

Breakpoints are agreed by international bodies (such as the Clinical & Laboratory Standards Institute [CLSI] and the European Committee on Antimicrobial Susceptibility Testing [EUCAST]), and are based on the bioavailability, pharmacokinetics, drug penetration and spectrum of activity of drugs in different species. It therefore follows that breakpoints are highly specific – breakpoints established for a drug in one species cannot be extrapolated to another species as the pharmacodynamics may differ and affect drug concentrations in the target tissue.

Using MICs to Predict the Response to Treatment

To explain this we'll work through an example. Look at the bacterial culture results in Figure 6.13. The results are for a *Pseudomonas aeruginosa* isolate from a case of otitis externa in a dog (isolated and tested by Idexx Laboratories, Wetherby, UK). The *Result* column reports whether the infection is likely to be *susceptible* (*sensitive*) or *resistant* to each antibiotic (we will look at *intermediate* results later). The next *MIC* column gives the actual MIC for each antibiotic for this isolate. The final *reference range* column shows the tested concentrations for each antibiotic, the breakpoints and the MIC.

Look at the letters under the reference range. Each individual letter refers to a single concentration within the tested range in doubling dilutions in µg/mL. In this example, the bacteria were grown in the presence of 0.25 µg/mL, 0.5 µg/mL, 1.0 µg/mL and 2.0 µg/mL enrofloxacin, 0.5 µg/mL, 1.0 µg/mL, 2.0 µg/mL and 4.0 µg/mL marbofloxacin and so on. The upper case letters refer to the actual MIC – in this case, the MIC

```
Isolate 1 : Pseudomonas aeruginosa

Antibiotic          Result        MIC      Reference Range
---------------     ------------  ------    --------------------
Enrofloxacin        Resistant     >=2       0.25  sssR      2
Marbofloxacin       Resistant     >=4       0.5   ssrR      4
Pot Sulphonamide    Resistant     >=320     10    sssrrR    320
Gentamicin          Resistant     >=16      0.5   ssssiR    16
Amikacin            Resistant     >=64      2     ssssiR    64
Ceftazidime         SENSITIVE     <=8       8     Sir       32
Piperacillin        SENSITIVE     <=8       8     Ssssrr    256
Carbenicillin       Intermediate  256       16    ssssIr    512
Ticarcillin         SENSITIVE     64        16    ssSrr     256
Tobramycin          SENSITIVE     4         0.5   sssSir    16
```

Figure 6.13 The antimicrobial susceptibility pattern showing minimum inhibitory concentrations (MICs) and breakpoints (from Idexx Laboratories, Wetherby, North Yorkshire) for a *Pseudomonas aeruginosa* isolate from a case of otitis externa in a dog. The accompanying text explains how to interpret MICs and breakpoints, how these can be used to select the most appropriate antimicrobial, and why these are not appropriate for topical therapy. *Source:* Nuttall 2013.

for enrofloxacin is more than or equal to 2.0 µg/mL (the highest tested concentration) and the MIC for carbenicillin is 256 µg/mL.

The letters under the reference range are 's' (susceptible), 'i' (intermediate – again, we'll look at this later) or 'r' (resistant). The change from 's' to 'r' is the breakpoint. If the MIC falls within the 's' range, then it is likely that standard systemic treatment will achieve a therapeutic concentration at the site of infection and the infection should respond to treatment. However, if the MIC falls within the 'r' range, then it is unlikely that the drug will attain a therapeutic concentration in the target tissue. Treatment is therefore unlikely to be successful and the infection should be regarded as resistant to that antibiotic.

In this example the infection has been reported as susceptible to four antibiotics – ceftazidime, pipericillin, ticarcillin and tobramycin. Which would be the most effective? It is important to look at where the MIC falls within the 's' zone. For ticarcillin, ceftazidime and tobramycin the MIC is only one dilution below the breakpoint. For piperacillin, in contrast, the MIC is at least four dilutions below the breakpoint. This *Pseudomonas* isolate is therefore more sensitive to pipercillin than it is to ticarcillin, tobramycin and ceftazidime. Variations in pharmacodynamics and/or problems with administration could lead to suboptimal concentrations of ticarcillin, ticarcillin, tobramycin and ceftazidime at the target site and treatment failure. This is less likely to occur with piperacillin, and this would be a better choice of drug for systemic treatment in this case.

Knowing the MIC can help you calculate the appropriate dose to attain a therapeutic concentration at the target tissue. This is easy if you know the concentration of the antimicrobial in a topical preparation, but you need to know some pharmacokinetic data to do this for systemic treatment (Box 6.1).

This *Pseudomonas* example illustrates another weakness of most commercial MIC tests – only a small range of concentrations is tested for each antibiotic. Here, the actual MIC is only known for carbenicillin, ticarcillin and tobramycin. Calculating an effective concentration and dose is impossible for the other antibiotics.

Box 6.1 Calculating drug doses using MIC data.

For a skin infection

MIC = 2 μg/mL

Required tissue concentration = 2 × 10 = 20 μg/mL

Plasma level at 10 mg/kg orally = 15 μg/mL

Skin concentration = 80% of plasma = 12 μg/mL

Dose required for this skin infection = (20/12) × 10 = >16.7 mg/kg

This example is for concentration-dependent antibiotics (e.g. fluoroquinolones and amino-glycosides) where the ratio between the maximum tissue concentration and MIC should be 10 or more. For time-dependent antibiotics (e.g. penicillins and cephalosporins) the level above MIC should be maintained for at least 70% of the dosing interval. The principles are the same but the calculation is harder as the half-life of the drug has to be taken into account.

Note that we have deliberately referred to the *infection* in this section and not the *bacteria*. The breakpoints only mean that the infection is likely or not likely respond to systemic treatment at standard doses. Changing the dose or route of administration violates the assumptions that the breakpoints are based on and makes the results difficult to interpret. In particular, breakpoints are meaningless with topical therapy (see later in this chapter).

The Problem of Intermediate Results

Intermediate susceptibility is sometimes used when the MIC or ZI is near to the limit of serum or tissue concentrations following standard doses. It can also be used as a 'buffer' to prevent classification errors associated with technical variables. Generally, these infections should be regarded as resistant to systemic treatment. However, an antibiotic may be successful if used topically, at a high dose and/or it concentrates in the target tissue, thereby exceeding the MIC.

Topical Therapy and Bacterial Culture

Bacterial culture and antibiotic susceptibility testing are much less helpful if you are considering topical treatment. Topical antibiotic treatment will typically result in mg/mL concentrations, compared to the μg/mL concentrations ranges used in antimicrobial susceptibility tests. Levels at the treated site may therefore greatly exceed the MIC, rendering breakpoints from *in vitro* tests meaningless and potentially misleading. For example, using the data above we would conclude that this *Pseudomonas* infection will be resistant to systemic enrofloxacin or marbofloxacin treatment. However, this infection could respond to topical therapy delivering concentrations of fluoroquinolone 1000 times that assumed by *in vitro* testing. The breakpoints in these tests refer to the infection following systemic therapy – they do not imply that the bacteria would *never* respond to that antibiotic.

Bacterial culture can still have a role in these situations, as knowing the species of bacteria can help you choose the most appropriate antibiotics based on their inherent susceptibility. For example, *Pseudomonas* species are inherently resistant to most beta-lactams (penicillins and cephalosporins) but susceptible to fluoroquinolones, amino-glycosides and certain anti-pseudomonal beta-lactams.

Why Doesn't the Clinical Response Match the *In Vitro* Test?

In vitro susceptibility tests do not necessarily predict the clinical outcome. There is a '90–50' rule – 90% of infections with susceptible bacteria respond to therapy, but infections with resistant isolates will respond to an 'inappropriate' antibiotic about 50% of the time (Box 6.2). It is important to treat the patient, not the susceptibility test. For example, if your patient is responding to amoxicillin but a subsequent test suggests that the bacteria are resistant to amoxicillin, do not change treatment – keep using amoxicillin, checking the clinical signs and cytology. Conversely, if your patient is not responding to an apparently appropriate drug, check administration and compliance, consider whether the drug can penetrate to the site of infection, check your cytology for other organisms and speak to the laboratory about further tests.

Other Things to Consider

Some antibiotics are indicative for the likely susceptibility of other antibiotics in the same class – see Table 6.1 for guidance on predicting antimicrobial susceptibility patterns.

The health of the patient, concurrent medication, underlying diseases and potential side effects (especially if using higher than recommended doses) must also be considered

---

Box 6.2 Mismatches between antimicrobial susceptibility tests and the clinical response.

- *In vitro* environment versus *in vivo* environment (inflammation and immunity, tissue responses, underlying diseases, blood flow, pharmacokinetics, drug penetration etc.)
- Compliance and administration
- Laboratory variation and error
- Course of treatment too short
- Culture is not representative of the infection
- There is not an bacterial infection
- Apparent *in vitro* susceptibility to beta-lactam drugs with some meticillin-resistant *Staphylococcus aureus* (MRSA), meticillin-resistant *Staphylococcus pseudintermedius* (MRSP) and extended spectrum beta-lactamase (ESBL) producing *Escherichia coli* should be checked – speak to your laboratory about tests for penicillin binding protein 2a (PBP2a) or PCR for *mec*A and ESBL genes (especially AmpC)
- MRSA and MRSP isolates showing apparent *in vitro* susceptibility to clindamycin should be checked for inducible clindamycin resistance (*erm* genes or an erythromycin D-zone test) to ensure that this drug will be effective
- Enrofloxacin is a pro-drug that is part-metabolised into ciprofloxacin – tests based on enrofloxacin or ciprofloxacin may not accurately reflect tissue levels of the two drugs in combination

Table 6.1 Predicting drug-specific antimicrobial susceptibility patterns using *in vitro* sensitivity tests.

Antimicrobial	Susceptibility patterns and predictions
Amikacin	Predicts resistance to other aminoglycosides; susceptibility does not imply susceptibility to gentamicin (see below)
Amoxicillin–clavulanate	ESBL-producing isolates sensitive to amoxicillin–clavulanate but resistant to cephalosporins AmpC-producing isolates are resistant to amoxicillin–clavulanate and cephalosporins
Ampicillin	Predicts susceptibility to amoxicillin in all bacteria and to penicillin in Gram-positive bacteria
Cephalexin	Predicts susceptibility to first- and second-generation cephalosporins (including cefovecin) ESBL- and AmpC-producing isolates are resistant (see note above for amoxicillin–clavulanate)
Cefoxitin	MRSA and MRSP are resistant EBSL-producing isolates are susceptible AmpC-producing isolates are resistant
Cefotaxime	Predicts susceptibility to all third-generation cephalosporins (not cefovecin)
Chloramphenicol	Predicts susceptibility to florfenicol
Clindamycin	Predicts susceptibility to all lincosamides (lincomycin) in Gram-positive bacteria; inducible resistance should be ruled out by susceptibility to erythromycin (see below) or PCR
Doxycycline	Predicts susceptibility to doxycycline in Gram-positive bacteria (including MRSA/MRSP) Specific susceptibility should be used with Gram-negative bacteria
Enrofloxacin or marbofloxacin	Predicts susceptibility to other fluoroquinolones in all bacteria except anaerobes (extended spectrum with pradofloxacin); enrofloxacin is part-metabolised into ciprofloxacin so *in vitro* susceptibility may not predict *in vivo* efficacy
Erythromycin	Predicts inducible resistance to lincosamides (lincomycin and clindamycin); do not use these drugs if the isolate is resistant to erythromycin
Gentamicin	Predicts susceptibility to other aminoglycosides; resistant isolates may still be susceptible to amikacin
Nitrofurantoin	Can be used to treat multidrug-resistant urinary tract infections
Sulphamethoxazole	Predicts susceptibility or resistance to all sulphonamides
Tetracycline	Predicts susceptibility to doxycycline in Gram-positive bacteria (including MRSA/MRSP) Specific susceptibility should be used with Gram-negative bacteria

ESBL = extended spectrum beta-lactamase; MRSA = meticillin-resistant *Staphylococcus aureus*; MRSP = meticillin-resistant *Staphylococcus pseudintermedius*; PCR = polymerase chain reaction.

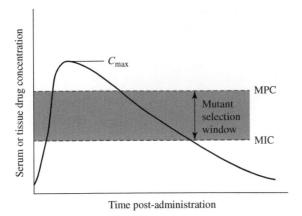

Figure 6.14 Mutant prevention concentration. *Source:* Drlica 2003. Reproduced with permission of Oxford University Press.

when selecting an appropriate antibiotic. The cost of the medication, frequency of dosing and owner compliance will also influence the choice or drug and formulation.

Mutant Prevention Concentration

Newer publications stress the importance of the mutant prevention concentration (MPC), which is the concentration that is effective in preventing selective proliferation of rare resistant mutants (Figure 6.14). The advantage of using this value to determine effective antibiotic dosages is that fewer resistant strains are expected to emerge, and antibiotic resistance is one of the major issues we face in medicine. The problem is that very high bacterial populations are required to identify the rare resistant mutants and the MPC (typically $>10^7$ bacteria compared to 10^5 bacteria used in MIC tests) and these tests are not yet commercially available.

Common Pitfalls for Bacterial Cultures

- The sampling site was not representative.
- Recent antibiotic or antibacterial use results in a false-negative culture.
- Topical disinfectant use prior to sampling results in false-negative culture.
- Contamination results in false-positive results.
- Subculturing in the laboratory is not representative of the *in vivo* bacterial population.
- Errors in interpreting the susceptibility results.

Wood's Lamp

Wood's lamp examination is a tool to find hairs infected with dermatophytes. A Wood's lamp is a source of ultraviolet (UV) light filtered through a cobalt or nickel filter, emitting a UV light of 253.7 nm wavelength. This light frequency makes the tryptophan metabolites of certain dermatophytes fluoresce. Many *Microsporum canis* (but not all) strains fluoresce and show up as apple green light (Figure 6.15). Other species that

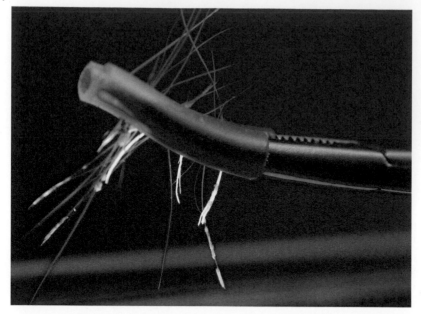

Figure 6.15 Apple green fluorescence along the hair shaft of hair obtained by trichography from a patient infected with dermatophytes. *Source:* Courtesy of F. Albanese.

may show up with this test include *M. distortum*, *M. audouinii* and *Trichophyton schoenleinii*, but most dermatophytes do not fluoresce at all.

Modern Wood's lamps emit stable UV light and do not need to be warmed up. However, it is important to wait a few minutes before conducting the examination to allow your eyes to adapt to the dark and increase the likelihood of seeing the fluorescence. There may also be a short delay before the fungal metabolites start to glow. The coat of the patient suspected of having a dermatophyte infection is then carefully examined in a completely dark room, which can take several minutes. Infected hair should show up as apple green fluorescing strands. False-positives are possible as scale, crust, some bacteria (e.g. *Pseudomonas* spp.) and some medications can fluoresce as well (although these normally fluoresce blue–white or dark green). Once fluorescing hairs have been identified, it is good practice to pluck these for direct microscopy or dermatophyte culture. Not all fluorescing hairs will be culture positive though, as the fluorescence may be residual in the absence of fungal growth or spores. Fluorescence of hairs on a slide can help guide direct microscopy. Permanent positive control slides can be made from infected cats for comparison.

Common Pitfalls

- The Wood's lamp was not used for long enough, or your eyes were not dark-adapted or the room was not dark enough resulting in a false-negative.
- Most dermatophyte species and strains do not fluoresce, leading to false-negative results.
- Scales, medication and certain bacteria can fluoresce leading to a false-positive result.
- Remember that Wood's lamps are a good rule in (highly specific) but not a good rule out (lower sensitivity).

Dermoscopy

Dermoscopy (see Chapter 4) may be useful in the diagnosis of dermatophytosis in cats and other species, although it takes some practice and experience to detect the infected hair shaft abnormalities (comma-like hairs). The dermascopic appearance of the skin and hairs is fairly specific for different fungal infections in humans. In one study, dermoscopy identified three cats with infected hairs not yet detectable by Wood's lamp. The technique could be particularly useful to identify hairs for direct microscopy and fungal culture. Again, the specificity seems to be high but the sensitivity can be low.

Fungal Culture Media

The two most commonly used dermatophyte culture media are dermatophyte test medium (DTM) and Sabouraud dextrose agar. Sabouraud dextrose agar contains agar, dextrose and peptones, and is suitable for dermatophytes, other fungi and filamentous bacteria, such as *Nocardia*. DTM is based on Sabouraud dextrose agar, with the addition of cycloheximide to suppress the growth of saprophytic fungi, gentamicin and chlor-tetracycline as antibiotics to inhibit bacteria growth, and phenol red as a pH indicator. The pH indicator is useful, as it enables the user to distinguish between the type of fungi cultured based on the preferred metabolism. Adding a drop of a vitamin B complex to the medium can be useful in cultures from horses, as *Trichophyton equinum* var. *equinum* requires niacin for growth.

DTM plates are much easier to use than the screw-top bottle agar slopes. A rapid sporulation medium is also available, which makes species identification easier as it encourages spore formation. The culture plates should be stored in the dark at 2–25 °C prior to use, and warmed to room temperature just before inoculation. The plate should be intact and not show any signs of contamination, drying, cracking, discolouration or excessive condensation. During the incubation period, the temperature should be maintained at 25–30 °C and 30% humidity. Ideally an incubator should be used to ensure minimal variation from these conditions, otherwise it may be better to submit the material to a reference laboratory. Some manufacturers allow full light exposure during the incubation period while some authors recommend protection from light to avoid UV-induced inhibition of fungal growth.

Interpreting Growth on Dermatophyte Test Media

On DTM, dermatophytes preferentially metabolise the proteins in the medium first and the alkaline by-products cause a red colour change. Most saprophytic fungi metabolise carbohydrates first, which results in acidic metabolites without a colour change. However, once the carbohydrates have been used up, saprophytic fungi can also utilise the proteins and a colour change occurs. It is therefore important to examine the DTM culture plate on a daily basis. If the colour change occurs within the first 7–10 days, when the colony is still relatively small, dermatophyte growth is most likely the reason for the pH change. However, if the colour changes after 7–10 days, and the colony is already relatively big, it is more likely that saprophytic fungi are present. In addition, dermatophytes form fluffy white to off-white colonies; slimy, smooth and/or pigmented colonies are likely to be contaminants. Be aware that *Trichophyton* species may not always induce a red colour change on DTM, although they will form typical fluffy white colonies. A stained tape-strip impression (using the basophilic stain only – see Chapter 1) of the colony will reveal characteristic spiral hyphae and flask-shaped spores and/or you can send a sample for culture on Sabouraud agar.

Identifying Common Fungal Pathogens

It can be very useful to speciate the dermatophyte implicated in a fungal infection as it gives more information about the source of infection. Dermatophyte test medium (DTM) is a good first indication that dermatophytes are the causative organisms in a patient's skin disease, although they are less useful to identify species of the fungus. In most cases DTM can reliably distinguish between a dermatophyte (Figure 6.16)

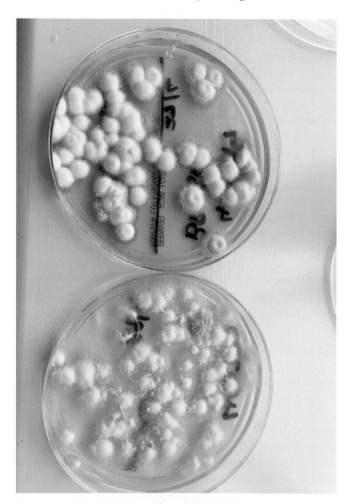

Figure 6.16 Obverse image of a culture of *Trichophyton mentagrophytes* (top) and *Microsporum canis* (bottom). *Source:* Courtesy of Stephen Steen.

and a contaminant (Figure 6.17), if used properly and examined on a daily basis. Once a dermatophyte has been cultured, this can either be subcultured on a Sabouraud plate in the practice (if this is commonly carried out) or sent to a commercial laboratory. Table 6.2 and Table 6.3 summarise diagnostic features of common dermatophyte species. Readers should be aware that pathogenic fungi are being reclassified according to recent molecular findings and that their nomenclature will change in the future. For example, dermatophytes are being classified in the genus *Arthoderma*, and the *Arthroderma otae* complex includes *M. canis*, *M. furrugineum*, *M. equimum* and *M. audouinii*.

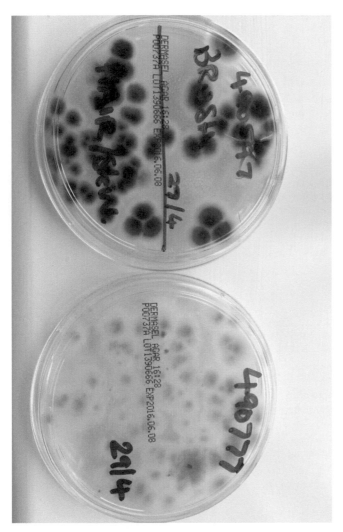

Figure 6.17 Reverse image of a culture of *Trichophyton mentagrophytes* (top) and *Microsporum canis* (bottom). *Source:* Courtesy of Stephen Steen.

Table 6.2   Identification of some dermatophyte species relevant for veterinary medicine.

Species	Incidence	Colony appearance	Reverse colony colour	Macroconidia	Microconidia
Microsporum canis	70% dogs 98% cats	Fluffy, white with golden yellow border, radial grooves	Yellow to brown	Six or more thick-walled cells with knob end, spiny	Pyriform (flame or pear shaped) to round, few, along hyphae
Microsporum gypseum	20% dogs 1% cats	Yellowish brown (cinnamon buff) with white border, mycelium fast spreading	Cream, tan or red brown	Thin walled, three to six cells, rounded ends, numerous	Clavate (club shaped)
Microsporum nanum	Pigs	White to buff, powdery	Orange turns to red–brown	Numerous, oval with thin spiny wall and one to three cells	Clavate, few
Trichophyton mentagrophytes	10% dogs 1% cats	Buff, powdery or white, downy	Brown to tan, dark red, yellow	Thin, cigar-shaped, smooth walls	Coiled, spiral hyphae, can be rare or numerous, round to pyriform
Trichophyton verrucosum	Cattle	White, yellow or grey, velvety, heaped smaller colonies	White or yellow	Rare, long, thin, smooth walled; chlamydospore chains	Rare, pyriform to clavate
Trichophyton equinum	Horse	Cream to tan, velvety	Yellow to red–brown	Rare, clavate, thin, smooth walled, three to five cells	Many on hyphae, pyriform to round

Table 6.3   Identifying common dermatophyte species.

Dermatophyte	Hyphae	Microconidia	Macroconidia
Microsporum canis	Straight	Club- to pear-shaped; along hyphae	Large, spindle-shaped, rough and thick-walled with terminal button; more than six cells
Microsporum gypseum	Straight	Club- to pear-shaped; along hyphae	Large, spindle-shaped, smooth and thin-walled without terminal button; fewer than six cells
Trichophyton mentagrophytes	Spiral	Grape-like clusters; flask-shaped	Long, cigar-shaped, smooth and thin-walled

Please note that macroconidia production by dermatophytes on DTM may be delayed or fail to occur. The other features are inconsistent and may be variable, and full identification should be made by a mycology laboratory using Sabouraud medium.

Detecting Unusual Fungal and Bacterial Organisms (e.g. Deep Fungal Infections and Mycobacteria)

Unusual, often deep and sometimes systemic fungal and bacterial infections are rarely encountered in small animal practice in the UK. They are more common in other parts of the world. Some infections, such as pythiosis, are restricted to certain geographic locations. It is important that you are aware of the local risk of infection, and ensure that you investigate this in suspicious cases (particularly those with granulomatous disease, nodules, draining sinus tracts and disseminated disease).

Many of these organisms are ubiquitous in the soil or are aquatic organisms, and are opportunistic infections only. Usually they are only found in immunosuppressed patients, e.g. dogs or cats on long-term therapy with ciclosporin, prednisolone and other immunosuppressive drugs. Organisms implicated include *Pythium* spp., *Rhizopus* spp., *Mucor* spp, *Absidia* spp., *Basidiobolus* spp., *Conidiobolus* spp., *Mortierella* spp., *Sporothrix* spp., *Lagenidium* spp., blastomycosis, histoplasmosis, aspergillosis, protothecosis etc.

Mycobacterial infections can also be found in domestic animals. Culture was thought to be essential to identify which species is implicated, but this can be slow and difficult, and requires specialist laboratory facilities. Cytology can be suggestive of mycobacteria infections (see Chapter 4) but biopsy may be needed to find the organisms. However, some cases may be Ziehl–Nielsen stain negative and even a positive stain will not differentiate the species involved. Polymerase chain reaction (PCR) techniques are available for some of the species, but may be limited – for example, in the UK the available tests will distinguish *Mycobacterium tuberculosis* complex from *M. avium* complex but will not distinguish species within these complexes (e.g. *M. microti* from *M. bovis*) or other types of mycobacteria. A whole-blood interferon gamma (IFNg) release assay (IGRA) can be used to help distinguish infections with environmental mycobacteria, avian TB (*Mycobacterium avium*), *Mycobacterium microti* and *Mycobacterium bovis* or *Mycobacterium tuberculosis* (Table 6.4).

Table 6.4 Whole-blood interferon gamma release assay (IGRA) for mycobacteria.

PPDA	PPDB	ESAT6/CFP10	Interpretation
Negative	Negative	Negative	Tuberculosis complex unlikely Avian complex unlikely Environmental mycobacteria possible if acid-fast bacteria in lesions
Positive	Negative	Negative	Tuberculosis complex unlikely Avian complex possible Environmental mycobacteria possible
Positive	Positive	Negative	Less pathogenic tuberculosis possible (most likely to be *Mycobacterium microti*)
Positive	Positive	Positive	Pathogenic tuberculosis complex (most likely to be *M. tuberculosis* or *M. bovis*)

IGRA involves incubating whole blood samples with specific mycobacterial antigens (PPDA = purified *M. avium* protein derivative; PPDB = purified *M. bovis* protein derivative; ESAT6 = 6 kDa early secretory antigenic target; CFP10 = 10 kDa culture filtrate protein antigen). Antigen-presenting cells process and present the antigens to antigen-specific T-cells inducing interferon gamma release.

Obviously, some species carry a high zoonotic risk and this needs to be discussed with the owner, and any material submitted to the laboratory with suspected mycobacterial infection needs to be marked as such, to enable personnel to take extra precautions.

Antifungal Susceptibility Testing

Fungal culture and antifungal drug susceptibility testing is available using microdilution, Kirby-Bauer disc and e-strip techniques. However, these are not routinely performed and are not generally available outside specialist fungal laboratories. In addition, susceptibility breakpoints for systemic treatment have not been established for all fungal pathogens (particularly in animals) and in some cases there is poor correlation between microdilution and disc-based methods. Clinicians are therefore strongly advised to contact the mycology laboratory before submitting samples for antifungal susceptibility tests.

7

Introduction to Histopathology

As we have already seen, most skin diseases cannot be identified on clinical appearance alone. Confirmation of the diagnosis relies on careful evaluation of the history, clinical signs and clinical data. Histopathology is the only test that allows the clinician to view what is actually happening in the skin at a cellular level. It can therefore be of huge value in confirming a diagnosis. Other advantages of histopathology compared to cytology and similar techniques include: greater sensitivity and specificity, as a much greater amount of tissue is harvested; assessment of tissue architecture and invasiveness of lesions; and assessment of the full thickness of the skin, including subcutaneous tissues.

Disadvantages of biopsy and histopathology, compared to cytology, include: it is more time consuming and invasive, often requiring sedation and local anaesthesia, or general anaesthesia; greater expense; and delayed results. Histopathology is not always diagnostic, as some diseases cause non-specific changes in the skin. It is also possible that poor site selection leads to non-specific and/or misleading results. Histopathology, like all tests in veterinary medicine, is only a snapshot in time and therefore not always diagnostic and it is important to warn the owners prior to performing the test that this may be the case.

Veterinary dermatohistopathology is a rapidly evolving, specialised field. It is important that samples are submitted to pathologists with an interest and experience in skin diseases of animals. Ideally, samples should be submitted to members of the International Society of Veterinary Dermatopathology (ISVD – https://www.isvd.org).

Indications for Performing a Biopsy

There are many indications for histopathology in veterinary dermatology. Although histopathology is never completely useless, the diagnostic yield is higher under certain circumstances than others. Certain primary lesions are unlikely to be associated with a diagnostic histopathology. Sometimes histopathology is useful to rule out certain conditions, but it will be most useful if the disease suspected by the clinician can only be diagnosed by biopsy, when the patient has not responded to seemingly appropriate therapy at adequate doses for a sufficient duration, when unusual lesions are present, when neoplastic lesions are suspected, when treatment of the suspected disease can be associated with adverse effects and in many cases of ulcerative disease. Some cases, where a persistent or unusual infection is suspected, may also benefit from submitting tissues samples both for histopathological analysis and for tissue culture.

Diagnostic Techniques in Veterinary Dermatology, First Edition. Ariane Neuber and Tim Nuttall.
© 2017 Ariane Neuber and Tim Nuttall. Published 2017 by John Wiley & Sons, Ltd.

Considerations Before Performing a Biopsy

Prior medical therapy can have an influence on the inflammatory infiltrate. If glucocorticoids have recently been administered, skin biopsies should ideally be delayed unless a life-threatening condition is suspected. As a guideline, prednisolone tablets should be withdrawn for about 2 weeks before performing skin biopsies. For injectable glucocorticoids the duration of action needs to be added to this. In contrast, antibiotic therapy is often helpful to avoid secondary bacterial infection masking the primary disease. However, in cases where deep infections are suspected and biopsy samples for tissue culture are planned, antibiotic therapy may need to be discontinued (see Chapter 5).

Site Selection

Correct site selection is important to maximise the clinical usefulness of biopsies. It is therefore important that clinicians learn to recognise and understand the significance of primary and secondary lesions. The gross skin lesions will not be evident once the biopsy specimen is taken and submitted. The pathologist relies on an accurate description of the clinical lesions to interpret the histopathology and make a diagnosis.

Generally speaking, you want to perform a biopsy on early lesions in inflammatory diseases before these are overlaid with non-specific secondary changes, such as ulceration, fibrosis and secondary infection etc. (Table 7.1). Atrophic, non-inflammatory diseases, in contrast, are best sampled at their fullest extent. These are not absolutes though, and in practice it may be better to take samples from a range of lesions. It is important, however, that these are submitted in separate pots that are clearly labelled, and that full clinical details (with digital or photogaphic images if possible) are also submitted. It is important to record the site of each biopsy so that the findings can be correlated to the precise clinical lesion. Knowing the site also helps the pathologist interpret the samples, as particular regions of the skin have distinctive histopathology and preferred reaction patterns.

Site Preparation

You will usually need to gently clip the hair, but should not otherwise prepare the skin. Any disturbance may remove surface features, and induce inflammatory changes that

Table 7.1 Primary and secondary skin lesions.

Primary lesions	Lesions that may be primary or secondary	Secondary lesions
Papule	Alopecia	Excoriation
Pustule or epidermal collarette	Scale	Lichenification
Vesicle or bulla	Crust	Erosions and ulcers
Plaque	Changes in pigmentation	Callus
Nodule	Comedones	Fissure
Wheal	Follicular casts	Scar
Macule or patch		

could mask subtle diagnostic pathology. The authors have yet to see any biopsy site become seriously infected or fail to heal as a result. The one exception is third phalanx amputation (see later in this chapter) – this involves entry into deep tissues and joint surfaces, and the digit should be surgically prepared. Hand washing, and sterile instruments and gloves should, however, be used with all biopsy techniques to minimise risks of contamination.

Biopsy Technique

Performing a skin biopsy is not technically difficult but has to be done carefully in order to avoid artefactual changes. Ideally the patient is sedated, for example with medetomidine and butorphanol or a similar combination. However, if performing a biopsy on the nose or some other areas on the head, a full general anaesthetic should be given. Some sites (e.g. digits) can be anaesthetised using regional nerve blocks.

1) After carefully choosing the biopsy sites, the hair is gently clipped if necessary. A circle can be drawn around the site with a permanent marker pen. Some dermatologists bisect this circle with a straight line along the direction of hair growth, which can help the pathologist correctly orientate the tissue block for sectioning along (and not across) the hair follicles.

2) If desired, a local anaesthetic can be injected underneath the sampling site to provide additional analgesia. Local anaesthetic should be injected into the subcutis rather than the dermis to avoid histopathological artefacts. Inserting the needle from outside the marked circle and redirecting under the biopsy site helps avoid any artefact from the needle track. The use of epinephrine may result in mast cell degranulation and can potentially affect dermal blood vessels; however, these changes are rarely of great importance. A volume of 0.5–1.0 mL is sufficient: large amounts of local anaesthetic can give the impression of dermal oedema or distort the tissue architecture.

3) Choose the biggest size biopsy punch possible for the tissue to be sampled. Haired skin on most body surfaces can usually be sampled with an 8-mm punch, whereas footpads (particularly on cats) and planum nasale biopsies may require the use of a 4- or 6-mm punch.

4) A biopsy punch is used to collect samples in a steady, firm, slow circular motion. It is important to rotate the biopsy punch in one direction only to avoid shear forces occurring and causing shearing artefacts. Some lesions, e.g. ulcers, lend themselves more to taking elliptical specimens with a scalpel blade. Firm pressure is needed to cut all the way to the subcutaneous adipose tissue in order to easily harvest the resulting tissue sample.

5) The sample is gently grasped with small forceps from underneath, as crush artefacts need to be avoided. The sample is then transferred into a pot and submerged in 10% buffered formalin for fixation during transport, or gently laid on a piece of cardboard or tongue depressor with the subcutaneous side touching the card and submerged attached to the cardboard/tongue depressor. This has the advantage that the direction of hair growth can be marked on the cardboard allowing the laboratory

technician to cut the skin in the desired plane. Placing the tissue sample onto cardboard or a tongue depressor is especially useful for elliptical samples as curling and distortion can otherwise occur.

6) The defect resulting in the skin at the biopsy site is then closed with an appropriate suture with a mattress, cross or single stitch and the suture should be removed about 10 days later. Wound complication post skin biopsies is extremely rare.

Punch biopsies largely harvest the epidermis and dermis, and only include variable amounts of the superficial subcutis. Punch biopsies may therefore not be representative of thicker and or deeper lesions. A wedge excision is usually preferred in these situations. Wedge excisions may also be useful where closure of a round punch biopsy site may deform the skin (e.g. nose, footpad, eyelid and ear). A 'double-punch' technique has also been described – a large-diameter punch is used to collect the epidermis and dermis, and a smaller diameter punch is then inserted into the biopsy site to sample deeper tissues. It can be difficult to achieve effective deep local anaesthesia without distorting the tissues in these cases so remote blocks (e.g. ring block, inverse L-block or direct nerve blocks) or a general anaesthetic should be used.

Third phalanx (P3) amputations are used for suspected symmetrical lupoid ony-chodystrophy and other digital problems. This is because the surrounding haired skin only reflects secondary inflammation and infection, with the representative changes only present in the periosteum or body of P3. A technique using a sharp 8-mm biopsy punch to shave off the lateral claw and underlying tissue down to the bone of P3 has been described, although the tissues may become fragmented and non-diagnostic. P3 amputation is usually diagnostic, although some care should be taken to select a digit early in the disease process without secondary infection and chronic change – look for lifting, splitting and (if visible) haemorrhage of the proximal claw plate. Owners are often resistant to this procedure, equating it to losing a fingertip, but they should be reassured that the cosmetic and functional outcome is good. Ideally, we would sample one of the dew claws (digit 1) or one of the least weight-bearing claws, but it is more important to select a claw that is most likely to give you a diagnosis. Many dermatologists will be happy to diagnose the disease based on the history, clinical examination and ruling out other differentials rather than pursuing this invasive diagnostic test.

As avian skin is very fragile, a special technique has been developed using transparent sticky tape applied to the skin surface prior to taking the sample. With the tape on the skin surface, the biopsy punch is used to cut both the tape and the skin in the same way as used for mammalian skin (Figure 7.1). The tape stops the sample from curling over (Figure 7.2). Curled samples are very difficult to cut and interpret.

Excessive squeezing of the sample can cause basophilic amorphous changes in the connective tissue and distortion of potential inflammatory infiltrates. Diathermy used to stop excessive bleeding can cause serious artefacts if used while the sample is still *in situ* during its use. A bizarre alteration of the cellular and nuclear architecture can be seen, as well as giving the connective tissues a homogenised eosinophilic appearance. If, despite careful handling, any crusts fall off, they should be submitted with the biopsy samples.

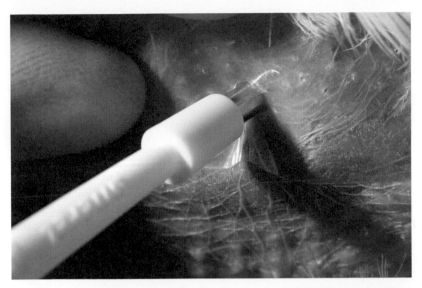

Figure 7.1 Biopsy technique for avian patients: clear sticky tape has been applied to the skin surface prior to sampling the site with a biopsy punch.

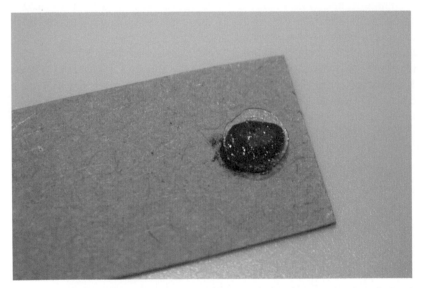

Figure 7.2 Biopsy technique for avian patients: the harvested skin punch with the clear sticky tape attached is laid on a piece of cardboard to avoid curling.

Submission of the Samples

The samples should be submitted in screw-topped containers, which are closed securely and preferably sealed with tape to prevent leakage. Biopsy specimens must be securely packaged, following IATA statutory regulations (further information can be found on the Royal Mail website). Each container should be marked with the owner's and animal's name and the biopsy site. The container needs to be accompanied by a short clinical history, including treatments and differential diagnoses. A lesion map is often helpful. The more information given, the easier it is for the pathologist to produce a good and helpful report.

Does the Histopathology Make Sense?

The histopathological changes should match the history, clinical signs and differential diagnosis. It is rare for histopathology to reveal a diagnosis out of the blue, although there are some changes that are non-specific and therefore less helpful in achieving a diagnosis. If the histopathology does not make sense, consider the following.

- Were the biopsy specimens representative? As discussed earlier, try to perform biopsies on active lesions and take several samples if unsure. Only a small percentage of the tissue sampled can actually be examined microscopically, so if the lesion is small, it may be missed during processing the sample. Important clues for the pathologist may be removed if the site has been surgically prepared, especially surface changes, such as crusts, pustules and bullae.
- Were the diagnostic features altered or overwhelmed? Do not prepare the biopsy site, use a careful technique, and avoid secondarily infected or excoriated sites. Secondary infection can overwhelm the features of many diseases, e.g. cutaneous lupus, so in some cases, a course of antibiotics prior to sampling may be indicated.
- Were the clinical lesions correctly identified and interpreted? Was the differential diagnosis list appropriate? Although the pathologist will not usually look at this section on the submission form prior to writing the description and morphological diagnosis, in order to review the sample with an open mind, all this information can be hugely helpful in the interpretation as many breed predispositions exist, the lesion distribution can be very helpful and the presence of certain types of lesions can be a useful feature.

If in doubt, contact the pathologist directly to discuss the case. Sometimes the examination of further or deeper sections or special stains may be useful or a second opinion from a different pathologist may be sought.

The Histopathology Report

It is important to learn to read and interpret all the histopathology report, not just the final diagnosis. The report will usually consist of:

- description of the findings in the epidermis, dermis and adnexae (and/or subcutis, claws etc. depending on the biopsy site);
- morphological diagnosis of the histopathology patterns – the pattern analysis (see later in this chapter);.
- clinical or aetiological diagnosis if possible;
- comments on the sections, possible underlying conditions, further investigation, treatment options, prognosis etc. as appropriate.

It is important, however, to remember that pathologists are not clinicians and it may be useful to speak to a dermatologist or consider referral in some cases, particularly in more unusual cases.

Basic Histopathological Terminology

It is important to have some familiarity with histopathological terminology. Many of the terms have very precise meanings, and understanding these greatly aids understanding and interpretation of the histopathology report.

Crusts

Crusts (Figure 7.3) are accumulations of dried exudates, consisting of variable numbers and amounts of keratinocytes, neutrophils and other inflammatory cells, red blood cells, microorganisms and proteinaceous debris. Depending on their composition they are classified as serous, cellular, neutrophilic or haemorrhagic (or combinations thereof). Pallisading crusts consist of alternate layers of different types. Microorganisms such as staphylococci, *Dermatophilus* and other bacteria, *Malassezia* and dermatophytes may be visible. Crusts should be distinguished from scaling caused by hyperkeratosis, although the two may occur together. Crusts are non-specific, but are most commonly seen with infections, parasites, pemphigus foliaceus and erosions or ulceration.

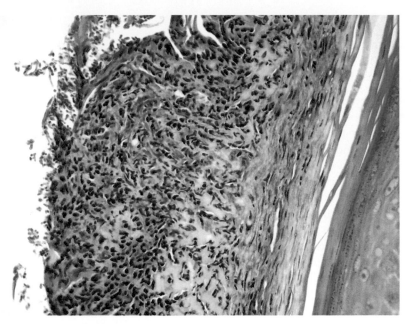

Figure 7.3 Neutrophilic crust with numerous *Malassezia* yeast visible on the top of the crust consisting predominantly of neutrophils. *Source:* Courtesy of D. Shearer.

Hyperkeratosis refers to thickening of the stratum corneum. Clinically apparent thickening of the skin (**lichenification**) is usually associated with a combination of hyperkeratosis and thickening of the living epidermis (**acanthosis**). This is a common, and fairly non-specific, finding in many skin conditions. Hyperkeratosis can be divided into several subtypes.

- Orthokeratotic hyperkeratosis – proliferation of non-nucleated keratinocytes. This is the most common form and is non-specific.
- Parakeratotic hyperkeratosis – proliferation of nucleated keratinocytes. Focal parakeratosis is fairly common with inflammation, especially trauma and erosion. More widespread parakeratosis is reasonably specific for metabolic conditions such as zinc-responsive dermatosis and superficial necrolytic dermatosis (or hepatocutaneous syndrome). Parakeratosis is usually associated with loss of the stratum granulosum (hypogranulosis).
- Basket weave hyperkeratosis is a loose arrangement of cornified cells in the stratum corneum. It is most common in milder and/or more acute conditions.
- Compact or lamellar hyperkeratosis is when the cornified cells are compacted into tight layers. It is usually associated with chronic inflammation, especially trauma, and severe scaling disorders, such as ichthyosis. Compact hyperkeratosis is usually associated with hyperplasia of the stratum granulosum (hypergranulosis).
- Dyskeratosis refers to abnormal, often disordered and premature keratinisation of the surface or follicular epidermis. It is uncommon but can be seen in severe inflammatory conditions, primary keratinisation disorders and squamous cell carcinoma.

Acanthosis or epidermal hyperplasia refers to thickening of the living epidermis. It is often associated with hyperkeratosis, and is a common, non-specific finding in many inflammatory dermatoses. There are a number of recognised subtypes.

- Regular – even thickening of the epidermis with a flat, regular dermo-epidermal junction.
- Irregular – irregular thickening of the epidermis with variable projections into the dermis (rete pegs) and folding of the dermo-epidermal junction. This is the most common form seen in cats and dogs.
- Psoriasiform – even thickening of the epidermis with regular rete peg formation and consistent folding of the dermo-epidermal junction. This is rare in dogs and cats, except at the nasal planum and foot pads, but is more common in large animals and humans.
- Papillated or papillomatous – uneven thickening of the epidermis with irregular surface projections and folding (i.e. like a papilloma). There is often irregular folding of the dermo-epidermal junction with projection of the dermis into the epidermis.
- Carcinomatous or pseudocarcinomatous – very irregular thickening of the epidermis and rete peg formation resembling invasive squamous cell carcinoma. This is uncommon in animals, but can be seen at the margins of chronic ulcers.

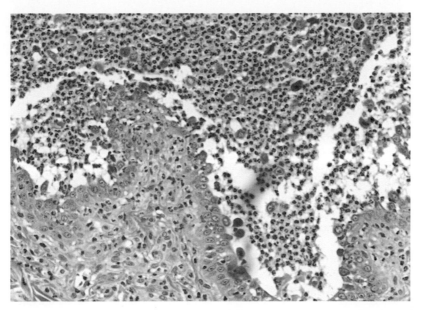

Figure 7.4 Exocytosis, spongiosis and intracellular oedema can be seen in this high-power photomicrograph of the epidermis of a dog with pemphigus foliaceus. *Source:* Courtesy of D. Shearer.

Epidermal Atrophy

Epidermal atrophy refers to specific thinning of the epidermis, which may or may not be associated with **dermal atrophy**. The structure of the stratum corneum and living epidermis is usually maintained. Thinning of the skin is uncommon, as the default reaction to most conditions is proliferation and thickening of the skin. Epidermal atrophy may be seen in cases of alopecia, especially endocrine or metabolic conditions.

Exocytosis

Exocytosis describes the migration of inflammatory cells into the epidermis (Figure 7.4). It is usually seen with spongiosis, and is a common, non-specific finding in inflammation.

Spongiosis

Spongiosis is intercellular oedema of the epidermis (Figure 7.4) that separates cells resulting in a 'spongy' appearance. In severe cases there may be intra-epidermal vesicles (also known as reticular degeneration). It is a common, non-specific finding in many inflammatory conditions.

Intracellular Oedema

Intracellular oedema should be differentiated from intercellular oedema or spongiosis. It results in cytoplasmic vacuolation and hydropic degeneration of cells. This is also known as ballooning degeneration, although this term is also used to describe the inclusion bodies and cytopathic effects seen in herpes and other viral infections. Hydropic degeneration is most commonly seen in the basal cell layer in immune-mediated conditions, but can also occur elsewhere in the epidermis. Severe, coalescing hydropic degeneration can lead to subepidermal clefts and dermo-epidermal separation.

Acantholytic Cells

Acantholytic cells (Figure 7.5) are rounded keratinocytes that have lost their intercellular adhesions. They are most commonly seen in vesicles or with neutrophils in pustules and crusts. They are most prominently seen in pemphigus foliaceus (Figure 7.6), but can occur in other conditions where keratinocyte separation occurs, such as pyoderma, dermatophytosis and dyskeratosis.

Epidermal Necrosis

Epidermal necrosis usually results in ulceration. There are some commonly described variants.

- Caseous necrosis when there is ill-defined, widespread cell death and degeneration of the epidermis and occasionally the superficial dermis, resulting in non-specific eosinophilic to basophilic debris. This may also be seen in overlying crusts. It is a non-specific finding, often as a result of trauma and severe inflammation.

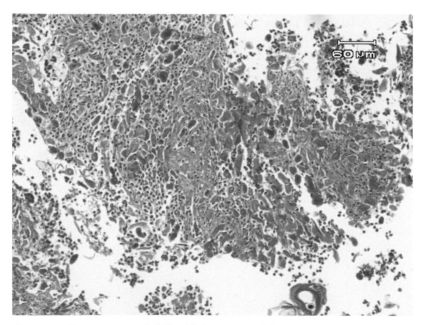

Figure 7.5 Numerous acantholytic cells in a neutrophilic pustule in a dog with pemphigus foliaceus. *Source:* Courtesy of D. Shearer.

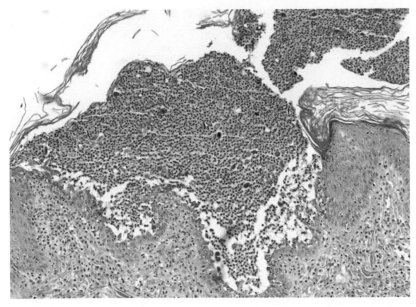

Figure 7.6 This sample shows a large pustule spanning multiple follicular ostiae with numerous acantholytic cells included in the neutrophilic inflammatory cells and debris. The sample was obtained from a dog with pemphigus foliaceus. *Source:* Courtesy of D. Shearer.

- Coagulative necrosis is more defined and more likely to involve both the epidermis and dermis, and occasionally overlying crust. It results in eosinophilic debris with 'ghost' cell outlines and pycnotic nuclear remnants. Coagulative necrosis is usually associated with physical injury, ischaemia or immune-mediated dermatoses.
- Necrolysis is a term used to describe coagulative necrosis of the epidermis only with no or minimal inflammation, e.g. toxic epidermal necrolysis.

Apoptosis

Apoptosis (Figure 7.7) refers to individual cell death within the epidermis. Apoptosis involves intracellular metabolic pathways and is distinct from necrosis, which is a non-metabolic process resulting from overwhelming cell damage. Apoptosis may be a physiological event or pathological, usually resulting from immune-mediated assault by cytotoxic T-cells. Apoptotic cells are usually eosinophilic, shrunken and surrounded by lymphocytes (satellitosis). They are eventually phagocytosed by neighbouring cells. Civatte bodies are apoptotic cells within the basal cell layer.

Pigmentary Incontinence

Pigmentary incontinence (Figure 7.7) is a term used to describe the release of melanin granules from the basal epidermis into the superficial dermis, where they are engulfed by macrophages. It is therefore associated with basal cell degeneration and interface dermatitis.

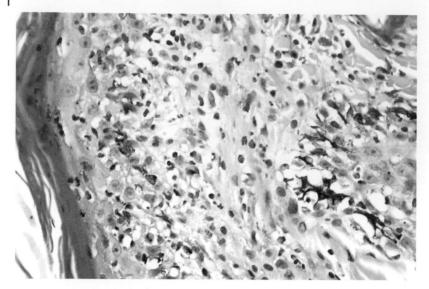

Figure 7.7 Apoptosis and pigmentary incontinence in a cat with erythema multiforme with a severe interface pattern. *Source:* Courtesy of D. Shearer.

Pattern Analysis

Pattern analysis is a widely used method of grouping and interpreting complex pathological changes within an individual into a series of inflammatory and other patterns. This greatly simplifies interpretation, as many patterns are associated with aetiological factors, enabling a diagnosis to be made or differential diagnosis and diagnostic plan (Table 7.2). Unfortunately, some of the more common reaction patterns are relatively non-specific. Major histopathological reaction patterns include:

- perivascular dermatitis (Figure 7.8, Figure 7.9);
- interface dermatitis (Figure 7.10, Figure 7.11);
- nodular dermatitis;
- diffuse dermatitis;
- intra-epidermal bullous or pustular dermatitis (Figure 7.12);
- subepidermal bullous or pustular dermatitis;
- vasculitis;
- folliculitis and/or furunculosis;
- panniculitis;
- atrophic.

Perivascular Dermatitis

This is the most common and least specific reaction pattern. There is normally dermal oedema with prominent blood vessels exhibiting margination and migration of inflammatory cells. These accumulate around the blood vessels, but there is no evidence of vasculitis (see later in this chapter). Epidermal involvement with

Table 7.2 Clinical signs of skin conditions and the associated histopathological patterns.

Clinical sign or lesion	Associated histopathological patterns
Pruritus	Intra-epidermal pustular or vesicular dermatitis Perivascular inflammatory infiltrate Nodular inflammatory infiltrate Interstitial to diffuse inflammatory infiltrate Folliculitis
Pustules	Intra-epidermal vesicular or pustular dermatitis Subepidermal pustules Crusting Perivascular dermatitis Folliculitis
Scaling/crusting	Intra- or subepidermal pustules or vesicles Perivascular dermatitis Folliculitis Hyperkeratosis (ortho- or parakeratotic)
Hyperpigmentation	Atrophic dermatopathy Perivascular dermatitis Folliculitis Diffuse to nodular dermatitis
Hypopigmentation	Interface dermatitis Nodular to diffuse dermatitis
Nodules	Diffuse to nodular dermatitis Folliculitis and/or furunculosis Panniculitis Vasculitis
Alopecia	Atrophic dermatosis Intra-epidermal pustular or vesicular dermatitis Perivascular dermatitis Folliculitis Interface dermatitis

acanthosis, spongiosis, hyperkeratosis, exocytosis and/or crusts is common. Perivascular dermatitis may be further classified as superficial (most common), mid or deep, depending on the depth of the blood vessels involved. Neutrophils are often associated with trauma or infection. Lymphocytes, macrophages and mast cells are common in most inflammatory infiltrates, and are particularly prominent in atopic dermatitis. Eosinophils suggest allergic or parasitic dermatoses, but degranulated cells may not be apparent without special staining.

Interface Dermatitis

Interface dermatitis is a pattern that involves hydropic degeneration and/or apoptosis of the basal cell layer with pigmentary incontinence. Interface dermatitis may be

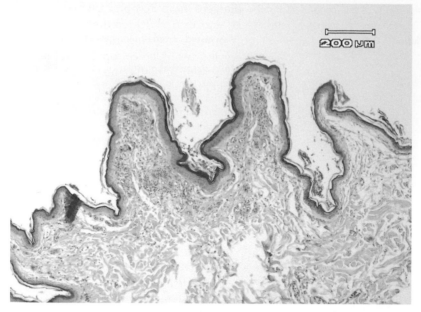

Figure 7.8 Low-power image of a perivascular dermatitis pattern. *Source:* Courtesy of D. Shearer.

cell-poor or cell-rich with a mononuclear cell infiltrate targeting the dermo-epidermal junction. This may be severe enough to obscure the junction and basal cell layer. Interface dermatitis usually supports a diagnosis of an immune-mediated, particularly lupus, condition.

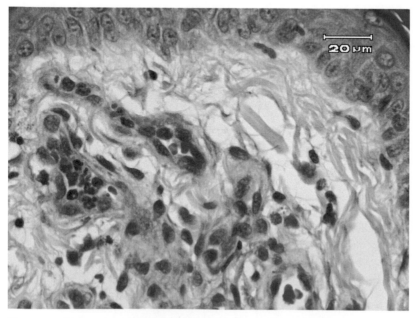

Figure 7.9 High-power image of a perivascular dermatitis pattern. *Source:* Courtesy of D. Shearer.

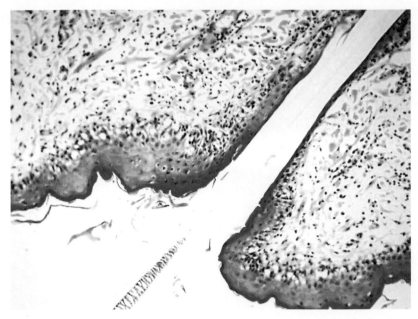

Figure 7.10 Low-power image of an interface pattern in a cat with thymoma-associated exfoliative dermatitis. *Source:* Courtesy of D. Shearer.

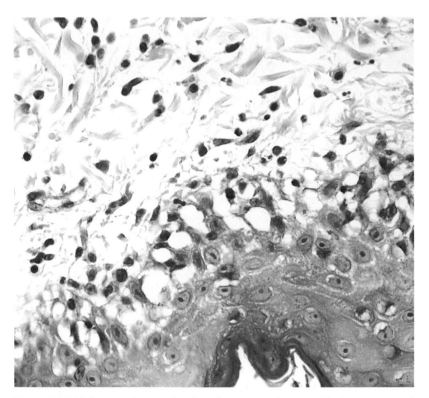

Figure 7.11 High-power image of an interface pattern in a cat with thymoma-associated exfoliative dermatitis. *Source:* Courtesy of D. Shearer.

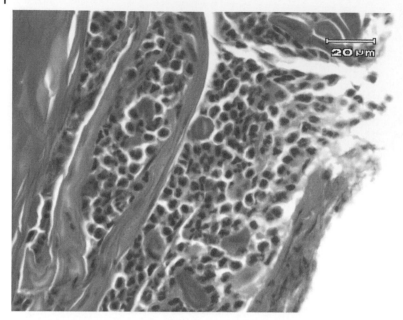

Figure 7.12 Footpad of a cat affected by pemphigus foliaceus. *Source:* Courtesy of D. Shearer.

Early cases of epitheliotropic lymphoma (mycosis fungoides) that obscure the dermo-epidermal junction may be confused with interface dermatitis. True interface dermatitis should also be differentiated from dense superficial mononuclear cell infiltrates without basal cell changes (often referred to as a lichenoid infiltrate or band). These are most commonly seen with superficial bacterial infections of the nasal planum and muco-cutaneous junctions (mucocutaneous pyoderma).

Nodular Dermatitis

Nodular dermatitis is characterised by well-defined, dense accumulations of inflammatory cells throughout the dermis. They may infiltrate into or efface other dermal structures. Nodules centred on hair follicle remnants and those in the subcutis usually indicate furunculosis and panniculitis respectively (see later in this chapter). The nature of the infiltrate often gives a clue to the aetiology:

- histiocytes and macrophages are usually associated with mycobacterial or fungal infections, foreign bodies and sebaceous adenitis (when targeting sebaceous glands);
- lymphocytic infiltrates can result from insect bites, vaccine and other drug reactions, idiopathic lymphocytosis and non-epitheliotropic lymphoma;
- neutrophils usually reflect bacterial infection, but can be a non-specific presence in most inflammatory reactions;
- eosinophils can be found in insect bites (e.g. mosquito bite hypersensitivity), other parasitic dermatoses and idiopathic eosinophilic granulomas.

Diffuse Dermatitis

A dense diffuse dermatitis usually results from a spreading and coalescing nodular dermatitis. A less dense diffuse dermatitis (also known as an interstitial dermatitis) usually results from a spreading and coalescing perivascular dermatitis.

Intra-Epidermal Bullous or Pustular Dermatitis

Bullae or vesicles are cell-poor, fluid-filled clefts within the epidermis. Pustules are essentially similar except that they are rich in inflammatory cells. They can result from intense spongiosis with or without exocytosis, acantholysis, intracellular oedema and cell degeneration and/or mechanical shearing forces. The lesions may be subcorneal (e.g. pemphigus foliaceus or pyoderma) or suprabasal (e.g. pemphigus vulgaris), and affect both the surface epidermis and hair follicle external root sheath.

The cell population can indicate the likely aetiology:

- neutrophils, often degenerate – pyoderma, especially if bacterial colonies can be identified;
- neutrophils, often non-degenerate, and acantholytic cells – pemphigus foliaceus;
- eosinophils – parasites, pemphigus foliaceus;
- macrophages – pyoderma, fungal infection;
- lymphocytes – hypersensitivity, epitheliotropic lymphoma.

Subepidermal Bullous or Pustular Dermatitis

Subepidermal bullous or pustular conditions (also known as subepidermal blistering diseases) are much less common. Most exhibit cell-poor vesicles with separation at the dermo-epidermal junction. This can be associated with immune-mediated or congenital diseases that affect the basal cell layer and basement membrane (e.g. epidermolysis bullosa acquisita, junctional epidermolysis bullosa, bullous pemphigoid and cutaneous lupus), severe dermal oedema, and physical, chemical or thermal trauma. Clefting can also be a shear artefact with poor biopsy technique, especially if the biopsy punch is blunt and/or rotated from side to side.

Vasculitis

This refers to specific inflammation of blood vessels and should not be confused with perivascular dermatitis (see earlier in this chapter). It is characterised by moderate to intense inflammation centred on blood vessels with margination, migration through the vessel wall and perivascular accumulation of cells. Some cases are associated with distinct inflammatory cell types, but the aetiological significance of this is not clear. There should also be definite involvement of the vessel wall with cell degeneration, nuclear 'dust', occasional endothelial cell hyperplasia and haemorrhage into the surrounding tissues. Mild vasculitis need not be associated with necrosis, although hair follicle atrophy can be seen. In more severe cases there may be thrombus formation and occlusion of blood vessels with necrosis of the vessel wall and surrounding tissues.

Folliculitis refers to inflammation of the hair follicle. Severe inflammation resulting in destruction and rupture of the hair follicle is termed furunculosis. This is essentially a type of nodular to diffuse dermatitis (see earlier in this chapter). Folliculitis may be further classified as:

- perifolliculitis – inflammation of the perifollicular dermis and blood vessels;
- mural folliculitis – inflammation of the external (outer) root sheath;
- luminal folliculitis – entire follicle and possibly also the hair shaft;
- bulbitis – inflammation targeting the hair bulb;
- sebaceous adenitis – inflammation targeting the sebaceous gland;
- hidradenitis – inflammation of the sweat glands.

The predominant cell type may yield clues to the aetiology:

- neutrophils, plasma cells and macrophages – bacterial folliculitis/furunculosis, bacterial colonies may be evident within the follicle and/or free in the dermis;
- eosinophils – parasites, especially mosquito bites;
- lymphocytes – idiopathic lymphocytic mural folliculitis, *Demodex*, dermatophytosis, epitheliotropic lymphoma, alopecia areata, pseudopelade;
- fungal hyphae and spores – dermatophytosis.

Panniculitis

This describes inflammation of the subcutaneous fatty tissues. This may be an extension of severe dermal inflammation, especially nodular dermatitis or furunculosis, vasculitis or necrosis. The predominant cell type may give an indication of the aetiology (see under Nodular dermatitis). Aetiological agents, such as foreign bodies, bacterial, mycobacteria or fungi, may be seen.

Atrophic

Unlike most other patterns, this is non-inflammatory. There may be combinations of epidermal, dermal, hair follicle and sebaceous atrophy. Epidermal and follicular hyperkeratosis may be present. This pattern is usually non-specific and associated with endocrinopathies or metabolic conditions, but more specific findings (e.g. calcinosis cutis in hyperadrenocorticism) may be present.

Hair Follicle Pathology

All the different anatomical structures that make up the hair follicle can be affected by inflammation. Therefore folliculitis is divided into: perifolliculitis (affecting the perifollicular vasculature), sebaceous adenitis (affecting the sebaceous glands), hidradenitis (affecting the apocrine sweat glands), mural folliculitis (affecting the outer root sheath), luminal folliculitis (affecting the hair follicle lumen) and bulbitis (affecting the hair bulb). If the inflammation is very severe, it can progress to

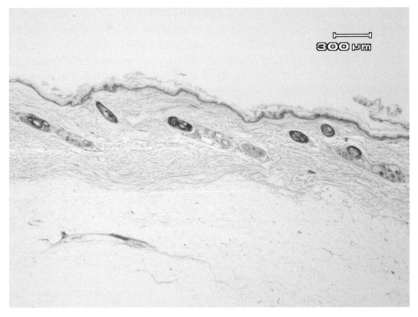

Figure 7.13 Low-power image of a dog diagnosed with alopecia X. *Source:* Courtesy of D. Shearer.

furunculosis: the follicle can rupture to release its contents into the tissue. This can lead to long-term complication due to free hair shafts in the tissue constituting foci for infection and eliciting a foreign body reaction even when the acute infection has been brought under control.

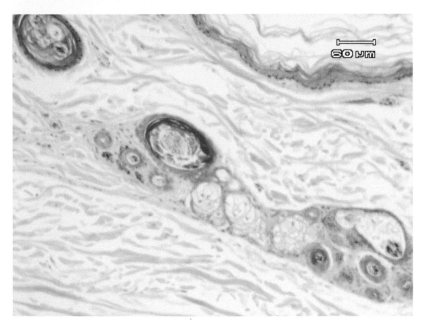

Figure 7.14 High-power image of a dog diagnosed with alopecia X. *Source:* Courtesy of D. Shearer.

Folliculitis can be caused by infections, such as bacterial folliculitis (often resulting in a neutrophilic inflammation) or dermatophytosis (lymphocytic inflammatory infiltrate predominating), parasitic skin disease, such as demodicosis (which is usually seen as a lymphoid mural folliculitis) or insect bite reaction (leading to an eosinophilic pattern of inflammation), or immune-mediated diseases, such as sebaceous adenitis and alopecia areata (seen as a lymphocytic bulbitis). Many non-inflammatory conditions can also affect the hair follicles, e.g. alopecia X, post-clipping alopecia, follicular dysplasias etc. Alopecia X, for example, is characterised by flame follicles histopathologically and in later stages the follicles can become distorted and dysplastic (Figure 7.13, Figure 7.14).

8

Allergy Testing

Pruritus is one of the most common reasons for pet owners to seek veterinary advice. The majority of cases are caused by parasitic or allergic skin diseases and are often complicated by microbial infections. The secondary infections need to be identified cytologically and treated successfully, before the primary disease can be diagnosed. Once parasitic dermatoses and, if indicated, rarer differential diagnoses have been ruled out in any given case of pruritic skin disease, an allergy work-up is indicated. Animals with cutaneous adverse food reactions (CAFR) or food-induced atopic dermatitis (FIAD) are often indistinguishable from atopic dermatitis (AD) associated with environmental allergens or the presumed non-allergic atopic-like dermatitis (ALD) based on historical and clinical features alone. Careful diet trials are therefore needed to identify animals where food plays a role in their skin disease.

The International Committee on Allergic Diseases in Animals (ICADA; www.icada. info) has defined canine AD as a genetically predisposed inflammatory and pruritic allergic skin disease with characteristic clinical features associated with IgE antibodies most commonly directed against environmental allergens. The same group has defined canine ALD as an inflammatory and pruritic skin disease with clinical features identical to those seen in canine AD in which an IgE response to environmental or other allergens cannot be documented. FIAD describes dogs with AD for whom food is one of the triggers for their disease.

The most important criteria for diagnosing an allergic skin disease are therefore historical and clinical features, which have been described by various authors. The most commonly accepted recent paper describing diagnostic criteria for canine atopic dermatitis was published by Favrot et al. in 2010 and has been summarised in Box 8.1. Only when a clinical diagnosis of atopic dermatitis has been made based on accepted diagnostic criteria, and all possible differential diagnoses have been ruled out, is allergy testing warranted. A diagnostic algorithm can be found in Figure 8.1 and a distribution of lesions for pattern analysis of pruritic diseases is given in Table 8.1.

Food Trials

As all cases of non-seasonal pruritus that are compatible with a clinical diagnosis of AD can potentially be exacerbated by food and/or non-food allergens, a food trial needs to be carried out to identify protein and/or carbohydrate sources that could trigger an adverse

Diagnostic Techniques in Veterinary Dermatology, First Edition. Ariane Neuber and Tim Nuttall.
© 2017 Ariane Neuber and Tim Nuttall. Published 2017 by John Wiley & Sons, Ltd.

Box 8.1 Diagnostic criteria for canine atopic dermatitis.

- Onset of signs under 3 years of age
- Dog living mostly indoors
- Glucocorticoid-responsive pruritus
- Pruritus *sine materia* at onset (i.e. non-lesional pruritus)
- Affected front feet
- Affected ear pinnae
- Non-affected ear margins
- Non-affected dorsolumbar area

A combination of five satisfied criteria has a sensitivity of 85% and a specificity of 79% to differentiate dogs with AD from dogs with chronic or recurrent pruritus without AD. Adding a sixth fulfilled parameter increases the specificity to 89% but decreases the sensitivity to 58%.

Source: Favrot C, Steffan J, Seewald W and others (2010) A prospective study on the clinical features of chronic canine atopic dermatitis and its diagnosis. *Veterinary Dermatology* 21, 23–30.

---

effect in the patient. These reactions may be associated with immunological or non-immunological pathways. There is a big overlap in food-induced and non-food-induced allergic skin disease, and recent research suggests that many 'food allergic' patients are a subgroup of AD termed FIAD. These animals should improve following dietary restriction, but will still have clinical signs associated with their inherent AD and/or environmental allergen exposure.

A dietary exclusion trial is the method recommended by most veterinary dermatologists to diagnose skin disease triggered by food. Alternative methods, such as intradermal allergy testing, patch testing and allergen-specific IgE testing at present have little value in the diagnosis of CAFR and FIAD, as they are neither sensitive nor specific and/or can be difficult to perform (see later in this chapter).

Food Antigens

Potentially any food can be an antigen, but the most frequent antigens in humans are eggs, cow's milk, nuts, fish, seafood, wheat and soy. The most common allergens in dogs include beef, wheat and milk, with chicken, egg, lamb and soy less common. Most dogs are react to more than one allergen, with an average of 2.4 in one study. This may reflect dietary habits rather than intrinsic allergenicity. Reactions to food additives are rare. There is no evidence that genetically modified (GM) foods are any more or less allergenic than 'native' foods.

The pattern of common reactive antigens in dogs seems to be changing. In 1996 the most common food antigen was beef (60%) with less common reactions to soy (32%), chicken (28%), milk (28%), corn (25%), wheat (24%) and egg (20%). This appeared to reflect common ingredients in pet foods at the time, and lamb and rice were commonly used in elimination diets. As commercial lamb and rice diets became more common, fish

Approach to a typical case of pruritus

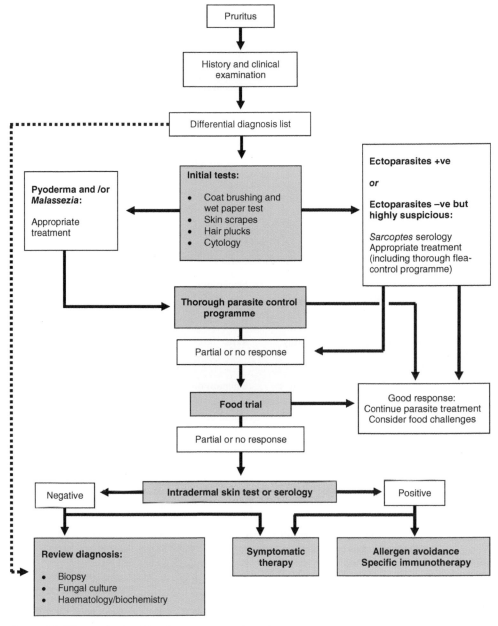

Figure 8.1 Diagnostic algorithm for non-seasonal pruritus.

Table 8.1 Lesion distribution of pruritic skin diseases in dogs.

Lesions	Differential diagnoses	Frequency	Other features
Face	Canine atopic dermatitis (food or environmentally induced)	Common	Other areas involved: axillae, paws, ears
	Malassezia lip-fold dermatitis	Uncommon	Secondary to allergic skin disease; breed predispositions: Basset Hound
	Otitis externa	Common	Otic discharge, malodour, head shaking, head tilt
	Otitis media	Uncommon	Otic discharge, malodour, head shaking, head tilt
	Behavioural disorders	Rare	History of stress, other behavioural problems
	Aujeszky's disease	Very rare	Sudden onset, violent self-trauma
Neck and shoulder	Fleas	Common	Fleas seen, inadequate flea control, multipet household, particularly with cats
	Chiari malformation; syringohydromelia	Uncommon	Strict breed predispositions brachicephalic breed (Cavalier Kind Charles Spaniel, Yorkshire Terrier, French Bulldog)
Distal limbs (not paws)	Peripheral neuropathy	Rare	Inherited in certain breeds (German Pointer, French Spaniel) or as post-traumatic issue
	Behavioural problem	Uncommon	History of stress, other behavioural problems
Tail base	Flea allergic dermatitis	Common	Fleas seen, inadequate flea control, multipet household, particularly with cats
Tip of the tail	Behavioural problem	Uncommon	History of stress, other behavioural problems
Flanks	Flea allergic dermatitis	Common	Fleas seen, inadequate flea control, multipet household, particularly with cats
	Canine atopic dermatitis (food or environmentally induced)	Common	Certain breed with unsual pattern of lesion distribution, e.g. Scandinavian breeds
	Behavioural problem	Uncommon	History of stress, other behavioural problems, Dobermann
Dorsum	Flea allergic dermatitis	Common	Fleas seen, inadequate flea control, multipet household, particularly with cats
	Lice	Uncommon	More likely in young or old or otherwise immunosuppressed dogs
	Herniated disc, vertebral pain	Common	Breed predispositions, e.g. Dachshund

Table 8.1 (*Continued*)

Lesions	Differential diagnoses	Frequency	Other features
Ventrum	Flea allergic dermatitis	Common	Fleas seen, inadequate flea control, multipet household, particularly with cats
	Canine atopic dermatitis (food or environmentally induced)	Common	Other areas involved: axillae, paws, ears
	Cystitis	Common	Inappropriate urination, blood in urine
Paws	Canine atopic dermatitis (food or environmentally induced)	Common	Other areas involved: axillae, paws, ears
	Malassezia dermatitis	Common	Secondary to allergic skin disease
	Interdigital furuncles	Common	Secondary to allergic skin disease
	Dermatophytosis of the footpads	Rare	Can cause ulceration of the pad

was more frequently used in trials. One result was that commercial fish-based diets became more popular, and recent studies have reported a high prevalence of reactions to herring and catfish.

Raw, Cooked and Processed Foods

There is no evidence that raw, cooked or processed foods are any more or less allergenic for any one individual. Protein allergens have complex primary (amino acid), secondary (alpha-helix and beta-sheets) and tertiary (three-dimensional [3D] folding) structures. Cooking, digestion and other processing may disrupt some epitopes but could also expose internal and previously hidden epitopes. The Maillard reaction occurs when amino acids and sugars combine at high temperatures to form melanoids. These may increase or decrease allergenicity of some foods, and may explain why some animals tolerate raw or home-cooked foods but not commercial diets (and vice versa).

Feeding a raw diet (BARF; biologically appropriate raw food or bones) has become very fashionable and most practices will be asked for advice on using these diets in animals with skin problems. Advocates of BARF diets claim that they are nutritionally superior to cooked and commercially available pet foods, as cooking and processing foods destroy enzymes and other nutrients. The nutritional significance of this is far from proven, and cooking or processing may increase digestibility and release nutrients. Where necessary, pet food manufacturers counteract this by enriching the diets with additional minerals and vitamins. Discussing all the pros and cons of this form of diet is beyond the scope of this book, however, if clients insist on feeding a BARF diet, advice should be sought from a veterinary nutritionist to ensure that the diet is fully balanced for long-term feeding. The owners also need to be aware of the potential for contamination with pathogens (e.g.

Salmonella, Escherichia coli, Clostridium spp., *Campylobacter*, and parasites), and the risk of disease in the pet, zoonotic conditions in the owners and the risk to the public due to faecal contamination.

Additions such as yeast, vegetables, starches, fats, lecithin and flavouring may contain proteins, although the level will vary widely. It is unknown what effect this has on the allergenicity of a food for a particular individual.

Owners are often very concerned (and confused) over grains and glutens in animal foods. Maize, rice and wheat proteins are in fact highly digestible. Glutens are proteins found in the grain family of wheat, spelt, barley and rye (but not oats, maize and rice). These proteins are used to bind and thicken foods ('glue' = gluten). Allergies to wheat glutens are recognised but should not be confused with coeliac disease, which is a rare and specific condition associated with a genetic susceptibility (most commonly in Irish Setters).

Taking a Dietary History

Prior to choosing a suitable exclusion diet, a detailed food history has to be established. It is important to ask not only about the main diet and treats but also about table scraps and fluid intake (e.g. just water or tea with milk). It is important to ask about foods and treats that may be given by friends, family and dog walkers outside the home. Flavoured tablets (such as wormers, heart worm medication, nutraceuticals etc.) may also contain food allergens and some will need to be discontinued during the exclusion diet. Getting a complete diet history is difficult, and is complicated by factors such as poor recall, uncertainty over the ingredients in commercial foods and treats, and lack of history in rehomed animals.

Diet Trial Options

There are several different ways in which the diet trial can be performed.

Home-Cooked Limited-Ingredient Diet

See Table 8.2. This trial involves identifying a novel protein and carbohydrate source (e.g. the patient has been fed a predominantly beef and rice based diet, with treats of pigs' ears and occasional pieces of toast and ham; therefore, fish and potatoes are suitable) that can be home cooked using fresh ingredients.

The meat and carbohydrate should be boiled, baked or microwaved at a ratio of about 1 : 2 (meat:carbohydrate) for dogs. In cats, pure meat or only little carbohydrate should be used. Excess fat can cause diarrhoea and should be removed. Minced and processed meat should be avoided, as the contents cannot be guaranteed. The cooked components are then processed together in a food processor to avoid the patient picking out individual bits. This mixture can then be portioned, bagged up and frozen or refrigerated until needed.

The amount of food required depends on the animal's weight, and is around 200 g protein and 400 g carbohydrate per 10 kg body weight daily. The animal's body weight should be monitored weekly during the diet trial, with adjustments to the amount fed if necessary. *Ad libitum* feeding is possible but may lead to food wastage, particularly in the summer.

Table 8.2 Protein and carbohydrate sources suitable for exclusion diet (depending on food history for each individual patient).

Protein	Carbohydrate
Chick peas	Barley
Crocodile	Butternut squash
Game meats	Carrots
Horse	Oats
Kangaroo	Peas
Ostrich	Potatoes
Pinto beans	Pumpkin
Pork	Quinoa
Rabbit	Rice
Salmon	Sweet potatoes
Tuna	Yams
White fish	

Home-cooked elimination diet recipe (makes 600 g):
200 g cooked protein source
400 g cooked carbohydrate source
1 teaspoon vegetable oil or olive oil
1.5 teaspoons dicalcium phosphate

Feed 600g/10kg/day. Note: not suitable for long-term use without further supplementation. Seek advice from a veterinary nutritionist if intended to be used long term

- **Advantages:** home-cooked novel protein and carbohydrate diet trials are still regarded as the 'gold standard', as there are no additives (such as colourants, flavourings, preservatives, vitamins and minerals) and contamination with other protein or carbohydrate sources can be ruled out.
- **Disadvantages:** it is important to make the owner aware of how time consuming this form of diet is, as many people cannot commit to cooking for their pet for the diet trial or longer. For large dogs the preparation time can be between 4 and 6 hours per week. The costs of the diet will vary depending on the ingredients, but may be significant (and more than commercial foods) for some exotic proteins. A few animals may refuse to go back to a commercial food following a home-cooked diet trial.

These basic home-cooked diets are not nutritionally balanced. The lack of certain vitamins, minerals and essential fatty acids should not cause a problem in otherwise healthy adult patients for the duration of the dietary trial, but these diets should not be used in growing animals and in patients with special nutritional needs due to another condition. A nutritionist should be consulted to balance diets for long-term feeding.

Commercial Limited-Ingredients Diet

See Table 8.3 and Table 8.4. A commercially available diet that contains a suitable novel protein and carbohydrate source can be chosen using the dietary history as for a home-cooked diet. This food is then fed exclusively for the duration of the diet trial.

Table 8.3 Selected commercially available exclusion diets for dogs (suitability needs to be determined for each individual patient).

Manufacturer/trade name	Wet/dry	Main ingredients	Full ingredients	Hydrolysed (H)/ limited ingredients (L)/skin care (SC)
Burns Dog Food Sensitive Duck and Rice	D	Rice, duck, oats, peas	Brown rice (63%), duck meal (22%), oats, peas, duck fat, sunflower oil, seaweed, vitamins and minerals	L
Burns Dog Food Sensitive Pork and Potato	D	Potato, maize, pork	Potato (35%), maize (27%), pork meal (17%), pea starch, peas, pork fat, seaweed, vitamins and minerals	L
Burns Dog Food Treats	D	Venison	Venison ears, hearts and tongues	L
Burns Dog Food Treats	D	Carrot	Carrot	L
Burns Dog Original Fish and Brown Rice	D	Fish, rice	Brown rice (60%), fish meal (20%), oats, peas, salmon oil, sunflower oil, seaweed, vitamins and minerals	L
Burns Dog Original Food Fish and Brown Rice	D	Rice, fish, oats, peas	Brown rice (60%), fish meal (20%), oats, peas, salmon oil, sunflower oil, seaweed, vitamins and minerals	L
Burns Dog Original Lamb and Brown Rice	D	Lamb, rice	Brown rice (58%), lamb meal (24%), oats, peas, sunflower oil, seaweed, vitamins and minerals	L
DECHRA Specific CDD Food Allergy Management	D	Rice, egg	Rice, eggs, minerals, pork fat, vitamins and trace elements, powdered cellulose, psyllium husk, methionine, sunflower oil, BHA, BHT	L
DECHRA Specific CDD-HY Food Allergy Management	D	Rice, hydrolysed salmon	Rice, rice protein, hydrolysed salmon protein, pork fat, minerals, vitamins and trace elements, powdered cellulose, sunflower oil, psyllium husk, BHA, BHT	L
DECHRA Specific CDW Food Allergy Management	W and D	Lamb, rice	Lamb, rice, sunflower oil, minerals, powdered cellulose, psyllium husk, vitamins and trace elements	L
Farmina Ultra Hypo®	D	Rice starch, hydrolysed fish	Rice starch, hydrolyzed fish protein, salmon oil, cellulose, potassium chloride, calcium carbonate, mono-dicalcium phosphate, salt, vitamins, choline chloride, beta-carotene, minerals, DL-methionine, taurine	H
Farmina Hypoallergenic Fish and Potato	D	Potato, fish	Potato, herring, salmon oil, cellulose, calcium carbonate, mono-dicalcium phosphate, salt, vitamins, choline chloride, minerals, taurine	L

(continued)

Product			Ingredients	
FarminaHypoallergenic Egg and Rice	D	Rice, egg	Rice, dehydrated egg product, salmon oil, cellulose, potassium chloride, calcium carbonate, mono-dicalcium phosphate, salt, vitamins, choline chloride, beta-carotene, minerals, taurine	L
Fish4Dogs Finest/Superior Adult Ocean White Fish	d	White fish, potato, pea, salmon	Ocean white fish (28%), potato (21%), pea flour (19%), salmon meal (11.2%), salmon oil (10.8%), beet pulp, brewers' yeast, minerals	
Fish4Dogs Finest/Superior Adult Salmon	D	Salmon, potato, pea	Salmon (27%), potato (21%), pea flour (19%), salmon meal (11.7%), salmon oil (10.7%), beet pulp, brewers' yeast, minerals	
Hill's d/d Duck and Rice dry	D	Duck, rice	Ground rice, duck meal, animal fat, hydrolysed chicken (low molecular weight), vegetable oil, cellulose, fish oil, potassium chloride, salt, potassium citrate, DL-methionine, taurine, calcium carbonate, vitamins and trace elements	L
Hill's d/d Duck Formula	W	Duck, potato	Water, duck, potato, duck liver, potato starch, soybean oil, powdered cellulose, dicalcium phosphate, fish oil, iodised salt, DL-methionine, calcium carbonate, taurine, vitamins (vitamin E supplement, ascorbic acid (source of vitamin C), thiamine mononitrate, niacin supplement, vitamin A supplement, calcium pantothenate, vitamin B12 supplement, pyridoxine hydrochloride, biotin, riboflavin supplement, vitamin D3 supplement, folic acid, menadione sodium bisulfite complex (source of vitamin K), Potassium chloride, choline chloride, minerals (zinc oxide, ferrous sulfate, manganous oxide, copper sulfate, cobalt carbonate, calcium iodate, sodium selenite), L-tryptophan, beta-carotene	L
Hill's d/d Egg and Rice dry	D	Egg, rice, hydrolysed chicken	Ground rice, dried whole egg, hydrolysed chicken (low molecular weight), vegetable oil, cellulose, animal fat, calcium carbonate, potassium citrate, dicalcium phosphate, fish oil, salt, potassium chloride, magnesium oxide, taurine, vitamins and trace elements. Contains EU approved antioxidant and preservative	L
Hill's d/d Lamb and Rice Formula	W	Lamb, rice	Rice, lamb, lamb liver, rice flour, cellulose powder, iron oxide, vegetable oil, fish oil, calcium carbonate, potassium chloride, dicalcium phosphate, taurine, vitamins and trace elements	L
Hill's d/d Salmon and Potato Formula	W	Salmon, potato	Salmon, dried potato, potato starch, potato protein extract, vegetable oil, fish oil, cellulose, dicalcium phosphate, iodised salt, DL-methionine, taurine, vitamins and trace elements	L

Table 8.3 (*Continued*)

Manufacturer/trade name	Wet/dry	Main ingredients	Full ingredients	Hydrolysed (H)/ limited ingredients (L)/skin care (SC)
Hill's d/d Salmon and Rice dry	D	Salmon, rice	Ground rice, salmon meal, animal fat, hydrolysed chicken (low molecular weight), vegetable oil, cellulose, potassium citrate, salt, fish oil, DL–methionine, potassium chloride, L-lysine hydrochloride, L–tryptophan, taurine, vitamins and trace elements	L
Hill's d/d Venison and potato Formula	W	Venison, potato	Venison, dried potato, potato starch, potato protein extract, vegetable oil, cellulose, fish oil, iodised salt, dicalcium phosphate, calcium carbonate, taurine, DL–methionine, L–tryptophan, vitamins and trace elements	L
Hill's z/d can	W	Hydrolysed chicken liver, maize starch	Chicken liver hydrolysate, maize starch, cellulose, vegetable oil, dicalcium phosphate, potassium citrate, calcium carbonate, DL–methionine, iodised salt, taurine, L–threonine, L–tryptophan, vitamins and trace elements	H
Hill's z/d	D	Hydrolysed chicken liver, maize starch	Maize starch, chicken liver hydrolysate, vegetable oil, cellulose, dicalcium phosphate, calcium carbonate, potassium chloride, salt, DL–methionine, taurine, vitamins and trace elements. Contains EU approved antioxidant	H
Iams/Eukanuba Dermatosis FP	D	Fish, potato	Potato, fish meal, animal fat, dried beet pulp (3.9%), fish digest, dicalcium phosphate, calcium carbonate, sodium hexametaphosphate, fructooligosaccharides (0.39%), potassium chloride	L
Iams/Eukanuba Dermatosis FP	W	Fish, potato	Catfish, herring meal, modified potato starch, maize oil, dried beet pulp, calcium carbonate, potassium chloride	L
Purina Veterinary Diet DRM	D	Hydrolysed pork, white fish, corn	Brewers' rice, salmon meal, trout, canola meal, animal fat preserved with mixed-tocopherols (form of Vitamin E), brewers' dried yeast, canola oil preserved with TBHQ, potassium chloride, fish oil, corn oil preserved with TBHQ, salt, choline chloride, zinc sulfate, taurine, ferrous sulfate, vitamin E supplement, manganese sulfate, ascorbic acid, niacin, calcium carbonate, beta-carotene, vitamin A supplement, calcium	H (pork) L (white fish)

Diet		Declared ingredients	Full ingredient list	
			pantothenate, thiamine mononitrate, copper sulfate, riboflavin supplement, vitamin B12 supplement, pyridoxine hydrochloride, folic acid, vitamin D3 supplement, calcium iodate, biotin, menadione sodium bisulfite complex (source of vitamin K activity), sodium selenite	H
Purina Veterinary Diet HA Hypoallergenic Canine	D	Hydrolysed soya protein, starch	Starch, hydrolysed soy protein isolate, vegetable oil, calcium phosphate, partially hydrogenated canola oil preserved with TBHQ, powdered cellulose, corn oil, potassium chloride, vegetable gums (gum arabic, guar gum), choline chloride, DL-methionine, salt, magnesium oxide, lecithin, taurine, zinc sulfate, ferrous sulfate, vitamin E supplement, manganese sulfate, niacin, calcium carbonate, vitamin A supplement, copper sulfate, calcium pantothenate, thiamine mononitrate, riboflavin supplement, garlic oil, vitamin D3 supplement, pyridoxine hydrochloride, folic acid, vitamin D3 supplement, calcium iodate, biotin, menadione sodium bisulfite complex (source of vitamin K activity), sodium selenite	
Royal Canin Canine Veterinary (Clinical) Diets Sensitivity Control Duck and Rice	W	Duck, rice	Meat and animal derivatives (duck 49%), cereals (rice 16%), minerals, derivatives of vegetable origin, oils and fats, various sugars, vitamin D3: 200 IU, E1 (Iron): 11 mg, E2 (iodine): 0.65 mg, E4 (copper): 4.5 mg, E5 (manganese): 3.5 mg, E6 (zinc): 33 mg.	L
Royal Canin Canine Veterinary (Clinical) Diets Skin Care Adult SK 23	D	Hydrolysed chicken, maize, whear rice, tapioca, soya	Maize, wheat gluten, rice, tapioca, animal fats, maize gluten, minerals, soya oil, beet pulp, fish oil, vegetable fibres, flax seed, hydrolysed animal proteins, fructo-oligo-saccharides, mono- and diglycerides of fatty acids esterified with citric acid, borage oil, marigold extract (source of lutein), vitamin A: 30100 IU, vitamin D3: 800 IU, E1 (iron): 56 mg, E2 (iodine): 5.6 mg, E4 (copper): 11 mg, E5 (manganese): 73 mg, E6 (zinc): 220 mg, E8 (selenium): 0.13 mg	SC
Royal Canin Canine Veterinary (Clinical) Diets Skin Care Adult Small Dog SKS 25	D	Maize, wheat, rice, tapioca, hydrolysed animal proteins	Maize, wheat gluten, rice, tapioca, animal fats, maize gluten, hydrolysed animal proteins, minerals, chicory pulp, soya oil, fish oil, flax seed, fructo-oligo-saccharides, mono- and diglycerides of fatty acids esterified with citric acid, borage oil, marigold extract (source of lutein), vitamin A: 30100 IU, vitamin D3: 800 IU, E1 (iron): 55 mg, E2 (iodine): 5.5 mg, E4 (copper): 11 mg, E5 (manganese): 72 mg, E6 (zinc): 215 mg, E8 (selenium): 0.1 mg	SC

(continued)

Table 8.3 (*Continued*)

Manufacturer/trade name	Wet/dry	Main ingredients	Full ingredients	Hydrolysed (H)/limited ingredients (L)/skin care (SC)
Royal Canin Canine Veterinary (Clinical) Diets Skin Care Junior Small Dog SKJ29	D	Maize, wheat, rice, soya, hydrolysed animal proteins	Rice, wheat gluten, animal fats, maize, maize gluten, minerals, hydrolysed animal proteins, soya protein isolate, beet pulp, soya oil, vegetable fibres, fish oil, flax seed, fructo-oligo-saccharides, borage oil, hydrolysed yeast (source of manno-oligo-saccharides), marigold extract (source of lutein), vitamin A: 24800 IU, vitamin D3: 800 IU, E1 (iron): 40 mg, E2 (iodine): 2.8 mg, E4 (copper): 11 mg, E5 (manganese): 53 mg, E6 (zinc): 202 mg, E8 (selenium): 0.1 mg	SC
Royal Canin Canine Veterinary (Clinical) Diets Anallergenic Dog Food	D	Feather hydrolysate, maize starch	Maize starch, feather hydrolysate with low molecular weight (source of L amino acids and oligopeptides), copra oil, soya oil, minerals, vegetable fibres, chicory pulp, fructo-oligo-saccharides, fish oil, mono- and diglycerides of fatty acids esterified with citric acid, animal fat, marigold extract (source of lutein), vitamins and trace elements	H
Royal Canin Canine Veterinary (Clinical) Diets Hypoallergenic Dog Food DR21 Dry Food	D	Hydrolysed soya protein, rice	Rice, hydrolysed soya protein isolate, animal fats, minerals, hydrolysed poultry liver, beet pulp, soya oil, fructo-oligo-saccharides, fish oil, borage oil, marigold extract (source of lutein), vitamins and trace elements	H
Royal Canin Canine Veterinary (Clinical) Diets Hypoallergenic Dog Food HME23 Moderate Calorie Dry Food	D	Hydrolysed soya protein, rice	Rice, hydrolysed soya protein isolate, animal fats, hydrolysed poultry liver, minerals, beet pulp, soya oil, fish oil, fructo-oligo-saccharides, borage oil, marigold extract (source of lutein), vitamins and trace elements	H
Royal Canin Canine Veterinary (Clinical) Diets Hypoallergenic Dog Food HSD24 Small Dog Dry Food	D	Hydrolysed soya protein, rice	Rice, hydrolysed soya protein isolate, animal fats, minerals, hydrolysed poultry liver, soya oil, beet pulp, fructo-oligo-saccharides, fish oil, borage oil, marigold extract (source of lutein), vitamins and trace elements	H

Product	Type	Ingredients	Composition	Class
Royal Canin Canine Veterinary (Clinical) Diets Hypoallergenic Dog Food	D	Hydrolysed soya protein, pea starch	Derivatives of vegetable origin (pea starch), vegetable protein extracts (hydrolysed soya protein), oils and fats, minerals, meat and animal derivatives (hydrolysed poultry liver), various sugars, vitamins and trace elements	H
Royal Canin Canine Veterinary (Clinical) Diets Hypoallergenic Dog Food	W	Hydrolysed soya protein, pea starch	Derivatives of vegetable origin (pea starch), vegetable protein extracts (hydrolysed soya protein), oils and fats, minerals, meat and animal derivatives (hydrolysed poultry liver), various sugars. Additives (per kg): Nutritional additives: vitamin A: 5000 IU, vitamin D3: 340 IU, E1 (iron): 25 mg, E2 (iodine): 2 mg, E4 (copper): 6 mg, E5 (manganese): 32 mg, E6 (zinc): 120 mg – Technological additives: pentasodium triphosphate: 3 g	H
Royal Canin Canine Veterinary (Clinical) Diets Sensitivity Control SC21Capelin and Tapioca	D	Capelin, duck hydrolysed poultry proteins, soya	tapioca, dehydrated duck meat, hydrolysed poultry proteins, vegetable fibres, animal fats, beet pulp, fish oil, soya oil, psyllium husks and seeds, minerals, fructo-oligo-saccharides, marigold extract (source of lutein), vitamin A: 25000 IU, vitamin D3: 800 IU, E1 (iron): 41 mg, E2 (iodine): 2.8 mg, E4 (copper): 10 mg, E5 (manganese): 54 mg, E6 (zinc): 203 mg, E8 (selenium): 0.1 mg - Preservatives - antioxidants	L
Royal Canin Canine Veterinary (Clinical) Diets Sensitivity Control Chicken and Rice	W	Chicken, rice	Meat and animal derivatives (chicken 52%), cereals (rice 12%), derivatives of vegetable origin, oils and fats, minerals, various sugars, vitamin D3: 135 IU, E1 (iron): 14 mg, E2 (iodine): 0.65 mg, E4 (copper): 4.5 mg, E5 (manganese): 4.5 mg, E6 (zinc): 44 mg	L
Wafcol	D	Fish, corn	Maize (57%), soya, fish meal (14%), sunflower oil, seaweed (3.4%), soya hulls, minerals, mannoligosaccharides (MOS 0.14%), vitamins, brewers' yeast	L
Wafcol	D	Salmon, potato	Potato (29%), salmon (24%), whole lupin, salmon meal (12%), seaweed (5%), potato starch (3%), salmon oil (2.5%), sunflower oil, salmon digest (1.8%), minerals, vitamins, mannan-oligosaccharides (2150 mg/kg), fructo-oligosaccharides (2150 mg/kg), glucosamine (340 mg/kg), methylsulfonylmethane (MSM 340 mg/kg), chondroitin (240 mg/kg)	L

Table 8.4 Selected commercially available exclusion diets for cats (suitability needs to be determined for each individual patient).

Manufacturer/trade name	Wet/dry	Main ingredients	Full ingredients	Hydrolysed (H)/limited ingredients (L)/skin care (SC)
Burns Cat Food Original Fish and Brown Rice	D	Rice, fish, maize	Brown rice (43%), fish meal (36%), maize, salmon oil, hydrolysed chicken livers, seaweed, vitamins and minerals	L/H (chicken livers)
DECHRA Specific Allergy Management Plus	D	Rice, hydrolysed salmon	Rice, hydrolysed salmon protein, rice protein, fish oil, minerals, powdered cellulose, pork fat, vitamins and trace elements, borage oil, psyllium husk, sunflower oil, taurine. Antioxidant: EC approved additives: BHA, BHT, ascorbyl palmitate, propyl gallate	H
DECHRA Specific Food Allergy Management	W/D	Lamb, rice	Lamb, rice, sunflower oil, minerals, psyllium husk, vitamins and trace elements, taurine, methionine	L
DECHRA Specific Food Allergy Management	D	Rice, hydrolysed salmon	Rice, hydrolysed salmon protein, rice protein, pork fat, minerals, powdered cellulose, vitamins and trace elements, psyllium husk, sunflower oil, taurine. Antioxidants: EC approved additives: BHA, BHT	H
FarminaUltraHypo®	D	Rice starch, hydrolysed fish	Rice starch, hydrolysed fish protein, fish oil, calcium carbonate, fructoligosaccharides, potassium chloride, calcium sulfatedihydrate, mono-dicalcium phosphate, sodium chloride, marigold extract (lutein), vitamins, minerals, choline chloride, beta-carotene, taurine, DL-methionine, L-carnitine, cellulose	H
Fish4Cats Finest Salmon	D	Salmon, sweet potato, cassava	Salmon meal (33%), fresh salmon (22%), sweet potato (17%), cassava (13%), salmon oil (8%), fish digest (2.5%), sunflower oil, yeast extract, malt extract, pea fibre, dried algae, dried cranberries, minerals	L
Fish4Cats Finest Mackerel	D	Salmon, mackerel, sweet potato, cassava	Salmon meal (33%), fresh mackerel (22%), sweet potato (17%), cassava (13%), salmon oil (8%), fish digest (2.5%), sunflower oil, yeast extract, malt extract, pea fibre, dried algae, dried cranberries, minerals	L

(*continued*)

Product	Form	Key ingredients	Ingredients	L/H
Fish4Cats Finest Sardine	D	Salmon, sardines, sweet potato, cassava	Salmon meal (33%), fresh sardine (22%), sweet potato (17%), cassava (13%), salmon oil (8%), fish digest (2.5%), sunflower oil, yeast extract, malt extract, pea fibre, dried algae, dried cranberries, minerals	L
Hill's d/d Venison and Green Pea	W/D	Venison, pea	Dehydrated peas, pea protein extract, animal fat, pea bran meal, venison meal, vegetable oil, fish oil, DL-methionine, calcium sulphate, hydrolysed chicken (low molecular weight), calcium carbonate, potassium chloride, salt, taurine, vitamins and trace elements. Contains EU approved antioxidant	L
Hill's d/d Duck Formula	W	Duck, pea	Water, duck, duck liver, ground green pea, powdered cellulose, soybean oil, pea protein concentrate, brewers dried yeast, fish oil, glucose, calcium carbonate, DL-methionine, dicalcium phosphate, taurine, l-cysteine, choline chloride, iron oxide, glycine, potassium chloride, iodized salt, vitamin E supplement, potassium citrate, thiamine mononitrate, ascorbic acid (source of vitamin C), zinc oxide, ferrous sulfate, thiamine hydrochloride, niacin, pyridoxine hydrochloride, beta-carotene, manganous oxide, calcium pantothenate, vitamin B12 supplement, riboflavin, biotin, vitamin D3 supplement, calcium iodate, folic acid, sodium selenite	L
Hill's z/d	D	Rice, chicken liver hydrolysate	Brewers' rice, rice protein concentrate, chicken liver hydrolysate, vegetable oil, minerals, dried chicken liver hydrolysate, cellulose, taurine, vitamins, trace elements and beta carotene. Contains EU approved antioxidant	H
Iams/Eukanuba Dermatosis LB	W	Lamb, barley	Lamb liver, lamb lung, lamb, barley, maize oil, dried beet pulp, dicalcium phosphate, calcium carbonate, potassium chloride, sodium chloride	L
Purina Veterinary Diet HA Hypoallergenic Feline	D	Hydrolysed soya protein, rice starch, hydrolysed chicken	Rice starch, hydrolysed soy protein isolate, partially hydrogenated canola oil preserved with TBHQ, hydrolyzed chicken liver, tricalcium phosphate, powdered cellulose, corn oil, hydrolyzed chicken, sodium bisulfate, DL-methionine, potassium chloride, choline chloride, tetra sodium pyrophosphate, L-Lysine monohydrochloride, phosphoric acid, salt, guar gum, taurine, lecithin, magnesium oxide, zinc sulfate, ferrous sulfate, Vitamin E supplement, manganese sulfate, niacin, calcium carbonate, citric acid, vitamin A supplement, calcium pantothenate, thiamine mononitrate, copper sulfate, BHA (a preservative), riboflavin supplement, vitamin B12 supplement, pyridoxine hydrochloride, folic acid, vitamin D3 supplement, calcium iodate, biotin, menadione sodium bisulfite complex (source of vitamin K activity), sodium selenite B-4575	H

Table 8.4 (*Continued*)

Manufacturer/trade name	Wet/dry	Main ingredients	Full ingredients	Hydrolysed (H)/ limited ingredients (L)/skin care (SC)
Royal Canin Feline Hypoallergenic DR25	D	Rice, hydrolysed soya protein, hydrolysesd chicken liver	Rice, hydrolysed soya protein isolate, animal fats, vegetable fibres, minerals, hydrolysed poultry liver, soya oil, beet pulp, fish oil, fructo-oligo-saccharides (FOS), borage oil, marigold extract (source of lutein).	H
Royal Canin Feline Sensitivity Control SC 27	D	Rice, duck	Rice, dehydrated duck meat, vegetable fibres, hydrolysed poultry proteins, animal fats, rice gluten, minerals, fish oil, soya oil, marigold extract (source of lutein). Additives (per kg): Nutritional additives: vitamin A: 24900 IU, vitamin D3: 800 IU, E1 (iron): 40 mg, E2 (iodine): 2.8 mg, E4 (copper): 9 mg, E5 (manganese): 54 mg, E6 (zinc): 202 mg, E8 (selenium): 0.1 mg – preservatives – antioxidants	L
Royal Canin Anallergenic	D	Hydrolysed chicken feathers; maize starch	Maize starch, chicken feather hydrolysate, copra oil, soya oil, vegetable fibre, fish oil, animal fats, chichory pulp, minerals, vitamins, fructo-oligo-saccharides, maltodextrin, marigold extract (lutein)	H

- **Advantages:** these diets are straightforward and convenient. They are nutritionally balanced and suitable for most animals during the diet trial and for long-term feeding. Costs vary according to the chosen diet but are usually moderate compared to routine feeding.
- **Disadvantages:** many diets are marketed as 'hypoallergenic', which can confuse owners. The recipes for many foods vary and labelling rules may not reflect this. Only major ingredients (>20% in the UK) must be declared, and minor ingredients may be grouped (e.g. cereals and cereal by-products, meats and meat by-products etc.). Ingredients are usually listed in decreasing order of the amount in the recipe, but ingredients present in small amounts may not be listed separately. Finally, studies using polymerase chain reaction (PCR) and bone analysis have found undeclared proteins in up to 80% of tested foods (many of which were 'restricted', 'hypoallergenic' or 'single' protein diets). This suggests that some batches of some diets would not be suitable to identify patients with CAFRs or FIAD. It is therefore important to choose a reputable food source.

Hydrolysed Diet

See Table 8.3 and Table 8.4. The proteins and, in some cases, carbohydrates in these foods have been hydrolysed into small fragments of amino acids and oligopeptides. In theory, reducing the molecular weight of these fragments to less than 10 kD renders them non-immunogenic and therefore suitable for diet trials. However, partial hydrolysation may result in the presence of varying amounts of larger peptides that could be allergenic. Cross-contamination during manufacture and inclusion of fats and other nutrients from other sources could also be a problem. One recent study used Western blots with canine sera to detect high molecular weight proteins (15–60 kD) in three hydrolysed foods (Royal Canin Anallergenic, Purina HA and Hill's z/d Low Allergen). Multiple proteins bound canine IgE, and one protein was identified as maize starch synthase. The necessary degree of hydrolysis probably depends on the allergenic protein and its epitopes. In human infants with severe milk allergy only single amino acid diets are considered non-allergenic. This is largely unknown in animals, but nearly 20% of dogs experimentally and naturally sensitised to chicken and soy have been shown to react to hydrolysed foods with these ingredients. It is therefore important to check the degree of hydrolysation of all the protein and carbohydrate sources in a diet. Recent studies suggest that the proteins should be fully hydrolysed to avoid reactions in animals previously exposed to the protein. Where possible, it would seem prudent to avoid using proteins and carbohydrates to which the animals have been exposed.

- **Advantages:** these diets are straightforward and convenient. They are nutritionally balanced and suitable for most animals during the diet trial and for long-term feeding. They are useful in animals where suitable novel proteins for home-cooked or commercial restricted protein diets cannot be identified.
- **Disadvantages:** the ingredients and degree of hydrolysis may not be suitable for all animals and may result in a missed diagnosis. Other problems with these foods can include constipation, diarrhoea, weight gain (they are often high in fats) and palatability. They are usually expensive compared to other diet trial options (although this will vary).

Length of the Diet Trial

Different authors suggest different minimum lengths for dietary trials, although a recent review of published studies advised 8 weeks. Gastrointestinal symptoms, when present, often respond within 2 weeks, whereas cutaneous manifestations can take up to 16 weeks to fully resolve (especially if there are chronic inflammatory changes and secondary infection). Owner compliance can be a problem with very long diet trial, but resolution of gastrointestinal signs can be used to encourage owners to persist. Conversely, a lack of response can be early indication that the diet trial will not be of benefit. Compliance with the trial should be looked at and, if good, consider using another food. The length of the trial can always be extended if there is doubt about the diagnosis.

Compliance

The success of any diet trial relies predominantly on client compliance. Compliance is a major issue due to the time it takes for the exclusion diet to improve the clinical signs, the fact that most animals (although figures vary) will not improve on the diet trial, the need to be strict, and the potential for other people to give unauthorised foods. The keys to successful diet trial are communication, contact and support.

Time spent explaining the purpose of the trial, ensuring that the owners' expectations are realistic, how to conduct the trial and tips on how to avoid pitfalls is certainly time well spent. For example, owners that know most dogs do not have a food allergy but understand the benefit of a diet trial in those that do are more likely to be compliant than those that believe the diet trial will 'cure' their dog.

Full written instructions and advice leaflets are invaluable. Clients will also appreciate follow-up emails and calls to check that the trial is going well. A diary to record pruritus scores, concurrent therapy, accidental food exposure etc. can be very helpful in focusing the owners on the food trial and evaluating the outcome.

Common pitfalls include those listed below.

- Small children dropping food during meals, which the patient can eat.
- Not all family members or other people caring for the patient are aware of the food trial and its importance or have the willpower to adhere to it.
- Other pets in the household that are fed a different diet resulting in the patient having access to an unsuitable food. If complete separation at feeding times is not possible, all pets (including pets of different species, e.g. cats and dogs) need to be fed the exclusion diet. In certain circumstances it may be possible to separate the patient and other pets in the house by using microchip-activated food bowls.
- Some flavouring in routine medications (e.g. heart worm preventatives, mineral or vitamin supplements etc.) can interfere with the dietary trial. They need to be checked for suitability or replaced by an alternative product if indicated.
- If the patient stays anywhere other than at home during the diet trial (e.g. in kennels during a holiday, for emergency treatment, with a dog sitter/walker during the day), the carers need to be informed of the diet and told which food is suitable.
- Scavenging should be avoided, if necessary, by restricting off-lead exercise and using muzzles.
- Cats with outdoor access may be able to hunt and/or be fed elsewhere. Where possible, cats should be kept indoors. However, this may lead to anxiety and behaviour changes.

A pragmatic approach to outdoor access may be necessary, although this means that diagnosis of CAFR may be missed.

Treats are often an important part of the companion animal bond and/or training aids. A 'no treat' approach is not acceptable in most cases. However, treats must not compromise the diet trial. Tips include:

- treat versions of some commercially available exclusion diets;
- using an appropriate dry food kibble in a Kong® or similar toy for treats and entertainment;
- canned foods can be removed from the can *en bloc*, sliced and hard baked in the oven for use as a treat;
- dried foods can be hydrated with water, mixed up, shaped and hard baked, giving a new shape, texture and flavour;
- foods used in restricted-ingredient diets can be made into treats (e.g. hard baking potatoes or other carbohydrate sources, liver or meat);
- small amounts of novel foods (e.g. sweet potato, kangaroo, ostrich, alligator etc.) can be similarly made into treats to supplement other diets. Small amounts can also be used to help improve the palatability of some diets.

In order to avoid gastrointestinal problems on changing the diet, regardless of the method chosen, the new food should be introduced gradually over a few days. Lower food intake for a few days will not affect healthy dogs, but inappetence is a concern in cats because of the potential for hepatic lipidosis.

Managing Animals During Food Trials

Concurrent antipruritic therapy can make interpreting the food trial much harder. In theory, it should be avoided but this can be difficult in animals that are still pruritic during the food trial. Ongoing pruritus is a common reason why owners give up. One possible solution is to allow the use of short courses of topical or oral glucocorticoids (prednisolone 0.5–1.0 mg/kg q24 h) or oral oclacitinib (0.4–0.6 mg/kg q12 h) for 3–5 days at the owner's discretion to manage unacceptable pruritus during the diet trial. This psychologically puts the owner in charge of the disease and improves compliance. Treatment can be noted in the food trial diary (see earlier, in Compliance) and carefully reviewed in light of the overall outcome.

Secondary microbial infections and ectoparasites can also have an influence on the outcome of the trial. If these are not adequately addressed an improvement may not be perceived, despite food playing a role in the primary disease, as the pruritus and inflammation due to the infection or ectoparasites may be severe enough to be constant and mask any benefit achieved by removing the food allergens. On the other hand, treatment of the infections or parasites may give the false impression that the improvement is due to the diet. Dietary challenge while continuing to control the infections and parasites is important in distinguishing the cause of the dermatitis.

Cross-Reaction Among Food Allergens

Some thought should be given to cross-reaction among food allergens, although there have only been a few studies on this in animals. Relatively few specific food allergens have been identified in dogs. IgE specific for bovine serum albumin has isolated in dogs clinically sensitised to beef. Other specific allergens include muscle phosphoglucomutase and bovine and ovine IgG. This may account for clinical cross-reactivity among foods – muscle phosphoglutamase is a ubiquitous mammalian protein, and ovine and bovine IgG have a close structural homology. Cross-reactions in dogs are known or suspected for: beef, lamb and cows' milk; chicken, turkey and duck; and among different types of fish.

It is reasonable to assume that proteins from species without a recent common ancestor are less likely to cross-react than those in closely related and recently evolved families. However, these need not be true for highly conserved proteins. Nevertheless, it can be helpful to refer to a Tree of Life or evolution chart (e.g. http://www.open.edu/openlearn/nature-environment/natural-history/tree-life) when selecting proteins for a diet trial.

It is important not to confuse 'exotic' with 'novel'. For example, cows, buffalo, bison and antelope are all members of the Bovidae family in the order Artiodactyla and share a fairly recent common ancestor. Progressively more distally related artiodactyls include deer (family Cervide) and pigs (family Suidae). Horses (order Perissodactyla) and rabbits (order Lagomorpha) are more distantly related still. Many owners, however, consider more familiar meat sources to be less exotic and less suitable for diet trials. Unfortunately, this is reflected in the marketing of some 'exotic' and 'hypoallergenic' pet foods.

Diet Challenge

It is important to conduct a dietary challenge using the original foodstuffs to prove that any improvement was in fact due to the diet rather than being coincidental, fluctuations in the environmental allergen load, or other measures put in place at the start of the dietary exclusion trial (such as treating secondary infections, using topical therapy or optimising the ectoparasite control measures).

Diet challenges can be done by feeding everything the patient received before the exclusion diet was introduced or by adding individual protein and carbohydrate sources to identify individual allergens. The latter method is the only way to determine precisely which meat or carbohydrate sources trigger a reaction. Whichever way this is done, most food-associated reactions occur within a few hours to a few days of introducing the offending food. However, each new food or group of foods needs to be given for at least 2 weeks before concluding that they do not trigger a reaction. Owners should watch their pet carefully for any exacerbation of pruritus, skin lesions and/or gastrointestinal problems. The exclusion diet should be restarted as soon as possible and fed until the condition has stabilised again before any other provocative tests are performed. Antipruritic drugs, ear cleansers and/or anti-emetics may be needed to achieve remission in some cases. Owners should be warned that there is a small risk of precipitating a more severe reaction (for example, *Pseudomonas* otitis).

Many dermatologists feel that this process needs to be repeatable and will perform two dietary challenges to ensure that the diagnosis is correct as any improvement and deterioration could be coincidental. Some owners, however, can be sufficiently worried about a relapse or so relieved that the problem is managed that they will refuse a food challenge and continue the exclusion diet. This is fine as long as the diet is balanced for long-term feeding. Alternatively, owners may just wish to test a few foods and treats that they wish to feed in the future.

Food-Allergen Serology and Patch Tests

Food allergen serology cannot be used to diagnose a CAFR or FIAD. Food-allergen-specific serology tests are widely used in first-opinion practice but dermatologists, in contrast, rarely use these tests. There are very few data confirming their specificity for food-allergen-specific IgG and IgE, and whether this is related to the clinical signs. Most tests have no published data and have not been validated. It is unclear whether these results are clinically significant or reflect dietary history. Not all adverse food reactions, moreover, may be immunological and/or involve IgE or IgG.

One study was carried out of food-allergen-specific serology by two different laboratories in healthy dogs, dogs with CAFR, with non-food-induced AD and dogs with miscellaneous skin diseases. There was no correlation between the two laboratories, and the IgG and IgE levels did not distinguish between the different groups of dogs. Two other studies (one using a food-specific IgE enzyme-linked immunosorbent assay (ELISA) and the other an IgE Western blot assay against commercial foods) showed that the positive predictive value (PPV) of these tests was roughly 30% – i.e. for every three dogs with a positive test only one dog has a food allergy and the other two are false-positives. In contrast, the negative predictive value (NPV) was about 80% – i.e. for every five dogs with negative serology, four will not react to the food but one will. These tests could therefore be used to predict which foods would be suitable for a food trial. However, with the author's prevalence figures for CAFR and FIAD, using serology alone to select foods for an exclusion diet would miss the diagnosis in 8% of pruritic dogs.

Patch testing with food extracts is more accurate than serology; the high NPV makes a response to a food with a negative reaction highly unlikely. However, the PPV is still low, making it difficult to interpret the clinical significance of positive tests. The results from carbohydrates were less reliable than those from proteins and the results from commercial foods were poor (possibly because of low and variable concentrations of the proteins in commercial foods). These tests could again be used to identify foods suitable for elimination diets but cannot be used to diagnose food allergy and they are difficult and time consuming to perform.

1) Gently clip a patch of skin.
2) Mark the test sites with indelible pen.
3) Apply the foods to the skin using Finn chambers; wet foods can be placed directly into the chamber, but dry foods should be mixed with some water to form a thick slurry.
4) Use an empty chamber as a negative control.
5) Tape the Finn chambers in place with an adhesive membrane and a body bandage; use collars, socks or boots if necessary to prevent trauma of the test sites.
6) Look for any inflammation of the test sites after 24–96 hours.

Allergy Testing for Environmental Allergens

When to Perform Allergy Testing for Environmental Allergens

With the advent of dermatological investigative profiles offered by many commercial laboratories, serum allergy testing has become very widely used and is one of the most misunderstood tests in veterinary dermatology.

Allergy testing is often performed to try to diagnose pruritic skin diseases, but it has no place in the investigation of the pruritic patient. It is merely a tool to identify the offending allergens in a patient diagnosed with AD for optimising allergen avoidance and, more importantly, to pick allergens for inclusion in allergen-specific immunotherapy (ASIT). Therefore, in every single pruritic patient, all possible differential diagnoses need to be ruled out first to reach a diagnosis of AD before embarking on allergy testing. Allergy testing is merely a step to help with the management of the case rather then a diagnostic test.

The question of whether intradermal allergen tests (IDTs) are better than *in vitro* allergen-specific serology tests is often asked but it is important to realise that they measure different aspects of the allergic response. IDTs have traditionally been regarded as the 'gold standard' as this is a functional assessment of mast-cell-bound IgE leading to mast cell releasebility and the subsequent cutaneous response to the inflammatory mediators. Allergen-specific serology, in contrast, just measures circulating allergen-specific IgE. Both have their advantages and disadvantages, but the key is to carefully evaluate the results in terms of likely exposure, clinical signs and history. ASIT can be just as successful using either method.

Allergen Selection

The principles of allergen selection are the same for IDTs and allergen-specific serology. Even though the laboratory largely sets allergen-specific serology panels you should make every effort to ensure that the allergens are relevant to your area. Allergen selection depends on the geographical location as different allergens are prevalent in different parts of the world. It is advisable to contact local veterinary schools, veterinary dermatologists, colleagues who perform tests on a regular basis and laboratories offering serum allergy tests. Other useful resources include textbooks, Wikipedia, Wikispecies, National Allergy Bureau (http://www.worldallergy.org/pollen/) and Polleninfo (http://www.polleninfo.org; European Union only).

Allergen panels should include the most relevant local allergens from: house dust and storage mites; epidermals (skin, hair, wool and fibres); pollens (tree, grass, weed and crops); insects; and moulds (Table 8.5). Where the exact species extract is unavailable, a closely related species (ideally same genus; at least the same family) can usually be used.

Allergen Extracts and Mixes

Most tests use single allergens to maximise sensitivity and specificity. Allergen mixes may cause false-positive irritant reactions if too concentrated, and false-negative reactions if the relevant allergen(s) in the mix are too diluted. However, it is likely that there is substantial cross-reaction between related allergens. For example, it is known that the house dust mites *Dermatophagoides pteronyssinus* and *D. farinae* strongly cross-react and that these share cross-reacting allergens with storage mites. It is likely that this also occurs with pollens, and a variable degree of cross-reaction has been shown with *Culicoides* and *Simulium* in horses. In the future, allergen mixes containing key cross-reacting allergens could be more commonly used. Component

Table 8.5 Selected allergens commonly tested for in serum allergen-specific IgE testing and intradermal allergy tests. Regional variability occurs (the allergens suggested are predominantly suitable for northern European regions). Some of the insect allergens are mostly useful in horses.

House dust and storage mites

Grain mite (*Lepidoglyphus destructor*)
House dust mite (*Dermatophagoides farinae*)
House dust mite (*Dermatophagoides pteronyssinus*)
Storage mite (*Acarus siro*)
Storage mite (*Tyrophagus putrsceantiae*)

Grass pollen

Bermuda grass (*Cynodon dactylon*)
Italian ryegrass (*Lolium multiflorum*)
Meadow fescue (*Festuca pratensis*)
Meadow grass (Kentucky blue grass) (*Poa pratensis*)
Orchard grass (*Dactylis glomerata*)
Perennial rye grass (*Lolium perenne*)
Couch grass (*Elymus repens*)
Sweet vernal grass (*Anthoxanthum odoratum*)
Timothy grass (*Phleum pratense*)
Yorkshire fog (*Holcus lanatus*)

Weed and flower pollen

Clover (*Trifolium*)
Dock (*Rumex obtusifolius*)
English plantain (*Plantago lanceolata*)
Lamb's quarter (*Chenopodium album*)
Mugwort (*Artemisia vulgaris*)
Ox-eye daisy (*Leucanthemum vulgare*)
Ragweed, short (*Ambrosia artemisifolia*)
Sheep sorrel (*Rumex acetosella*)
Stinging nettle (*Urtica dioica*)
Wall pellitory (*Parietaria officinalis*)

Tree pollen

Alder (*Alnus* spp.)
Beech (*Fagus sylvatica*)
Birch (*Betula populifolia*)
Cedar (*Chameacyparis* spp.)
Cypress (*Cupressus* spp.)
Elm (*Ulmus* spp.)
Hazel (*Corylus avellana*)
Maple (*Acer pseudoplantanus*)
Oak (*Quercus* spp.)
Olive/Ash (*Olea europaea/Fraxinus excelsior*)
Poplar (*Populus* spp.)
Willow (*Salix caprea*)
Scot's pine (*Pinus sylvestris*)
Elder (*Sambucus nigra*)

(continued)

Table 8.5 *(Continued)*

Fungi

Alternaria alternata
Aspergillus fumigatus
Cladosporium herbarum
Malassezia
Penicillium spp.
Mucor mucedo

Crops

Maize (*Zea mays*)
Oats (*Avena sativa*)
Rape (*Brassica napus*)
Wheat (*Triticum aestivum*)

Insects

Blackfly (*Simulium* spp.)
Cockroach (*Periplaneta americana*; subgenera of *Blattaria*)
Flea
Horsefly (*Tabanus* spp.), stable fly (*Stomoxys* spp), midges (*Culicoides* spp.)
Mosquito (*Aedes communis*; subgenera of *Culex*)

---

resolved diagnostic tests that use the exact allergenic proteins rather than crude extracts may also become available.

It is important to review test results as part of your clinical audit procedure. The frequency and pattern of positive results should be evaluated to identify poorly reactive allergens. These can be replaced with more relevant allergens or the testing concentration can be revised.

Drug Withdrawal Periods

Drugs that may interfere with IDTs and ASIS must be withdrawn before testing (Table 8.6). The International Committee on Allergic Diseases of Animals (ICADA) recently conducted an evidence-based review of studies on anti-allergic drug withdrawal times and proposed optimal withdrawal times prior to IDTs and ASIS. However, the number of studies available for review was small and each study only reported the effect of medication of certain allergens and often the treatment duration was relatively short. For example, there were only five studies that examined the effect of short-acting glucocorticoids on IDTs and three of those five papers related to flea allergens rather than house dust and storage mites, moulds, epithelia or pollens. The lack of studies examining the effects of topical glucocorticoids and antihistamines on ASIS, furthermore, makes it difficult to make firm recommendations for withdrawal of these drugs.

Optimum withdrawal times have not been established in detail for every allergen and duration of drug intervention and will vary enormously for each allergen and each compound, and possibly even in each patient. In the absence of a large number of

Table 8.6   Proposed drug withdrawal times prior to allergy tests.

Drug	IDTs	ASIS
Antihistamines	7 days	None
Topical glucocorticoids	14 days	None
Short-acting oral glucocorticoids	14 days	None
Long-acting injectable glucocorticoids	28 days	28 days
Ciclosporin, oclacitinib, pentoxifylline, essential fatty acids (EFAs) and high-EFA diets	None	None

Adapted from Olivry T, Saridomichelakis M, International Committee on Atopic. *Diseases of Animals* (2013) Evidence-based guidelines for anti-allergic drug withdrawal times before allergen-specific intradermal and IgE serological tests in dogs. *Veterinary Dermatology* 24, 225.

published studies examining these factors, many dermatologists recommend at least 2 weeks for antihistamines and essential fatty acids and 4 weeks plus the duration of action for glucocorticoid preparations. In individual cases this may need to be adjusted, however, after discussion with the owners. Moreover, withdrawal periods may need to be longer in animals showing signs of iatrogenic hyperadrenocorticism.

Intradermal Allergy Testing

Intradermal allergy testing in a patient with proven AD demonstrates the presence of environmental hypersensitivity based on cutaneous reactivity to the injected allergens. Due to the expense and tine involved with purchasing and preparing the allergens, IDTs are only cost effective in practices with a dermatologically biased case load. The clinician performing this procedure needs to have considerable experience to interpret the test results. Therefore, IDTs are mainly performed by veterinary dermatologists with postgraduate qualifications in the discipline.

IDTs are often described as the 'gold standard' to determine which allergens elicit the hypersensitivity response in the patient. However, unlike in human medicine where World Health Organization controlled standardised allergen solutions are available, the allergen extracts used in veterinary medicine vary and there is no evidence of the superiority of any extracts over others. Concentrated aqueous extracts can be purchased for immunotherapy and IDTs when diluted. Alternatively, ready-made testing dilutions can be obtained. Published studies confirming optimum concentrations are sparse and lacking for many extracts. Recent consensus guidelines for IDTs have been published (Table 8.7).

Allergens loose potency over time, and strict adherence to expiry dates is essential. Allergens should be kept refrigerated (taking care to avoid freezing). Allergens diluted to testing strength are stable for up to 8 weeks in glass vials and up to 2 weeks in plastic syringes.

IDT Procedure

IDTs are usually performed under sedation and suitable agents include xylazine, medetomidine, tiletamine/zolazepam (in cats), and halothane or isoflurane (although

Table 8.7 Recommended allergen concentrations for intradermal allergen tests (IDTs).

	Standard dilutions for IDTs	Revised dilutions for IDTs
Histamine (positive control)	1:1 000 000 w/v	1:10 000 w/v
House dust and storage mites	250 PNU/ml 1:50 000 w/v	100–200 PNU/mL (*Dermatophagoides pteronyssinus*) 75 PNU/mL (*D. farinae, Tyrophagus putresceantiae* and *Lepidoglyphus destructor*) 50 PNU/mL (*Acarus siro* and *Blomia tropicalis*)
Epidermal extracts	250–500 PNU/mL	1250 PNU/mL
Insects	1000 PNU/mL	1750 PNU/mL
Whole flea extract	1:1000 w/v	1:500 w/v
Pollens	1000 PNU/mL	1000–8000 PNU/mL

w/v = weight to volume; PNU = protein nitrogen units.
Adapted from Hensel P, Santoro D, Favrot C, Hill P, Griffin C (2015) Canine atopic dermatitis: detailed guidelines for diagnosis and allergen identification. *BMC Veterinary Research* 11, 196. DOI 10.1186/s12917-015-0515-5.

one author has seen these drugs inhibit IDTs in dogs). Ketamine/diazepam, oxymorphone, acepromazine and propofol, however, can affect skin reactivity. Sedated animals should be monitored carefully, and oxygen and suitable resuscitation equipment should be available.

Once the patient has been sedated it is placed in lateral recumbency and skin in the test area gently shaved but not prepared surgically (Figure 8.2). Permanent marker is used to make rows of dots to mark where the injections are placed (Figure 8.3). The procedure is

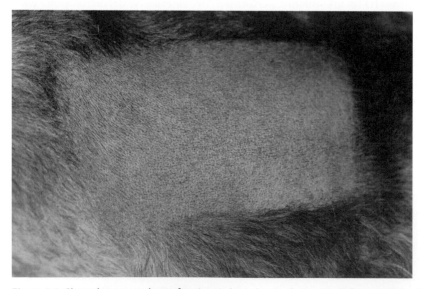

Figure 8.2 Shaved areas on chest of patient in lateral recumbency ready for intradermal allergy testing.

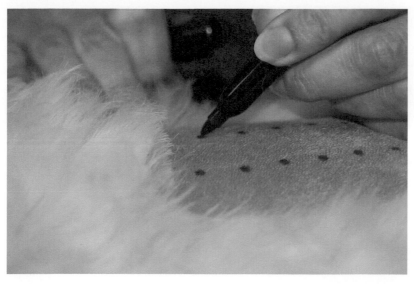

Figure 8.3 A permanent marker is used to place rows of dots on the shaved area to mark the test sites for each injection.

similar in horses except that standing sedation is used, and the injections are given in the lateral neck. This seems to give more reproducible reactions than other sites.

The allergen solutions should be drawn up in separate syringes (0.3–1.0 mL with 25–27-gauge needles) to allow accurate dosing and intradermal injections with as little trauma as possible (Figure 8.4). These should be allowed to warm to room temperature before use. Separate syringes and needles should be used for each patient.

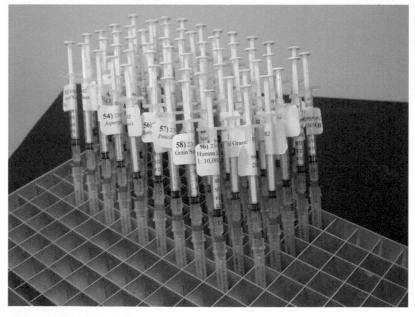

Figure 8.4 Intradermal allergy test kit drawn up in 1-mL syringes and marked appropriately.

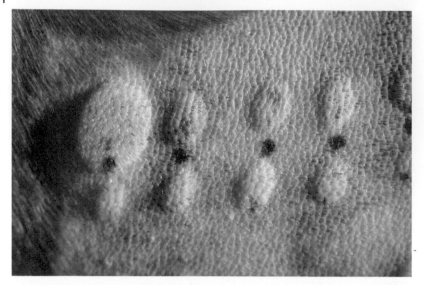

Figure 8.5 Intradermal allergy testing. The top left injection is the positive control (histamine), the negative control (diluent) is next to it on the right.

The positive and negative control solutions are injected first, followed by the individual allergen solutions (Figure 8.5). All injections need to be given intradermally, requiring very superficial injections resulting in a 'bleb' on the skin surface (Figure 8.6). Gently pulling the skin tight during the injection and making sure that the bevel is up and the needle goes in almost parallel to the epidermis, ensures that the injections are placed

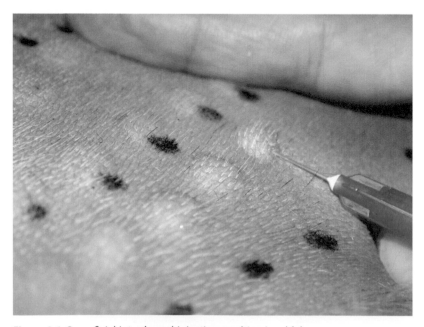

Figure 8.6 Superficial intradermal injection resulting in a bleb.

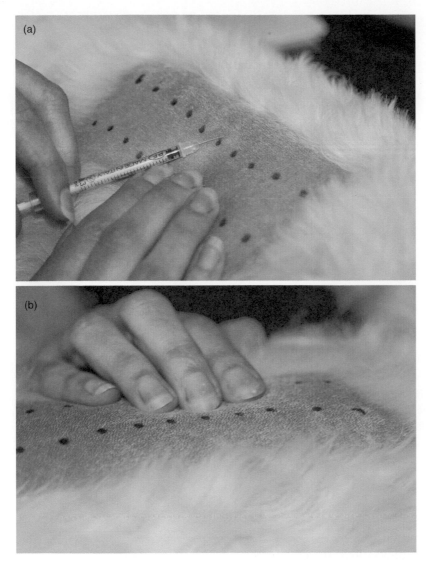

Figure 8.7 (a, b) Intradermal allergy testing – pressure is applied to stretch the skin slightly downwards to facilitate the superficial intradermal injection technique.

intradermally rather than subcutaneously (Figure 8.7). After correct placement, there is some resistance to injection and a characteristic 'bleb' is seen. There is no resistance to subcutaneous injections and no 'bleb' forms. If in doubt, withdraw, reposition slightly and inject again. Roughly 0.05–0.1 mL is injected at each site – it is most important to ensure that all the 'blebs' are the same size initially. This makes interpreting the results much more straightforward.

Positive reactions are usually seen within about 15 minutes of injecting (Figure 8.8, Figure 8.9, Figure 8.10). Reactions can be evaluated subjectively by interpreting the size of the wheal, the turgidity, the intensity and size of erythema and the steepness of the edge. By convention, the positive control is given a score of 4 and the negative control a

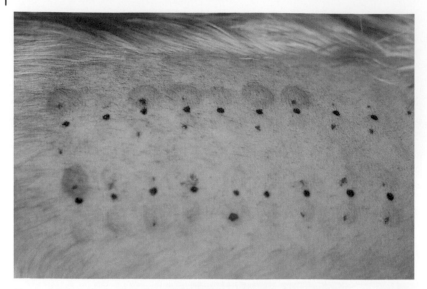

Figure 8.8 Intradermal allergy testing – the top left injection represents the positive control, the injection just to the right is the negative control and various positive reactions can be seen on the first row (different house dust and storage mites) and the third row (*Malassezia* spp.).

score of 0. The allergen test sites are scored 0 to 4 in comparison to the controls; scores of 2 or greater are considered positive. Objective measurements of the size of the reactions are also possible (positives are greater than or equal to the mean diameter of the control sites), but these do not take parameters other than the size into account and may therefore miss some positive reactions.

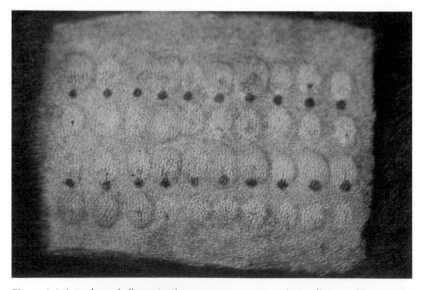

Figure 8.9 Intradermal allergy testing – numerous strong immediate positive reactions to house dust mites and various pollens in a black Labrador Retriever with pruritus.

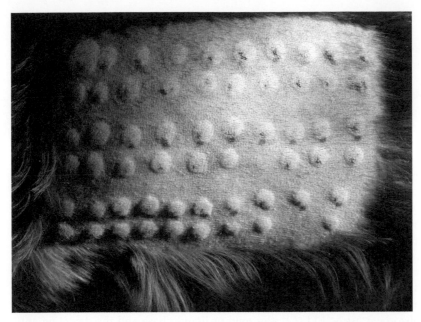

Figure 8.10 Intradermal allergy testing revealing a very strong histamine response and various small reactions to pollens.

IDT reactions (particularly in cats) may be very short lived and have to be assessed while finishing off the remaining allergen injections. For this reason, 4.4 mg/kg of 10% fluorescein can be injected intravenously after the initial reading of the test result in cats. This should enhance the reactions under ultraviolet (UV) light (Figure 8.11).

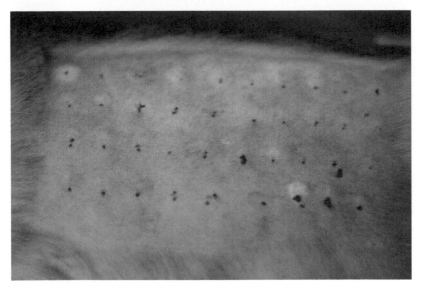

Figure 8.11 Intradermal allergy testing with fluorescein in a cat. The positive reactions are highlighted by the fluorescent dye. *Source*: Courtesy of Charlie Walker.

Allergen-Specific Serology

Many veterinary laboratories offer allergen-specific IgE serum testing (ASIS). These can be in the form of a 'screening' test using one or more different panels of mixed allergens (e.g. indoor/outdoor, or dust mites, tree pollens, grass pollens, moulds, epithelia etc.) or can use more extensive panels of individual allergens from these groups. By using mixtures of flea, HDM and pollen allergens, the Heska Allercept E-screen® immunodot assay has been shown to reliably predict whether an IDT or ASIS would be positive or negative to individual allergens in these groups. However, screening tests with mixed allergens do not identify individual allergens and therefore do not replace complete IDT or ASIS testing. Moreover, they cannot be used to make a diagnosis of AD.

The advantage of this form of ASIS is that it is readily available, requires no specialist training and equipment, and that the different assays appear less prone to changes caused by medication.

There are many different assays on the market and discussing every single one of them in detail is beyond the scope of this book. It is important to gather as much information as possible before deciding which laboratory to use – look for published data, ask about validation and quality control, and discuss these with experienced colleagues. Differences include the source of allergens, the detection method (radio-immuno-assay [RIA]; enzyme linked immunosorbent assay [ELISA]), the solid or liquid phase and the detecting antibodies (monoclonal, polyclonal, oligoclonal [mixed monoclonals] or recombinant FcεRIα [high-affinity IgR receptor]). It is crucial that the assay is able to reliably distinguish between IgE and IgG, which is circulating in far greater quantities and not relevant for the allergic reaction. Clinicians should take great care in selecting a laboratory, as a recent study in the US revealed extremely poor correlation between four commercial ASIS tests.

Measuring allergen-specific IgE does not discriminate between allergens that are relevant for the disease and result in inflammation on a cutaneous level and allergens that merely induce circulating IgE with no effect on cutaneous mast cells and cutaneous inflammation. Despite this, success rates with ASIT are largely comparable when this is based on IDTs or ASIS. The success of immunotherapy will depend on various factors, such as control of flare factors, and there is a study that shows that patients managed by an experienced dermatologist tend to respond better.

Skin Prick Testing

Skin prick tests (SPTs) are widely used in humans. A drop of the allergen extract is placed on the skin and a fixed length stylet is inserted through the drop and into the dermis. SPTs are quicker and easier to perform than IDTs. Recent studies have demonstrated reproducible sensitive and specific reactions in dogs following SPT with control solutions and allergen extracts. Dogs accepted the SPTs without sedation. SPTs need further validation to optimise testing concentrations, but could become more widely used in the future.

Allergy Tests for *Malassezia* and Staphylococci

Extracts for IDTs and ASIS tests are available to test for hypersensitivity reactions are widely available. There is good evidence that some dogs with AD become sensitised to their own *Malassezia* organisms and that this is clinically relevant to their disease. The evidence for staphylococcal hypersensitivity is less good, but it is likely that this also occurs. These tests may be therefore be useful in identifying animals that might benefit from intensive antimicrobial therapy. However, it is not yet known whether inclusion of *Malassezia* or staphylococcal extracts in ASIT is beneficial.

Patch Testing

Patch testing in human patients suspected of suffering from contact allergies is usually performed by applying a small amount of potentially allergenic substances mixed with an inert carrier into a metal chamber (Finn chamber), which is subsequently fixed to the patient's back with adhesive tape and bandages.

The same approach can be used in animals. Fractious animals may need sedation, although it is usually possible to perform a patch test in conscious animals. The test area is gently shaved, but is not otherwise prepared. Finn chambers containing the suspect substances and appropriate controls are applied to the skin and held in place with adhesive covers and bandages. It is possible to suspend solid substances in Vaseline® or similar. Allergen extracts are available, but these have not been validated in animals.

It is much more difficult to keep the allergen chambers in position for long enough to elicit a meaningful response (usually 24–96 hours) in animals than in humans, and this test is rarely performed in practice. In addition, there are no studies confirming which concentrations of allergens are suitable for demonstrating truly allergic rather than irritant reactions. However, preliminary studies confirming that epicutanous application

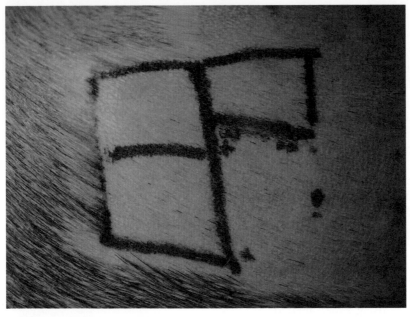

Figure 8.12 Open patch testing to grass extract in a dog with reported pedal dermatitis after walking on freshly cut grass.

of allergen solutions can elicit an inflammatory reaction 24–96 hours later, provide evidence that this may be a useful tool for research purposes.

Open patch testing can also be used, when allergen solutions are applied directly onto the skin and the area is observed for immediate or late phase and delayed reactions (Figure 8.12). This can be useful with suspected reactions to ear cleaners, shampoos and other topical medications.

As mentioned earlier, patch testing may also be useful in choosing ingredients for an elimination diet in dogs with suspected CAFR.

9

Immune-Mediated Skin Diseases

Immune-mediated skin diseases, with the exemption of hypersensitivity disorders, are relatively uncommon conditions. The immune system protects the body from external threats by distinguishing self from non-self and attacking foreign antigens. However, under certain circumstances the immune system fails to detect self as self and mounts an abnormal immune response against certain cells, tissues or substances in the body. Immunosuppressive treatments are therefore used to decrease the inappropriate immune response.

Depending on the condition, the patient may present with pustules, ulceration, nasal planum lesions, footpad disease or in some cases multi-systemic disease, which includes skin lesions. Many of these patients may benefit from being referred to a dermatologist or internal medicine specialist, depending on the clinical signs and their severity. However, a few tests are described in this chapter to give the reader an overview of the tests available. Diagnostic steps include:

- looking at the signalment, taking a good history and doing a thorough clinical examination;
- cytology (see Chapter 5);
- biopsy and histopathology (see Chapter 7);
- immunohistochemistry;
- haematology, biochemistry, serology and urinalysis;
- anti-nuclear antibody tests.

Prior to considering specialised laboratory techniques, a thorough history and clinical examination are crucial. Routine tests to rule out non-immune-mediated differential diagnoses are also important – these may include skin scrapings, cytology, hair plucks and fungal culture. For pustular and crusting diseases, differential diagnoses for pemphigus foliaceus include bacterial folliculitis, impetigo, dermatophytosis, keratinisation defects, pemphigus erythematosus and demodicosis. Deep skin scrapings can rule out demodicosis, cytology can reveal evidence of bacterial infection pointing towards a bacterial infection or acantholytic cells, which are compatible with a diagnosis of pemphigus foliaceus (Table 9.1), and a fungal culture needs to be performed to rule out dermatophytosis, which can produce lesions that are macroscopically and histo-pathologically difficult to distinguish from pemphigus foliaceus. Cytology can be highly suggestive of pemphigus foliaceus (Figure 9.1) or more consistent with a bacterial infection (Figure 9.2). In some cases, large numbers of eosinophils can also be found on

Diagnostic Techniques in Veterinary Dermatology, First Edition. Ariane Neuber and Tim Nuttall.
© 2017 Ariane Neuber and Tim Nuttall. Published 2017 by John Wiley & Sons, Ltd.

Table 9.1 Comparison of cytological features of pemphigus foliaceus and bacterial pyoderma.

Cytological finding	Pemphigus foliaceus	Bacterial pyoderma
Cells	Non-degenerative neutrophils or mildly degenerative neutrophils	Degenerative neutrophils
	Acantholytic cells	Acantholytic cells: only very rarely in very deep pyoderma
Organisms	Lack of significant infection	Intra- and/or extracellular bacteria

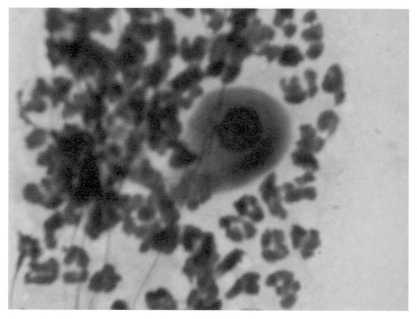

Figure 9.1 Photomicrograph of an impression smear from a patient with pemphigus foliaceus. There are numerous neutrophils, with some mild signs of degeneration in the majority, and an acantholytic cell. There are some nuclear strands, representing nuclear material from burst neutrophils.

cytology (Figure 9.3). However, cytology is non-specific in most cases of immune-mediated skin diseases.

Skin Biopsy and Histopathology

Biopsy of skin lesions is very important and in many cases diagnostic. It is therefore the mainstay of diagnosis of autoimmune diseases in veterinary dermatology.

The correct choice of the best sampling sites is crucial to select representative lesions and maximise the likelihood of a diagnosis. Ulceration, necrosis, secondary infection and prior treatment can make the diagnosis difficult. Early lesions are most likely to yield a

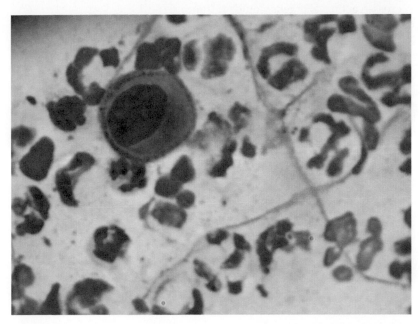

Figure 9.2 Numerous highly degenerate neutrophils in a photomicrograph of an impression smear taken from the skin of a dog with a deep pyoderma. Some intracellular cocci are visible. A large round cell with a round nucleus and neutrophilic plasma is visible. This most likely represents a keratinocyte that has lost attachment with the surrounding cells due to the severity of the infection.

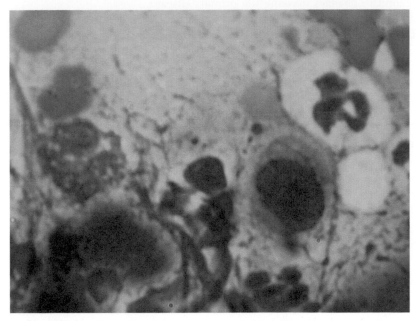

Figure 9.3 An eosinophil, a neutrophil, an acantholytic cell, nuclear strands, erythrocytes and a proteinaceous background on the cytological image of an impression smear of a dog with pemphigus foliaceus.

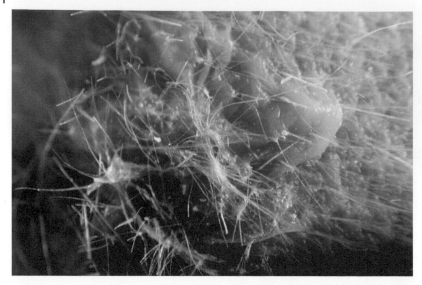

Figure 9.4 Close-up of a large intact pustule spanning several follicular units in a dog with pemphigus foliaceus.

diagnosis, and the history and clinical signs should alert clinicians to the possibility of an immune-mediated disease and prompt biopsy. In cases where secondary infection has been demonstrated, the patient should receive a course of antibiotics prior to sampling to avoid the secondary changes masking the primary disease.

A list of differential diagnoses based on the clinical and historical features of the patient helps to identify the most suitable lesions for sampling, as some lesions are more diagnostic than others. Early lesions include macules, papules, pustules, loss of pigment, haemorrhage, and intact nodules, vesicles and bullae. For example, the hallmark of pemphigus foliaceus is large pustules spanning several follicles (Figure 9.4) with associated acantholytic cells. With time these rupture and develop into large, tightly adherent crusts (Figure 9.5). Therefore, choosing intact pustules or large crusts will enhance the chance of obtaining a diagnostic sample with features characteristic of the disease (Box 9.1; Figure 9.6). Pemphigus erythematosus shows similar histopathological features (Box 9.2; Figure 9.7). Paraneoplastic pemphigus (Box 9.3) is histologically a crossover between the more superficial forms of pemphigus and the deeper pemphigus vulgaris (Box 9.4; Figure 9.8, Figure 9.9). In cutaneous lupus erythematosus, on the other hand, pigmentary incontinence and basal cell degeneration are major histopathological features, so choosing a biopsy site that is depigmenting and showing macroscopic signs of inflammation is more likely to result in a diagnosis than sampling an ulcerated area (Figure 9.10). See Table 9.2.

Punch biopsies are suitable for superficial and/or diffuse lesions. Deep wedge biopsies are better for lesions that involve the deep dermis or subcutaneous tissues. Elliptical wedges are also effective for spanning the margins of ulcers and may be more appropriate for sites needing careful closure to avoid deformation (e.g. pads, nasal planum, ears etc.). Third phalanx (P3) amputations are necessary for symmetrical lupoid onychodystrophy. Most laboratories will examine at least three samples, so clinicians can collect several

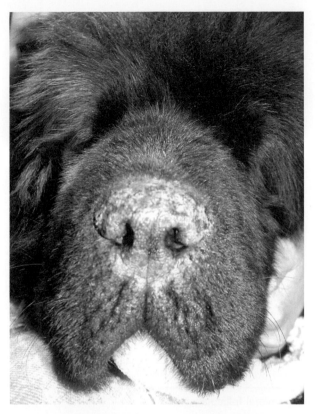

Figure 9.5 Large, tightly adherent crusts on the dorsal edge of the planum nasale and spanning onto the bridge of the nose in a dog with pemphigus foliaceus.

Box 9.1 Histological signs of pemphigus foliaceus.

Large subcorneal pustules spanning several follicular units
Non-degenerate neutrophils
Acantholytic cells
Secondary pyoderma can be present
Pustules may extend into follicular epithelium

Care to rule out dermatophytosis (PAS stain if suspected)
If apoptosis is present, consider drug reaction or pemphigus erythematosus

---

different lesions if unsure (more, including clinically normal skin, may be necessary in some cases).

It may be worth freezing some tissue for potential polymerase chain reaction (PCR) or submitting a piece for microbiology to investigate the possibility of a deep and unusual infection in pyogranulomatous or granulomatous lesions.

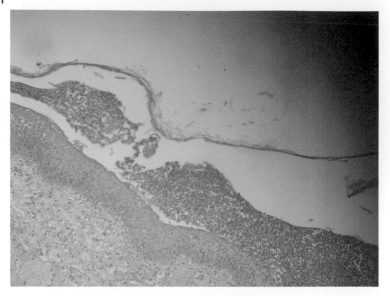

Figure 9.6 Photomicrograph of a skin biopsy specimen taken from a patient with canine pemphigus foliaceus. Note the size of the pustule, spanning several follicular units. Three are numerous neutrophils and acantholytic cells contained in the pustule.

Box 9.2 Histopathological features of pemphigus erythematosus.

Large subcorneal pustules spanning several follicular units
Non-degenerate neutrophils
Acantholytic cells
Interface dermatitis
Basal cell damage
Secondary pyoderma can be present

Immunostaining

Immunohistochemistry or immunofluorescence can be used to detect the presence of antibodies, complement and cells targeting self-antigens. Briefly, direct immunostaining techniques employ specific regents directly on sections from the affected skin, whereas indirect immunostaining involves incubating serum from affected animals with an appropriate substrate to demonstrate binding of circulating antibodies or other components. The sensitivity and specificity of the indirect approach relies on using appropriate and validated substrates (e.g. neonatal mouse skin, canine footpad, salt-split canine skin etc.) and reagents. These techniques were restricted to specialist centres and limited to IgG, IgM, IgA or complement factor C3. However, the advent of automated staining, immunoperoxidase labelling and much wider panels of specific antisera have made these techniques rapid, affordable and accurate even in formalin-

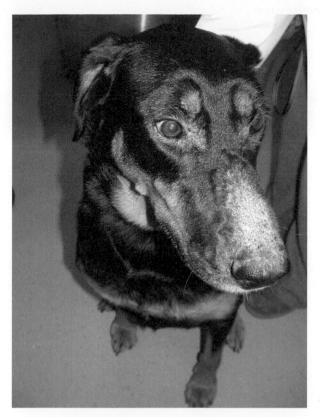

Figure 9.7 The face of a Dobermann with pemphigus erythematosus. Note the alopecia and crusting on the bridge of the nose and dorsal planum nasale.

Box 9.3 Histological features of paraneoplastic pemphigus.

Suprabasilar cleft
Rows of basal cells seen (tombstones)
Hair follicles may be involved
Intra-epidermal pustules (throughout epidermis)
Significant apoptosis

Box 9.4 Histopathological features of pemphigus vulgaris.

Supra-basilar clefting
Rows of 'naked' basal cells seen (tombstones)
Hair follicles may be involved

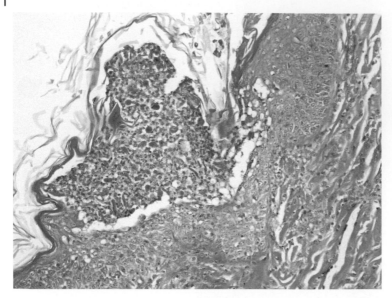

Figure 9.8 Photomicrograph of the histopathological specimen of the skin of a dog with pemphigus vulgaris.

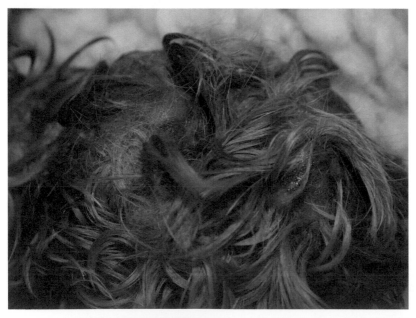

Figure 9.9 A pad of a patient with pemphigus vulgaris. There is severe ulceration of the footpad; the patient showed similar lesions on all mucocutaneous junctions.

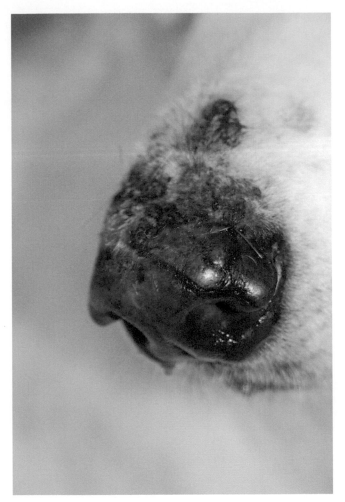

Figure 9.10 The planum nasale of a German Shepherd Dog with cutaneous lupus erythematosus. Note the loss of cobblestone appearance and the depigmentation of the previously black nose. There is also some crusting on the dorsal edge of the planum nasale, where it meets the haired skin on the bridge of the nose.

fixed samples. Immunogold techniques (with gold particles coupled to the antibody) are similarly used for transmission electron microscopy.

Immunostaining should not be used to replace conventional histopathology, but it can be useful to confirm the diagnosis in equivocal cases and/or where differentiating conditions is impossible with histopathology (e.g. in autoimmune subepidermal blistering diseases [AISBDs]). For example, 80% of sera from dogs with pemphigus foliaceus have positive indirect immunostaining with intercellular, top-heavy, web-like patterns most common. IgG4 antibodies are most common in the pemphigus foliaceus sera. With direct staining about 50% of biopsy specimens from animals with pemphigus foliaceus show deposition of immunoglobulins or complement between keratinocytes, and biopsy specimens from animals with lupus show deposits at the basement membrane zone

Table 9.2 Histopathological descriptions in immune-mediated skin diseases.

Histopathological descriptions		Disease
Acantholysis	Loss of intra-epidermal keratinocyte adhesion	PF
Interface dermatitis	Hydropic degeneration and apoptosis of basal keratinocytes with (cell-rich) or without (cell-poor) a lichenoid band, pigmentary incontinence and/or basement membrane thickening	DLE, GDLE, VCLE, ECLE, MCLE, SLE, SLO, pemphigus erythematosus
Lichenoid band	Subepidermal mononuclear cell infiltrate	See above
Hyperkeratosis	Chronic inflammation; scaling	ECLE, GDLE, SA, Pveg
Suprabasal apoptosis	Death of individual cells in epidermis; often surrounded by T-cells (satellitosis)	MCLE, EM, vasculopathy
Vasculitis	Specific inflammation of blood vessel walls; perivascular cuffing and microhaemorrhage	Vasculitis; lupus vasculitis
Vasculopathy	Changes consistent with ischaemia (e.g. endothelial swelling and degeneration, perivascular mononuclear cells, collagen necrosis, oedema, hair follicle atrophy)	Vasculitis
Necrosis	Full-thickness loss of epidermis +/− dermis	Vasculitis, SJS/TEN
Nodular dermatitis	Pyogranulomatous	Sterile pyogranuloma
	Histiocytic	Cutaneous histiocytosis
	Lymphocytic	Vaccine reactions
Intraepidermal pustules	Acanthocytes; neutrophils and/or eosinophils	PF
Suprabasilar clefts	Dermo-epidermal vesicles and separation above the basement membrane; acantholytic cells attached to basement membrane (PV)	PV, bullous SLE, VCLE
Subepidermal clefts	Dermo-epidermal vesicles and separation below the basement membrane	BP, EBA, MMP, other AISBDs
Folliculitis	Outer root sheath	Mural folliculitis
	Hair follicle bulb (bulbitis)	AA
	Isthmus	Pseudopelade

DLE = discoid lupus erythematosus; GDLE = generalised DLE; VCLE = vesicular cutaneous LE; ECLE = exfoliative CLE; MCLE = mucocutaneous LE; SLE = systemic LE; SLO = symmetric lupoid onychodystrophy; PF = pemphigus foliaceus; PV = pemphigus vulgaris; Pveg = pemphigus vegetans; SA = sebaceous adenititis; AA = alopecia areata; BP = bullous pemphigoid; EBA = epidermolysis bullosa acquisita; MMP = mucous membrane pemphigoid; AISBDs = autoimmune subepidermal blistering diseases; EM = erythema multiforme; SJS = Stevens–Johnson syndrome; TEN = toxic epidermal necrolysis.

(lupus band). AISBDs usually show linear deposition of immunoglobulins along the basement membrane. Natural clefts or salt-split skin can be used to show the depth of separation. In EBA IgG binds the superficial dermis in clefts and to the dermal side of salt-split skin. In mucous membrane pemphigoid and the other rare AISBDs, the immunostaining is below the cleft. However, false-positives can be seen in chronic inflammation with leaking of serum immunoglobulin into the epidermis and other tissues (especially in nasal and footpad biopsy specimens).

Most laboratories will perform these tests on formalin-fixed tissues. Michel's fixative, which should reliably preserve the specimen for 7–14 days provided the pH is maintained at 7.0–7.2, may be preferred in some cases – check with the histopathology laboratory before performing the biopsies (they will normally supply the required medium).

Specific Serology Tests

Modern laboratory techniques have recently vastly improved the diagnostic methods used in human dermatology. Knowing the major target antigens will allow the development of similar enzyme-linked immunosorbent assays (ELISAs) to help diagnose some conditions. For example, IgG serology for Dsc1 is consistently positive in dogs with pemphigus foliaceus and negative in dogs with exfoliative staphylococcal pyoderma, and there is a recently developed canine Dsg3 ELISA to help in the diagnosis of canine pemphigus vulgaris. Titres may correlate with clinical severity and could, in theory, be used to monitor disease progression. These and similar tests will become more common in the future.

Anti-Nuclear Antibody Test

Anti-nuclear antibodies (ANA) are antibodies against epitopes in the nucleus such as histones and single- and double-stranded DNA. The test employs an indirect immuno-fluorescence method. A species-specific fluorescent antibody is used to detect antibodies against nuclear components in the patient's serum. Sequential dilutions of the patient's serum are incubated with Hep2 cells, a rat liver cell-line. If antibodies against nuclear components are present, they will bind to the nuclei of the substrate and can then be detected with the labelled antibody. The pattern obtained in the serial dilutions is compared with a positive and negative control sample to detect the ANA titre. Different patterns, such as homogeneous, speckled, rim or nucleolar, have been described but they are not as specific for different autoimmune diseases in dogs as they are in humans.

Positive ANA titres are used to support a diagnosis of systemic lupus erythematosus (SLE), but positive ANA titres can also be found in dogs with infectious conditions such as vector-borne diseases (e.g. *Bartonella* spp., *Leishmania* spp. and *Ehrlichia* spp.). Other situations that can lead to false-positive titres are liver disease, lymphoma, non-specific latex agglutination, drug therapy (e.g. griseofulvin and antibiotics such as sulphonamides) and other immune-mediated diseases. Two to ten percent of normal dogs also have a positive ANA titre. A positive titre must therefore be critically reviewed and correlated with the clinical signs present in the given patient. Glucocorticoid therapy and non-species-specific antiglobulin can cause false-negative results.

Coomb's Tests

Coomb's testing is useful in the diagnosis of immune-mediated haemolytic anaemia (IHA) and is referenced in this book, as this may be a feature in cases of SLE. Two different tests, the direct and indirect Coomb's test are available. The direct Coomb's test is the more useful of the two and detects anti-erythrocyte antibodies (AEABs) that are attached to red blood cells, whereas the indirect test detects AEABs in the patient's serum. Given that the majority of the AEABs are bound to erythrocytes, the risk of false-negatives in the direct Coomb's test is much lower and the test is therefore more sensitive than the indirect test.

In a direct Coomb's test the erythrocytes are washed and incubated with the Coomb's reagent. This can be monovalent (directed at IgG, IgM or complement) or polyvalent (directed against several of them) and must be species specific. AEABs cause cross-linking, which results in visible agglutination of the cells in a positive test. Very large levels of AEABs can lead to a false-negative result due to the prozone effect, and many laboratories conduct serial dilutions to avoid this. Different temperatures can also affect the number of positive results achieved. The test result is usually reported as positive or negative as there is no clear correlation between the titre and the disease severity or outcome. False-positives can occur due to non-specific binding, damaged erythrocytes adsorbing serum proteins, post blood transfusion, infections, neoplasia and drug therapy. False-negatives can occur due to incorrect (species) antiserum, incorrect test temperature, very low levels of AEABs, IgA-mediated disease, aged samples and immunosuppressive drugs. Fresh EDTA blood is required, but some laboratories also request air-dried blood smears, as the presence of spherocytes in the smear can still be suggestive of IHA even if the direct Coomb's test is negative.

For indirect Coomb's testing, erythrocytes from a normal dog are incubated with patient serum for 30 minutes and the test subsequently performed as described above. As most AEABs are erythrocyte bound, this test is much less sensitive and false-negatives are very common.

Anti-Platelet Antibodies

Again, this test is mentioned in this textbook as immune-mediated thrombocytopenia (ITP) can be a part of canine SLE. Similar to ANA and Coomb's tests, a positive result can also be seen in patients with infectious diseases. The platelet factor 3 test commonly mentioned in the older literature is no longer available as it was unreliable. Direct immunofluorescence methods, similar to those described earlier in this chapter, detect IgG on megakaryocytes. However, this is neither particularly sensitive nor specific. Some referral laboratories offer flow cytometric tests detecting anti-platelet antibodies with monoclonal or polyclonal fluorescent labelled species-specific antibodies that express the test result as a percentage of platelets coated with IgG. The percentage of coated platelets increases with aging of the blood sample, which needs to be taken into EDTA tubes and submitted as soon as possible.

Rheumatoid Factor

Rheumatoid factor (RF) is a non-specific autoantibody with an unknown target, which may be found in a number of inflammatory, infectious and neoplastic diseases. It is particularly found in cases of rheumatoid arthritis. In humans, patients classically have either rheumatoid arthritis with a positive RF and negative ANA or arthritis due to a connective tissue disease (SLE) with a positive ANA and negative RF. However, in practice the situation is not always as clear-cut and dogs with immune-mediated arthritis can have none, both or one of the two autoantibodies. Separated serum or heparinised plasma are usually used for this test.

Cold Agglutinin Titres

Cold agglutinin disease is a form of immune-mediated anaemia. It is a condition in which proteins that precipitate from serum and plasma (cryoglobulins and cryofibrinogens respectively) associated with immunoglobulins (usually IgM) directed against erythrocytes, result in cold-induced skin lesions.

Autohaemagglutination can be diagnostic for the disease. Blood collected in heparin or EDTA is cooled on a slide; autoagglutination indicates that the condition may be present. The agglutination should be reversible by warming and accentuated by cooling to 0 °C. Cold agglutinin testing consists of performing two Coomb's tests, one at body temperature (37 °C) and one at 0 °C.

Urinary Protein

SLE frequently involves immune-complex glomerulonephritis, which can result in elevated urinary protein levels. However, other forms of renal damage and urinary tract infections will also lead to increased urinary protein. Testing usually involves commercial test strips, giving a semi-quantitative reading within a few seconds of applying a drop of urine to the strip. Urinary protein:creatine ratios provide a more accurate quantitative assessment of urinary protein levels that are unaffected by the urine concentration. Other skin diseases that can lead to increased urinary protein include scabies, lymphocytic thyroiditis and feline leukaemia virus (FeLV) infection.

Other Tests

Haematology, biochemistry, urinalysis and other tests may be appropriate in multi-systemic disorders. Diagnostic imaging may detect internal neoplasia and blood cultures may be necessary if sepsis is suspected. In appropriate cases and areas, tests for viruses (e.g. feline immunodeficiency virus [FIV], FeLV and feline infectious peritonitis [FIP] in cats, equine viral arteritis [EVA] and equine infectious anaemia [EIA]), rickettsias (e.g. Rocky Mountain spotted fever, erlichiosis, borreliosis etc.) or *Leishmania* by serology or PCR should be considered.

Many treatments for immune-mediated skin diseases can have serious adverse effects and routine blood and urine tests are important for monitoring. It is important to collect pretreatment samples for haematology, biochemistry and urinalysis to provide a baseline to assess the effects of treatment.

10

Endocrine and Metabolic Skin Diseases

Endocrine skin diseases are relatively common in small animal practice, although thyroid disease may be overdiagnosed. Some of these cases start showing mild clinical signs a long time before the disease can be diagnosed with laboratory methods. It is important to monitor the progression of the clinical signs. Tests may need to be repeated after a suitable time until a diagnosis can finally be made.

Clinical Signs Associated with Endocrinopathies

Canine Hypothyroidism

Dogs with hypothyroidism most commonly present with skin changes such as alopecia (Figure 10.1 and Figure 10.2), recurrent pyoderma (Figure 10.3), dorsal scaling, 'tragic' facial expression (due to thickening of the skin on the face, Figure 10.4), seborrhoea, 'rat tail' (Figure 10.5), loss of coat quality, coat discolouration, obesity and lethargy or listlessness, with each patient showing a different combination of clinical signs. Cardiovascular changes (low heart rate), neurological problems (polyneuropathy, focal neuropathy, central nervous problems resulting in ataxia, hemiparesis, hypermetria, head tilt, circling and cranial nerve changes, and hypothyroid coma [very rare]) and ocular disease (corneal dystrophy and lipid deposits) have also been reported. Trichograms often show telogenisation, i.e. most or all hair is in telogen (Figure 10.6).

Feline Hyperthyroidism

Cats with hyperthyroidism are usually older and present with weight loss, increased appetite, hyperexcitability, polydipsia, polyuria and palpable enlargement of the thyroid gland. Gastrointestinal signs are also common and may include vomiting, diarrhoea and increased faecal volume. Cardiovascular signs include tachycardia, systolic murmurs, dyspnoea, cardiomegaly and congestive heart failure. Some affected cats may display pruritus or behaviour associated with hyperaesthesia. Approximately 10% of cats present with an 'apathetic' form, which is usually associated with concurrent renal failure, heart failure or other problems.

Diagnostic Techniques in Veterinary Dermatology, First Edition. Ariane Neuber and Tim Nuttall.
© 2017 Ariane Neuber and Tim Nuttall. Published 2017 by John Wiley & Sons, Ltd.

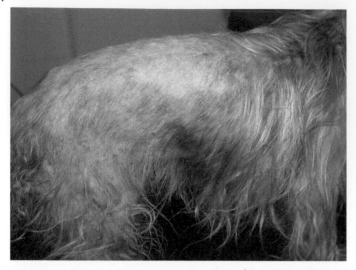

Figure 10.1 Caudo-dorsal and generalised alopecia in a Yorkshire Terrier with hypothyroidism.

Hyperadrenocorticism

Dogs with hyperadrenocorticism usually present with signs associated with excessive cortisol levels rather than problems with the mass secreting the hormone. Clinical signs such as polyuria/polydipsia, polyphagia, lethargy, abdominal distension, hepatomegaly, muscle atrophy and dermatological changes (bilateral truncal alopecia, generalised coat thinning, development of a 'rat tail' (Figure 10.7), calcinosis cutis (Figure 10.8), thinning of the skin, often with prominent blood vessels and hyperpigmentation) are most commonly seen. Cats are rarely diagnosed with hyperadrenocorticism but can present with skin fragility (Figure 10.9).

Sertoli Cell Tumours

Sertoli cell tumours often result in cutaneous atrophy and clinical signs similar to hyperadrenocorticism. However, the raised oestrogen levels can cause more specific clinical signs such as gynaecomastia, attractiveness to male dogs and linear preputial erythema.

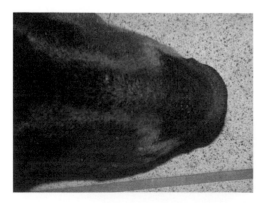

Figure 10.2 Partial alopecia on the bridge of the nose in a Dobermann with hypothyroidism.

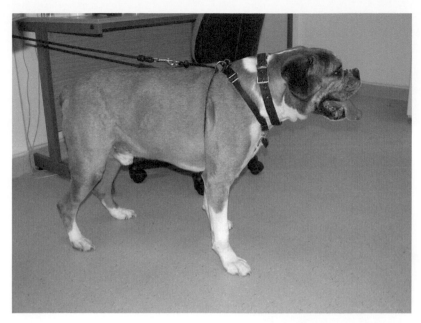

Figure 10.3 Circular alopecia and obesity in a Boxer with pyoderma secondary to hypothyroidism.

Approach to Diagnosis

There is no single test that can diagnose any of the hormonal diseases and it is important to perform tests in the context of the clinical situation rather than as a blanket screening test. In particular, specific endocrine tests should only be performed when their use is supported by the clinical presentation and basic screening tests.

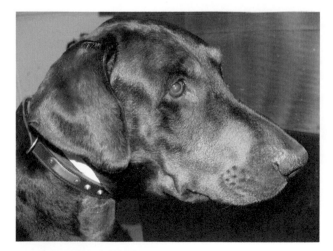

Figure 10.4 'Tragic' facial expression in a Dobermann with hypothyroidism.

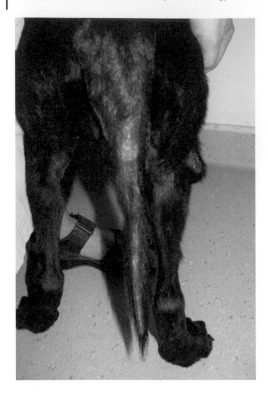

Figure 10.5 'Rat tail' in a Labrador Retriever with hypothyroidism.

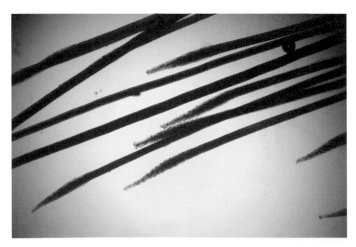

Figure 10.6 Telogenisation of the hair in a trichogram from a dog diagnosed with hypothyroidism.

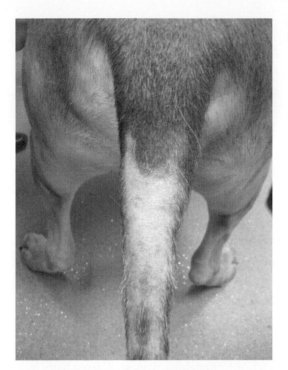

Figure 10.7 'Rat tail' in a dog with hyperadrenocorticism.

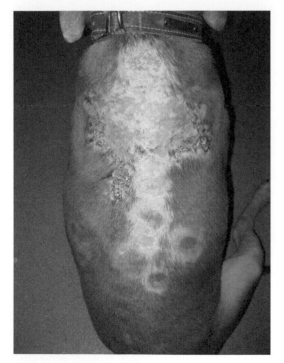

Figure 10.8 Extensive alopecia and areas showing erosions and calcinosis cutis in a Staffordshire Bull Terrier with iatrogenic Cushing's disease due to long-term glucocorticoid therapy for atopic dermatitis.

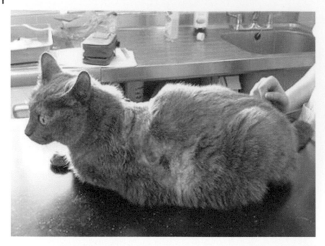

Figure 10.9 Cat with Cushing's disease leading to skin fragility and non-healing wounds.

Hair Plucks

Hair plucks (see Chapter 3) are often overlooked, but are very useful in assessing cases of alopecia. Complete telogenisation with intact hair tips indicates that the hairs are not being replaced; this is consistent with endocrine or metabolic disease. Anagen hairs with broken tips or abnormal shafts indicate that the coat is growing and that the hair loss is more likely to be associated with pruritus, inflammation, infection or follicular dysplasia. However, this should be interpreted with some care as breed and season-specific patterns of anagen to telogen ratios have not been established.

Routine Haematology and Biochemistry

Routine haematology and biochemistry testing are often overlooked but are very important diagnostic tests in suspected cases of hormonal disease and should be performed in all canine patients of suspected endocrine disease prior to specific hormonal tests. In feline patients with suspected hyperthyroidism, haematology is not particularly useful, although certain changes can be seen in some patients.

Haematology

The haematological picture of dogs with hypothyroidism is very different to that of patients with hyperadrenocorticism (HAC).

Hypothyroidism

In about a third of dogs with hypothyroidism, decreased blood oxygen consumption and decreased erythropoietin (leading to decreased erythrocyte production in the bone marrow) lead to a mild normocytic, normochromic, non-regenerative anaemia. Leptocytes (target cells) may develop due to the increased blood lipid levels leading to lipid accumulation in the cell membrane of the red blood cells.

Hyperadrenocorticism

A stress leucogram is the hallmark of canine HAC – this involves an absolute or relative lymphopenia, eosinopenia, neutrophilia, monocytosis, erythrocytosis and thrombocytosis. These features are due to steroid lymphycytolysis, eosinophil bone marrow sequestration, and reduced neutrophil and monocyte capillary margination and diapedesis. Glucocorticoids stimulate the bone marrow, mildly elevating erythrocyte and thrombocyte counts.

Other Conditions

Cats with hyperthyroidism can show mild to moderate erythrocytosis with increased haemoglobin concentration and packed cell volume (PCV), and macrocytotic erythrocytes. Anaemia is much less common, but can be associated with nutrient deficiencies (low iron levels) and bone marrow exhaustion. This can be accompanied by Heinz body formation and large thrombocytes. However, in most cats with hyperthyroidism, the anaemia is caused by something other than the thyroid disease. A stress leucogram (neutrophilia, lymphopenia and eosinophilia) is also a common finding.

Most other endocrine and metabolic conditions do not result in any specific haematological changes, although anaemia may be seen with canine Sertoli cell tumours and associated with underlying conditions in anagen defluxion or telogen effluvium.

Biochemistry

The biochemical analysis also reveals subtle differences and is worth doing to increase or decrease suspicion of a hormonal disease.

Hypothyroidism

Cholesterol and trigycerides are both affected in hypothyroidism. In about 80% of dogs with hypothyroidism there is a reduction of lipid degradation and lipid synthesis, but as the degradation is more severely affected, the net result is a lipid increase. About 80% of dogs with hypothyroidism exhibit hypercholesterolaemia, with increases to greater than 20 mmol/L not uncommon. Although hypercholestrolaemia is non-specific, increases to this extent are rare and should prompt consideration of hypothyroidism.

Decreases in the clearance of creatine kinase (CK) are commonly seen in hypothyroidism patients, but this change is neither sensitive nor specific enough to be very useful in the diagnosis of this disease. Changes in liver enzymes are similarly non-specific, as mild increases are very common in many non-thyroidal illnesses (NTIs), although very marked changes in alkaline phosphatase (ALP) are more likely to be found in patients with HAC rather than hypothyroidism.

Fructosamine in the high reference range or just above can be found in many cases of hypothyroidism and this may be a low-cost and easy test to give supportive evidence for the disease. After exclusion of cases of diabetes mellitus (DM), which is usually associated with more marked changes in fructosamines, the diagnostic specificity can reach over 80%. The increase in fructosamine in hypothyroidism is caused by increased protein turnover rather than lack of glycaemic control.

Hyperadrenocorticism

The most common biochemical change in canine HAC is an increase in alkaline phosphatase (ALP). A marked increase up to 5–40 times the reference range can be found in over 90% of cases. This change is neither 100% sensitive, nor 100% specific, however, as other diseases can also lead to a marked increase. The increase is caused because of a specific glucocorticoid-induced isoenzyme. Alanine aminotransferase (ALT) and bile acids can also be mildly increased, but this is usually only a mild change and not very sensitive or specific. It is probably caused by liver damage due to glycogen storage in the liver cells (steroid hepatopathy).

Cholesterol and triglycerides are often elevated due to increased lipolysis. Cholesterol is often above 8 mmol/L but it is also commonly raised in other diseases, such as hypothyroidism, DM, protein-losing nephropathy and cholestatic liver disease, which may be differential diagnoses.

Glucose can be increased or at the high end of the reference range. A number of patients with HAC develop overt DM (about 10%), probably induced by exhaustion of the pancreatic islet cells due to the glucocorticoid antagonism of insulin via gluconeogenic effects.

Urea and creatinine can both be low normal or slightly decreased as an effect of the polyuria caused by glucocorticoids.

Feline Hyperthyroidism

Cats with hyperthyroidism often show increases in ALT, aspartate aminotransferase (AST), ALP and lactate dehydrogenase (LDH). These changes are thought to be caused by a direct toxic effect of the thyroid hormones and return to normal upon successful therapy of the thyroid disease.

The increased glomerular filtration rate can result in decreased creatinine and urea nitrogen (BUN) levels. This may be compounded by decreased formation and/or a loss of muscle mass. However, azotaemia is found in about 20% of cases, which is comparable in age-matched cats without hypothyroidism. This can be compounded by the increase in protein metabolism and hypertension. Hypokalaemia can be found in patients with muscle weakness. Glycaemia can occur due to an increased stress response in hyperthyroid cats when collecting a blood sample. Phosphataemia can occur in about a third of these patients, even without evidence of azotaemia.

Urine Analysis

Urine analysis is not important in the diagnosis of hypothyroidism but may be useful to investigate other differential diagnoses and other alopecic conditions.

Hyperadrenocorticism

Urine glucose is present if the HAC is associated with DM and is usually mild. Specific gravity (SG) is usually low (<1.015 or even hyposthenuric, <1.008) as long as there is free access to water. In most cases anti-diuretic hormone (ADH) production is not reduced, unless there is a macroadenoma in pituitary-dependent HAC that is compressing the posterior lobe of the pituitary gland. Most dogs with HAC are therefore able to concentrate their urine if water is withheld.

Proteinuria is found in about 45% of patients with untreated HAC without a urinary tract infection, possibly due to hypertension. However, in about 50% of dogs with HAC, urinary tract infections occur due to urine retention as muscle weakness prevents complete emptying of the bladder. The infection is often 'silent', as the anti-inflammatory effects of the glucocorticoids suppress the symptoms. If unrecognised and untreated, an ascending infection can cause pyelonephritis. Cystocentesis followed by urinary culture is therefore useful in recognising this complication.

Feline Hyperthyroidism

Urinalysis is usually unremarkable but can be useful to distinguish similar conditions, such as diabetes mellitus, from hyperthyroidism. Urine SG is variable, but low SG can be indicative of concurrent renal disease. Proteinuria is common and needs to be confirmed by measuring the urinary protein:creatinine ratio. This change resolves with successful therapy. Urinary tract infections are common and cystocentesis followed by culture and sensitivity testing is indicated.

Analysis of Thyroid Function for Dogs with Suspected Hypothyroidism

Prior to testing for hypothyroidism it is important to rule out NTIs and the use of drugs that decrease total T4 (TT4), such as steroids, barbiturates, non-steroidal anti-inflammatory drugs and sulphonamides. It is beneficial to postpone thyroid testing until these drugs clear the body. Although the time needed for the effects to subside varies with the agent and individual, it often takes 6 weeks for thyroid function to return to normal. Equally, ruling out NTIs and treating or stabilising these conditions prior to assessing thyroid function is very important.

Different forms of thyroid hormones circulate in the body (Figure 10.10), and there is a number of parameters that can be used in the diagnosis of hypothyroidism. However,

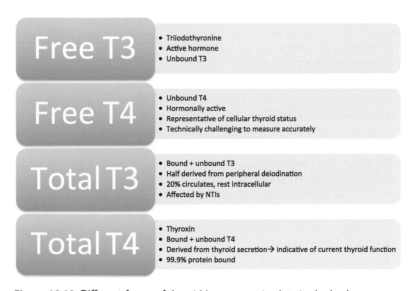

Free T3
- Triiodothyronine
- Active hormone
- Unbound T3

Free T4
- Unbound T4
- Hormonally active
- Representative of cellular thyroid status
- Technically challenging to measure accurately

Total T3
- Bound + unbound T3
- Half derived from peripheral deiodination
- 20% circulates, rest intracellular
- Affected by NTIs

Total T4
- Thyroxin
- Bound + unbound T4
- Derived from thyroid secretion→ indicative of current thyroid function
- 99.9% protein bound

Figure 10.10 Different forms of thyroid hormones circulate in the body.

none of them are very sensitive as well as specific, and combinations of different values are used to improve the diagnostic power. Basal serum values of total T4 (TT4), free T4 (fT4ed), total T3 (TT3), canine thyroid-stimulating hormone (cTSH) and occasionally free T3 (fT3) and reverse T3 (rT3) can be measured. Autoantibodies to T4 and T3 can competitively interfere in the hormone assays and their determination may be relevant in specific cases.

Total T4

All circulating TT4 is derived from thyroid secretion and therefore most indicative of current thyroid function. The majority (99.9%) of TT4 is bound to protein or lipoprotein and acts as a reservoir, leaving only a small percentage unbound and hormonally active. In the diagnosis of hypothyroidism, TT4 shows a sensitivity of about 95% and a specificity of approximately 70% – in other words there are few false-negative results but false-positive results are frequent. TT4 is therefore often used in conjunction with cTSH to achieve better diagnostic power.

TT4 can be low for a variety of reasons including hypothyroidism, NTI and drug therapy. There are also random fluctuations in T4 levels, marked breed differences and reduced levels with aging.

Increased T4 level above the reference range, particularly with a concurrent increase in TSH, is suspicious of circulating T4 autoantibodies (T4AAs) as they interfere with the test leading to falsely high values. More problematic is where TT4 is in the reference range due to T4AAs having lifted subnormal values into the normal range. T4AA testing is not as readily available as other thyroid tests but is also not indicated nearly as often.

Hypothyroidism is reported to be the most common endocrine disorder of dogs, and up to 80% of cases result from autoimmune (lymphocytic) thyroiditis. It is heritable and identification in a breeding animal is important.

- Advantages: this is an easy, inexpensive and readily available test. A resting T4 value in the higher two thirds of the normal reference range makes a diagnosis of hypo-thyroidism unlikely.
- Disadvantages: the definition of 'normal' varies:
  - laboratory factors: the normal thyroid range varies between laboratories and among tests;
  - age and breed: puppies have higher basal thyroid levels than adults; geriatrics have lower basal thyroid levels than adults; large and giant breeds have lower basal thyroid levels; sighthounds have much lower basal thyroid levels;
  - circulating hormones: glucocorticoids and oestrogen lead to lower T4 levels, and progesterone to higher T4 levels;
  - concurrent medication: corticosteroids, sulphonamides, iodine supplementation (kelp and seaweed) and phenobarbital all decrease resting total T4.

Free T4

Only the unbound fraction of T4 is hormonally active and therefore fT4 is theoretically a more representative assessment of cellular thyroid status. This is less affected by NTIs and drug therapy than TT4 and decreased values are therefore more specific for the diagnosis of hypothyroidism. However, the accurate assessment of the truly free fraction is technically challenging. The current method is the so-called equilibrium dialysis (fT4ed), which takes longer and costs more as it is a two-step test. The first step consists of dialysis of the sample across a membrane, which is impermeable to T4 antibodies and T4 binding proteins. The dialysate is subsequently analysed with a radio-immuno-assay (RIA) for T4. The specificity for this test is around 90% and the sensitivity approximately 80%.

Total T3

Only half of the TT3 circulating results from thyroid synthesis and the rest is derived from peripheral deiodination of T4. Peripheral deiodination is affected further by NTIs. T4 to some extend is a pro-hormone as T3 is three to five times more hormonally active. Only 20% of T3 circulates in the blood stream and the rest is intracellular. Due to a large overlap of values between euthyroid and hypothyroid dogs, this test offers no practical advantages and it is rarely used.

Canine Thyroid-Stimulating Hormone

In euthyroid dogs cTSH controls secretion of thyroid hormone through a negative feedback mechanism. Primary hypothyroidism leads to loss of negative feedback and increased levels of cTSH. It is therefore a useful first-line test in combination with TT4 or fT4ed to distinguish hypothyroidism from euthyroid sick syndrome due to NTI. If cTSH and TT4 are within reference range, the dog is most likely euthyroid. If cTSH is normal and TT4 decreased, the patient probably suffers from NTI or drug-associated decreased TT4. However, 20–40% of hypothyroidism patients also have normal cTSH, and in cases where the clinical suspicion is high, repeat testing or second-line testing (e.g. thyroglobulin autoantibodies [TgAA] or T4/T3 AA) may be indicated. If TT4 is low and cTSH high, the patient is most likely hypothyroid. If cTSH is high and TT4 within reference range, the patient may have early hypothyroidism and may benefit from repeat testing in a few months, may be recovering from NTI or have had recent steroid or sulphonamide therapy. This reinforces the importance of ruling out NTIs and taking a thorough drug history before embarking on thyroid testing.

- Advantages: an elevated cTSH value is supportive of hypothyroidism.
- Disadvantages: a large percentage of hypothyroid dogs have a normal TSH value.

The cTSH test has 70% predictability for primary hypothyroidism in dogs compared to 95% in people. Dogs regulate the pituitary–thyroid–hypothalamic axis via another pathway with growth hormone, and both false-negatives and false-positives occur.

Thyroglobulin Autoantibodies

Thyroglobulin is a high molecular weight glycoprotein component of the thyroid gland. Dogs with lymphocytic thyroiditis commonly show elevated circulating TgAAs as thyroglobulin is exposed during destruction of the thyroid cells. A negative result does not rule out hypothyroidism, but a positive result is a strong indication of thyroid disease (albeit not a measure of thyroid function). Positive results are more commonly found in hypothyroidism patients of certain breeds (e.g. Old English Sheepdogs, English Setters, Basenjis, Boxers, Golden Retrievers, Shetland Sheepdogs and Dalmatians) and in young or middle-aged patients. Positive results in clinically normal dogs can be used to identify dogs predisposed to hypothyroidism, although more extensive studies are needed to confirm the exact predictive value of this test.

Dynamic Thyroid Function Tests

Traditionally the TSH-response test was regarded as the gold-standard test. This test was carried out by injecting bovine TSH intravenously in a supra-physiological dose resulting in maximum stimulation of the thyroid gland. The TT4 values were measured before and after TSH administration. Although this is a very reliable test to assess the functional reserve of the thyroid gland, bovine TSH is no longer available. Recombinant human TSH is very expensive and difficult to obtain, and improvements in other thyroid tests have made dynamic functions tests less important. As an alternative, thyroid-releasing hormone (TRH) response testing was recommended, but this test is less reliable than the combined use of baseline tests and is therefore obsolete.

Therapeutic Trial

Therapeutic trials should only be used as a last resort in cases with a high clinical suspicion that have repeatedly been tested with equivocal results. If a therapeutic trial is deemed appropriate, written targets should be set to thoroughly evaluate an adequate response. Withdrawal of thyroid supplementation should lead to recurrence of the clinical signs, which should again respond to repeat supplementation. Only if clinical signs resolve with thyroid supplementation, recur following withdrawal and again respond fully to supplementation, can a diagnosis of hypothyroidism be made.

Summary

Many clinicians choose TT4 and cTSH as their first-line tests, with fT4, TgAAs and T4AAs used as second-line tests in specific situations. A complete thyroid test could include the following: T4, free T4, T3, free T3, TgAA (important if breeding or for breeds at risk for thyroiditis), and T3 and T4 autoantibodies (T3AA and T4AA). If necessary, discuss the pros and cons of these tests in specific cases with a specialist or the laboratory.

Analysis of Thyroid Function for Cats with Suspected Hyperthyroidism

In cats with overt clinical disease the diagnosis of hyperthyroidism is relatively straight-forward. Basal total thyroid hormone concentrations are readily accessible and cheap. RIA methodology is considered the gold standard, although automated and in-house techniques are becoming more popular and correlate reasonably well with RIA analysis (the specific reference ranges for each test must be used). These tests tend to be cheaper, making them very popular, although in-house TT4 may produce discordant results. However, as patients now tend to be presented much earlier in the development of the disease, reaching a diagnosis can be more challenging as borderline and discordant results are more common and care should be taken to check the results and rule out other conditions.

Total T3/Total T4

These are widely used and are the most reliable tests for the diagnosis of hyperthyroidism in cats. RIA-based tests are the most accurate, but in-house and automated systems are increasingly accurate and can be an acceptable alternative. However, severe NTI can suppress total T3 and total T4 values, and there are random fluctuations in thyroid hormone levels. Hyperthyroidism cannot therefore be ruled out on a single measurement alone. Cats with TT4 levels of less than 25 nmol/L are unlikely to have hyperthyroidism, but further tests should be considered for cats with TT4 levels of 25–50 nmol/L with suggestive clinical signs.

Free T4 by Equilibrium Dialysis

FT4ed is more consistently elevated in cats with hyperthyroidism and this is therefore the more sensitive test. However, the test is not widely available, is expensive and is prone to errors due to incorrect sample handling. Furthermore, 6–20% of euthyroid sick cats have elevated values, making it less specific. The results of free T4 tests should not be used on their own to diagnose hyperthyroidism and should interpreted in conjunction with a total T4 measurement (which makes total T4 alone the most cost-effective screening test). High normal TT4 and high fT4 is consistent with hyperthyroidism, whereas a low/low normal TT4 and high fT4 is consistent with NTI. If appropriate, you can manage the NTI and reassess TT4 and fT4 in 4–6 weeks.

TSH

A feline-specific TSH assay is not currently available and the canine test has poor sensitivity for the feline TSH. However, in certain situations it may be a valuable additional test (e.g. in occult hyperthyroidism in patients with compatible clinical signs, lack of demonstrable non-thyroidal illness and total and free T4 in the upper reference range; to diagnose hypothyroidism in cats after radio-I^{131} treatment or surgery; in patients with subclinical hyperthyroidism; and to exclude hyperthyroidism in cats with a high normal total T4). In the absence of a feline-specific assay, the canine test is used, although it is prudent to contact the laboratory prior to testing to discuss suitability of the method used.

Dynamic Tests

The T3 suppression test is most useful in ruling out hyperthyroidism rather than in diagnosing it. The TSH response test is poorly diagnostic and is considered obsolete. The TRH response test is easier to perform than the TSH response test, but transient adverse effects following TRH administration and the inability to distinguish between sick euthyroid and hyperthyroid patients limit the diagnostic value.

Tests to Confirm Hyperadrenocorticism

Diagnosing hyperadrenocorticism (HAC) is an art as well as a science, as there is no single test that answers the question of whether the patient is suffering from the condition or not.

All the pieces of the puzzle, i.e. the history, signalment, clinical signs and physical examination, have to fit in order to reach a high suspicion of HAC, which can then be confirmed with laboratory testing. Dynamic tests for HAC should not be used as screening tests for all patients with just one compatible clinical sign. They are only useful and live up to their published levels of sensitivity and specificity if the clinician in charge of the case has a very high suspicion of the disease based on the available data.

Cortisol-based tests are not useful for adrenal tumours in ferrets as these are typically associated with an overproduction of sex hormones, rather than cortisol. In addition, plasma levels of androstenedione, oestradiol and 17-hydroxyprogesterone do not reliably differentiate intact female ferrets, ferrets with an ovarian tumour and ferrets with HAC. Adrenal ultrasonography (see Chapter 12) is preferred for diagnosis of HAC in ferrets (which is often associated with pruritus rather than alopecia).

Baseline Cortisol Measurement

Determination of baseline serum or plasma cortisol levels does not require freezing as long as the samples are kept below 20 °C and processed within 8 days. Cortisol levels fluctuate significantly during the day, as well as with stress, non-adrenal illness and with age. Therefore, single point measurements of blood cortisol levels do not distinguish patients with HAC from patients with other problems or normal animals.

Urinary Cortisol:Creatinine Ratio (UCCR)

This is the only single point assay that is useful in the investigation of HAC. However, it is more useful in ruling out the disease as the positive predictive value is low (about 87%), whereas the negative predictive value is high (close to 100%). Urine should be collected in the morning in the patient's usual environment to avoid stress interference. The levels of cortisol and creatinine are measured and the ratio determined. Normal dogs typically show low values (this varies from laboratory to laboratory but is usually less than 10). Dogs with HAC have very high values (often over 300), although there is a big overlap with non-adrenal disease and stress. Some clinicians ask owners to collect morning urine samples on three consecutive days, keep the samples in the fridge and submit a sample consisting of equal aliquots from each day pooled in one tube. This gives a better overview of adrenal function over a few days and is less prone to influences of stress etc. Adrenal tumours, in particular, may secrete cortisol irregularly, so a single sample may not detect a randomly secreting adrenal tumour.

Dynamic Testing

As the overlap between normal, HAC and non-adrenal/pituitary disease is very high, there is no single ideal test for HAC and several tests may need to be performed to reach a diagnosis. False-positive and false-negative results can occur with all of the tests. Due to its speed and ease, many clinicians perform an adrenocorticotropic hormone (ACTH) stimulation test in the first instance. This is also the test of choice for monitoring of therapy as well as the investigation of Addison's disease and iatrogenic Cushing's disease.

Low-dose dexamethasone suppression testing (LDDST) has traditionally been perceived to be more sensitive than ACTH testing, but it takes much longer and is more affected by stress and non-adrenal/pituitary illness. More recently, a study comparing LDDST and ACTH stimulation testing in dogs with HAC and normal dogs revealed sensitivity values of 96% and 95% respectively. The specificity, however, was 91% for the ACTH stimulation test and 76% for the LDDST, making the positive predictive value of ACTH stimulation tests much better.

Ideally, patients with known non-adrenal/pituitary illness should have HAC testing delayed until these other conditions have been treated. In some patients repeat tests are necessary before a diagnosis can be reached. This is the single most important aspect in the investigation of HAC and in interpreting any test results.

Measurement of 17-hydroxyprogesterone (17OHP) can be useful in cases of 'atypical' HAC and in the investigation of alopecia X. This is because some adrenocortical tumours release steroid precursors rather than cortisol into the bloodstream, resulting in a 'flat-line, mid-range' cortisol response to ACTH testing. This test may also be useful in cases where a strong clinical suspicion of HAC is not confirmed with adrenal testing.

ACTH Stimulation Test

ACTH stimulation tests are convenient as only two samples 1–2 hours apart are required. A basal blood sample is followed by intravenous or intramuscular injection of 0.25 mg or 5 μg/kg synthetic ACTH (tetracosactide, Synacthen®, Cortrosyn®) and a post-stimulation sample obtained 1 hour later. If ACTH gel is used, the post-stimulation sample is collected 2 hours after administration of 2.2 IU/kg ACTH gel. Both samples are carefully labelled with the patient's details and time obtained, and submitted to the laboratory. Values vary with the laboratory, but as a guide normal dogs show an elevation of up to 450 nmol/L. Dogs with pituitary-dependent HAC (PDH) often show a normal pre-stimulation value with an exaggerated post-ACTH response above 600 nmol/L and often more than 1000 nmol/L (Figure 10.11). Dogs with adrenal tumours can have elevated pre-stimulation values of above 250 nmol/L and show no significant elevation

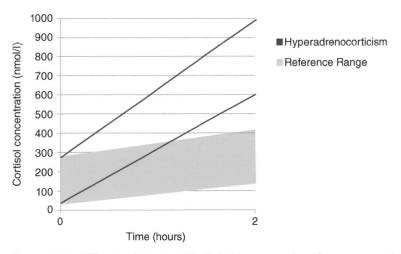

Figure 10.11 ACTH stimulation test. The light blue area is the reference range. The red lines show an exaggerated stimulation suggestive of Cushing's disease.

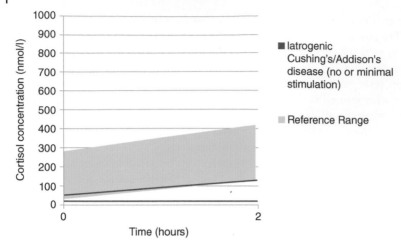

Figure 10.12 ACTH stimulation test. The light blue area is the reference range. The red lines show highly suppressed or even non-existing stimulation suggestive of iatrogenic Cushing's disease or Addison's disease.

post ACTH injection. However, as this is not a diagnostic finding, a LDDST should be performed to confirm this. Dogs suffering from iatrogenic HAC or hypoadrenocorticism will show no or hardly any stimulation (Figure 10.12). However, if there is stimulation up to the normal level and/or the first sample shows a low cortisol level (Figure 10.13), an alternative test (LDDST) should be performed and/or the ACTH stimulation test repeated a few months later.

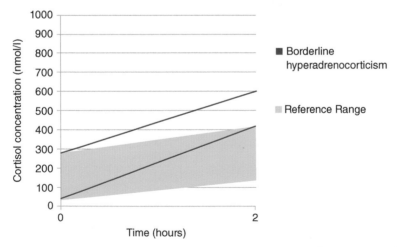

Figure 10.13 ACTH stimulation test. The light blue area is the reference range. The red lines show a significant stimulation, albeit within the reference range, following a low first value compatible with Cushing's disease. An alternative test should be performed in this situation.

Low-Dose Dexamethasone Suppression Test (LDDST)

LDDSTs are more time consuming than ACTH stimulation tests. A basal blood sample is followed by injection of 0.01 mg/kg of dexamethasone intravenously. Two further samples are then obtained: the first 3 or 4 hours (varies with the laboratory) and the second 8 hours later. Failure to suppress cortisol levels below 50% of baseline at 3 or 4 hours and 40 mmol/L at 8 hours is suggestive of HAC. Suppression below 50% of baseline at 3 or 4 hours but not 8 hours is consistent with pituitary-dependent HAC (PDH) (Figure 10.14). Minimal or no suppression is consistent with an adrenal tumour, but further discriminatory tests are indicated to rule out PDH.

17-Hydroxyprogesterone

17-OHP can be assayed alongside cortisol in an ACTH stimulation test. In cases with few clinical signs suggestive of HAC, 17OHP below 4.5 nmol/L can be used to rule out the disease. However, dogs with non-adrenal neoplasia and healthy female dogs in oestrus, dioestrus and pregnancy may have elevated 17OHP in response to ACTH stimulation testing. As for all endocrine tests, the results need to be interpreted with caution and always in the context of the patient's clinical signs.

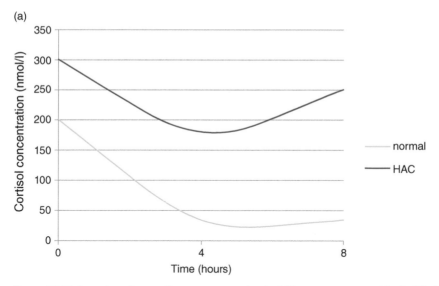

Figure 10.14 Low-dose dexamethasone suppression test. Figures a-e represent typical findings on low dose dexamethasone suppression tests (LDDSTs). The blue curve represents a patient that does not have hyperadrenocorticism (HAC). The red line shows the different possible responses to the test in patients with HAC. (a) The patient has minimal suppression at 4 hours and an increase in the cortisol level to around the original value at 8 hours. This patient could be suffering from pituitary-dependent HAC (PDH) or adrenal-dependent HAC (ADH). Further tests are needed to distinguish between these two conditions. (b) The patient shows no suppression and, again, could be suffering from PDH or ADH and further tests are needed to distinguish between them. (c) The patient shows mild suppression at 4 hours and a further mild suppression at 8 hours. Again, the patient could be suffering from PDH or ADH and further tests are needed to confirm the diagnosis. (d) A small number of patients suffering from HAC show a curve similar to that of normal dogs. A negative LDDST cannot rule out HAC completely. (e) There is suppression of cortisol levels at 4 hours and the levels 'escape' back to baseline at 8 hours. This can seen in patients with PDH. (*Continued*)

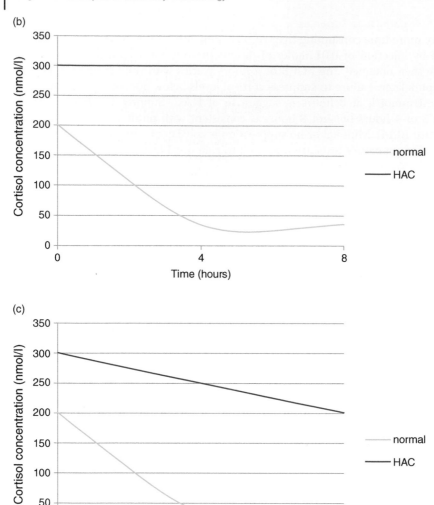

Figure 10.14 (*Continued*)

(d)

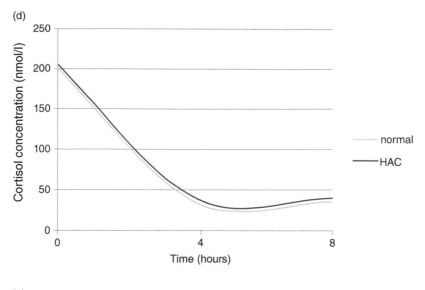

(e)

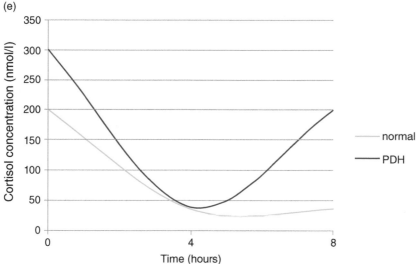

Figure 10.14 (*Continued*)

Urinary Cortisol:Creatinine Ratio with Dexamethasone Suppression Test

In dogs that are very stressed or difficult to sample, this test may be useful as it is carried out in the calm home environment. Morning urine is collected on two consecutive days and kept in labelled tubes in the fridge. Immediately after obtaining the second sample, dexamethasone tablets at a dose of 0.1 mg/kg are administered. Dexamethasone administration is repeated at the same dose 8 and 16 hours after the first dose. A further morning urine sample is collected the following day and all samples are submitted separately for UCCR analysis.

The UCCR in normal dogs should be less than 30 in all the samples. A UCCR above 30 in the pre-dexamethasone samples is consistent with HAC (often the value is well above 300). Dexamethasone administration suppresses UCCR by 50% in patients with PDH. Further tests are indicated to distinguish between PDH and ADH if suppression is less than 50%.

Tests to Distinguish Adrenal- and Pituitary-Dependent Hyperadrenocorticism

Once a diagnosis of HAC has been made, it may be important to distinguish between pituitary-dependent (PDH) and adrenal-dependent (ADH) HAC, as the treatment and prognosis differ between the two. The high-dose dexamethasone suppression test (HDDST) was historically the only test available to distinguish ADH from PDH in cases that could not be differentiated on a LDDST. More recently ultrasonography or magnetic resonance imaging (MRI) have been used to detect adrenal tumours (see Chapter 12), MRI imaging has been used to identify pituitary lesions (see chapter 12) and endogenous ACTH assays have become available commercially. As with all of the tests described, they always have to be interpreted in the context of the patient's clinical signs and hormone testing, as an adrenal or pituitary gland mass may not necessarily be a functional tumour.

High-Dose Dexamethasone Suppression Test (HDDST)

This test is only useful in dogs with confirmed HAC as high doses of dexamethasone will suppress the pituitary–adrenal axis in most normal dogs as well as in most dogs with PDH. The drawbacks of this test are the long duration and the possibility that further tests might be indicated, making endogenous ACTH testing or advanced imaging techniques attractive alternatives. Also, the accuracy of this test has recently been questioned and, with the availability of alternative, more reliable methods, the HDDST has become obsolete. The test is conducted in a similar way to the LDDST, except the dose of dexamethasone injected is tenfold higher (0.1 mg/kg). Suppression greater than 50% indicates PDH, with less profound suppression due to ADH or 'dexamethasone-resistant' PDH, making further tests necessary.

Endogenous ACTH

Again, this test is only useful in patients that have already been diagnosed with HAC based on other tests as it cannot distinguish between normal dogs and dogs with HAC. As endogenous ACTH levels fluctuate during the day, overlap with normal values occurs in some cases. Repeat sampling would increase the sensitivity, but this is rarely done due to cost and complexity. Measurement of endogenous ACTH requires specific sample collection and handling as well as carefully performed RIA testing. The blood should be collected into a chilled or frozen syringe and transferred into a cooled EDTA or cooled Aprotinin EDTA tube, which is kept on ice. This is then gently mixed and centrifuged as quickly as possible, ideally in a chilled centrifuge. The resulting plasma is transferred into a specialised chilled plastic tube (Figure 10.15) and frozen until dispatch with an ice pack. Most laboratories that perform the assay will upon request supply a special collection and dispatch pack for this test. Dogs with PDH show normal to elevated (>40 pg/mL) endogenous ACTH levels, and dogs with PDH have low levels or undetectable (<20 pg/mL) levels.

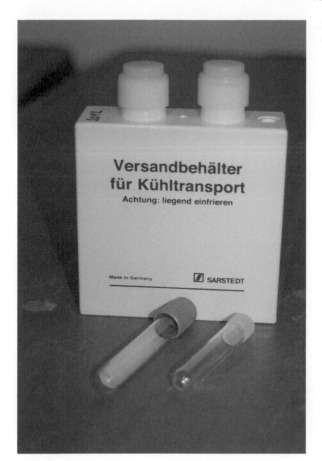

Figure 10.15 Endogenous ACTH sampling kit.

Feline Hyperadrenocorticism

Hyperadrenocorticism (HAC) is rare in the cat. Roughly 75–80% of cases are PDH and 20–25% have adrenal tumours (of which 60–70% are benign adenomas). Iatrogenic disease is possible, and there are rare reports of sex-hormone-secreting adrenal tumours.

The clinical appearance differs from dogs, with polydipsia/polyuria less likely to occur unless there is concurrent diabetes mellitus. A potbellied appearance and skin thinning are more commonly reported; in some circumstance the skin atrophy can lead to extreme fragility with spontaneous tearing or tearing following minimal trauma (e.g. scruffing). Other coat changes include colour change, dullness, seborrhoea, scaling, matting and (less commonly) alopecia. *Demodex* and infections secondary to HAC are also seen in cats (Figure 10.16). Many cases (80–90%) will develop diabetes mellitus later on in the disease. Other clinical signs include neurological abnormalities, plantigrade stance, hepatomegaly and muscle atrophy.

As the number of reported cases is low, knowledge about sensitivity and specificity of the tests available is scarce and is mainly extrapolated from normal cats and dogs with HAC.

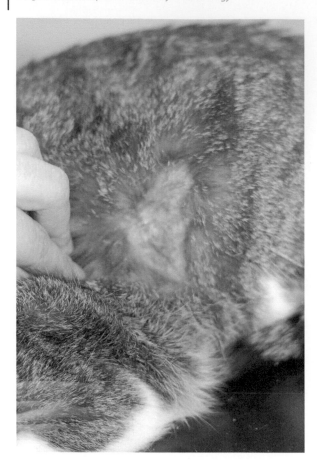

Figure 10.16 Feline demodicosis secondary to hyperadrenocorticism.

ACTH Stimulation Test

The test is slightly modified for the investigation of feline HAC. The basal blood sample is is followed by intravenous injection of 0.125 mg of synthetic ACTH and two further blood samples, 1 and 3 hours after ACTH administration. This test is less sensitive than in dogs (35–40%) and false-positives may be due to non-adrenal illness.

Feline Combined High-Dose Dexamethasone/ACTH Test

This test combines suppression with dexamethasone and stimulation with ACTH, and using the two endpoints may be more accurate than ACTH stimulation testing alone. A basal blood sample is followed by injection of 0.1 mg/kg dexamethasone. Two hours later a second sample is obtained and followed by injection of 0.125 mg of synthetic ACTH intravenously. The third and last sample is collected 1 hour after ACTH administration. It is important to accurately label all the samples with patient details and time. Normal cats should show 50% suppression in the post-dexamethasone sample and ACTH stimulation up to 400 nmol/L. Cats suffering from HAC exhibit little suppression after dexamethasone and exaggerated stimulation after ACTH.

Feline Endogenous ACTH

This test can be used in cats diagnosed with HAC to differentiate between PDH and ADH, similar to the situation in the dog.

Urinary Creatinine:Cortisol Ratio

The high negative predictive value of this test makes it very useful to rule out HAC. Non-absorbent litter, such as plastic or glass beads, can be useful to obtain samples in the home environment.

Urinary Cortisol:Creatinine Ratio with Dexamethasone Suppression Test

This test is conducted and interpreted in the same way as described for dogs.

Other Tests

Abdominal ultrasonography can be used to assess the adrenal glands as in dogs. This can also be helpful to check for local adrenal tumour expansion and infiltration, and metastasis to the abdominal organs. Computed tomography (CT) or MRI can also be used to assess pituitary lesions as in dogs.

Sex Hormone Assays

RIAs to detect oestrogens are available commercially and may be useful for cases of suspected male feminisation syndrome or other sex-hormone-related dermatoses. However, most laboratories only test for one type of oestrogen (e.g. oestradiol or oestrone), explaining the low number of cases with functional Sertoli cell tumour shown to have high oestrogen blood levels. There are also assays to detect a range of other oestrogen, androgen and progesterone hormones. However, as levels fluctuate markedly during the day, between neutered and intact animals, and between individuals, establishing reference ranges is difficult. Serum, plasma or whole blood can be submitted for testing if indicated. However, skin changes associated with Sertoli cell tumours, hyperandrogenism and hyperoestrogenism are best diagnosed by demonstrating neoplastic or hyperplastic changes in the gonads. Hyperoestrogenism can cause anaemia or pancytopenia, especially in dogs and ferrets.

There are several follicular dysplasia-like alopecic conditions that have been associated with abnormal gonadal–adrenal steroid hormone metabolism, which may result in altered levels of sex hormones and/or steroid precursors. Alopecia X has been associated with increased 17-hydroxyprogesterone and other adrenal steroid hormones (including progesterone, 17-hydroxyprogesterone, oestradiol, androstene-dione and aldosterone). The diagnosis of alopecia X is suggested by demonstrating an increase in 17-hydroxyprogesterone post-ACTH administration, and it has appeared to respond to treatment with deslorelin and trilostane. Despite this, the interpretation of these results is complex and their relationship to skin and other conditions is controversial. Values may vary with breed and there is no clear causal association with alopecia. Clinicians should therefore use the results of these tests with care. Dermatologists do not rely on these tests to achieve the diagnosis, looking instead at the whole picture, including signalment, history, clinical signs and histopathology, before considering these assays.

Miscellaneous Endocrine and Metabolic Tests

Growth Hormone and Plasma Insulin-Like Growth Factor 1

Measurement of growth hormone (GH) is useful in the diagnosis of hypopituitarism caused by hypothalamic or pituitary deficiencies, which can be congenital or acquired (e.g. infectious, neoplastic or traumatic). Pituitary dwarfism and acromegaly are diseases in dogs and cats that are characterised by low and high levels of GH respectively. However, GH assay is not commercially available and, as plasma insulin-like growth factor 1 (IGF-1) levels correlate very closely, this test is used instead. The results must be interpreted in view of the clinical situation. Submitting sibling samples is helpful in the interpretation of test results when diagnosing pituitary dwarfism.

Amino Acid Levels

Patients with suspected hepatocutaneous syndrome (also known as necrolytic migratory erythema, superficial necrolytic dermatitis or metabolic epidermal necrosis) show a normocytic, normochromic, non-regenerative anaemia, elevated liver enzymes, increased post-prandial bile acids, borderline or frank hyperglycaemia, and may have a positive ANA. If the clinical signs are compatible with the disease (Figure 10.17, Figure 10.18, Figure 10.19), the diagnosis is supported by routine tests, histopathology is compatible and ultrasonography reveals the characteristic

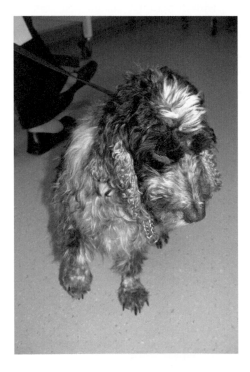

Figure 10.17 Cocker Spaniel with hepatocutaneous syndrome. The patient was depressed, reluctant to walk due to paw pad lesions and had lesions on most mucocutaneous junctions.

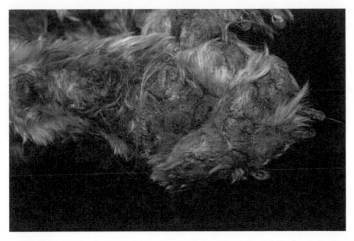

Figure 10.18 Ulceration of the paw pads and interdigital *Malassezia* dermatitis in a Cocker Spaniel with hepatocutaneous syndrome.

'honey-comb' pattern of the liver or pancreatic neoplasia, measurement of amino acid levels and glucagon may be useful. Glucagon assays may also be helpful in cases associated with glucagonomas, although these are less common. Heparinised whole blood or plasma needs to be submitted for this test. These tests have limited availability.

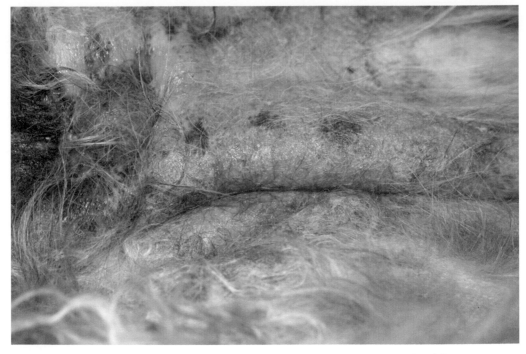

Figure 10.19 Ulceration of the perivulvar region and inner thighs in a Cocker Spaniel with hepato-cutaneous syndrome.

11

Infectious Diseases

Infectious skin diseases are becoming more and more relevant with globalisation leading to increasing numbers of pets travelling. More exotic diseases need to be a consideration when faced with a patient with skin disease. Nevertheless, by far the most common skin and ear infections involve staphylococci, *Malassezia* and (less frequently) other commensal or transient organisms, which can be identified by the cytology or culture techniques discussed in other chapters. The more unusual infections need more specialised laboratory methods, which we will describe here. Important clues that a more unusual infection, possibly non-indigenous to your region, may be present come from taking a thorough history, including questions about travel.

Laboratory Techniques

Polymerase Chain Reaction

Polymerase chain reaction (PCR) (Figure 11.1) is a method that is indispensable in research and routine diagnostic laboratories. It relies on amplification of single copies of DNA by thermal cycling, using primers and DNA polymerase. Specific primers allow targeted replication of the DNA that is of specific interest. PCR only requires very small amounts of DNA from the patient, allowing earlier diagnosis and treatment. However, this extreme sensitivity can come at the cost of lower specificity and the results must be carefully assessed to avoid a false-positive diagnosis. Other problems include DNA contamination, poor preservation of DNA in samples, and operator and laboratory error.

The process involves thermal DNA melting of the DNA double helix to expose the individual DNA strands, which then act as templates for the replication process. This leads to an exponential amplification, making it possible to detect very small numbers of DNA molecules, such as in the early stages of infection or neoplasia, or detection of slow-growing organisms that are hard to culture (e.g. mycobacteria). The amplified DNA segments are then electrophoretically separated, transferred onto a membrane and hybridised with labelled probes, which can be demonstrated by fluorescence or radiography. This is called a Southern blot, named after Edwin Southern (similar techniques are used to detect and quantify RNA [Northern blots; Figure 11.2] and proteins [Western blots]). Real-time quantitative (q)PCR techniques allow precise quantification of the

Diagnostic Techniques in Veterinary Dermatology, First Edition. Ariane Neuber and Tim Nuttall.
© 2017 Ariane Neuber and Tim Nuttall. Published 2017 by John Wiley & Sons, Ltd.

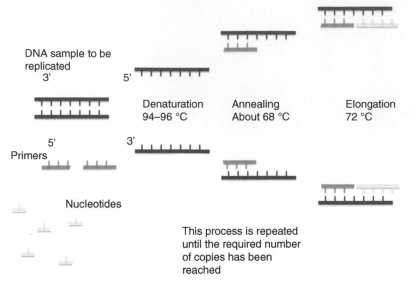

DNA sample to be
replicated
3'   5'

Primers
5'   3'

Nucleotides

Denaturation   Annealing   Elongation
94–96 °C   About 68 °C   72 °C

This process is repeated
until the required number
of copies has been
reached

Figure 11.1 Schematic representation of the polymerase chain reaction (PCR) process. The stages of denaturation, annealing and elongation are typically repeated 20–40 times to reach an adequate sample.

amount of DNA in the sample. More recent advances allow amplification of multiple targets in a single sample.

Serology

Serology is a widely used tool to detect antibody formation in response to infections, parasite infestations or hypersensitivity reactions. Serum is assayed for the presence of antibodies with different methods, including enzyme-linked immunosorbent assay (ELISA), radio-immuno-assay (RIA), agglutination, precipitation, complement-fixation test and fluorescent antibodies.

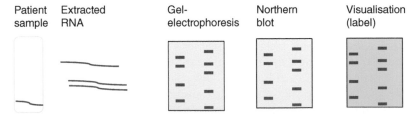

Patient   Extracted   Gel-   Northern   Visualisation
sample   RNA   electrophoresis   blot   (label)

Figure 11.2 Schematic representation of a Northern blot test. The RNA from the patient sample is extracted. The RNA is subjected to electrophoresis to sort the RNA fragments according to size. The RNA is then transferred to a membrane from the gel. It is labelled with a probe and can be visualised with varying techniques, depending on the probe used.

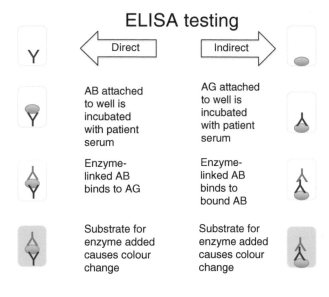

ELISA testing

Direct

AB attached to well is incubated with patient serum

Enzyme-linked AB binds to AG

Substrate for enzyme added causes colour change

Indirect

AG attached to well is incubated with patient serum

Enzyme-linked AB binds to bound AB

Substrate for enzyme added causes colour change

Figure 11.3 Schematic represen-tation of the ELISA technique. In a **direct ELISA** test the well is coated with an antibody (AB) specific for the antigen in question. Patient serum is added and incubated. After wash steps an enzyme-labelled antibody specific for the antigen (AG) is added. Following further wash steps the substrate for the enzyme is added and a colour change can be seen. An **indirect ELISA** starts with a plate that is coated with the antigen rather an antibody. In this test, antigen-spe-cific antibodies are detected in the patient serum, hence it is an indirect method. Patient serum is added and incubated. After wash steps an enzyme-labelled antibody specific for the patient antibody is added. Following further wash steps the substrate for the enzyme is added and a colour change can be seen.

ELISA

ELISA or enzyme-linked immunosorbent assay (Figure 11.3) is a method to detect and semiquantify the presence of antigens or antibodies in serum. A specific binding protein (an antigen to detect patient antibodies, or an antibody to detect patient antigen) is immobilised on a solid surface by incubation on a plastic well. Ready-made kits prepared with the solid protein are available for many diseases. Liquid phase tests are also used, but these are less common. The well is then incubated with the patient serum, whole blood or other fluids. After washing gently with a buffer solution to remove unbound or non-specifically bound antibodies, a detection reagent (an antibody specific to the patient's bound antibody or antigen attached to an enzyme by bioconjugation) is added. After a further incubation period and gentle washing, the enzyme's substrate is added, resulting in a colour change that is proportional to the amount of the patient's antibody or antigen bound to the target.

The results may be expressed in several ways. Allergy tests normally report the absolute optical density values or a corrected class score. Tests for infectious disease normally report a titre, which is the highest serum dilution at which a colour change is still detectable. A high titre (e.g. 1:1000) corresponds to high antibody or antigen levels, and a low titre (e.g. 1:20) to low levels.

Radio-immuno-assay

RIA requires specialised equipment and licensing for the radioactive agents, and ELISAs are used more frequently. However, due to its low cost, sensitivity, specificity and robust nature, RIA still regarded as the gold-standard test for some conditions. ELISAs are much faster, often taking only a few minutes to a few hours, than RIA, which typically takes several days. For RIA, a specific amount of antigen is labelled with a radioactive isotope, often gamma-radioactive iodine. A predetermined amount of antigen-specific antibody is mixed with this labelled antigen, leading to specific binding. When patient serum is added, quantitative competition occurs and some of the radiolabelled ('hot') antibodies are displaced. Bound and unbound antibodies are separated and the radio-activity of the unbound antigens in the supernatant is measured in a gamma counter. By measuring serial dilutions, the concentration in the patient's serum can be determined mathematically.

Agglutination

The word agglutination is derived from Latin *agglutinare* (to glue), and is used to describe clumping of cells in the presence of antibodies. This can be used as a rapid diagnostic test for the presence of bacteria (Figure 11.4). Cross-matching of blood types and Coomb's tests also fall into this category of testing.

Precipitation

In this test, soluble antibodies react with soluble antigens and at optimum concentra-tions lattice formation occurs, leading to a visible band of precipitation (Figure 11.5).

Complement-Fixation Test

This test is useful when only small amounts of antibodies are present in the patient's serum. It is a two-step test involving complement fixation and detection (Figure 11.6). First, complement and antigen specific for the antibody tested for are added to the serum. If the antibody in question is present, it will specifically bind the antigen and fix the complement. After an incubation period, erythrocytes and species-specific anti-erythrocyte antibodies are added. If the complement has been bound in the first

Agglutination

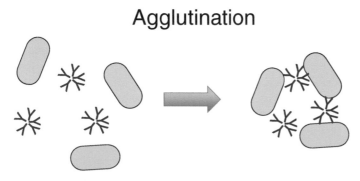

Figure 11.4 Schematic representation of agglutination used to detect antibodies or antigen in a patient's sample (e.g. serum, saliva etc.). In **direct agglutination**, latex beads are coated with antigen and incubated with the sample. If the sample forms an agglutinate (clots), the test is positive. In an **indirect agglutination test**, the beads are coated with a specific antibody instead.

Precipitation

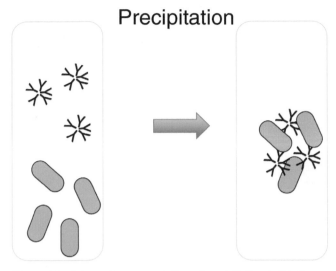

Figure 11.5 Schematic representation of precipitation. In this figure **direct precipitation** is represented. Patient serum with antibodies is added to a tube of antigen. If they are present in approximately equal numbers, precipitation occurs.

Complement fixation

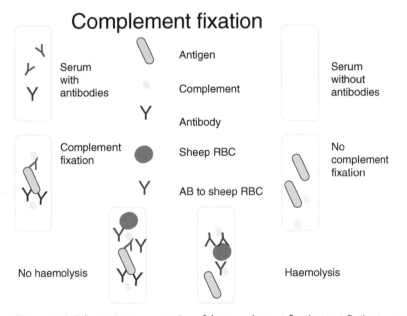

Figure 11.6 Schematic representation of the complement-fixation test. Patient serum is incubated with complement and the antigen in question. If the patient serum contains antigen-specific antibodies, complement is bound in an antigen–antibody–complement reaction. When sheep red blood cells (RBC) and antibodies (AB) are added, complement is not available for a further reaction: no haemolysis occurs. If the patient serum does not contain the antigen-specific antibodies, no complement fixation occurs and complement is therefore available for reaction with the sheep RBC and AB to sheep RBC added in the second step: haemolysis occurs.

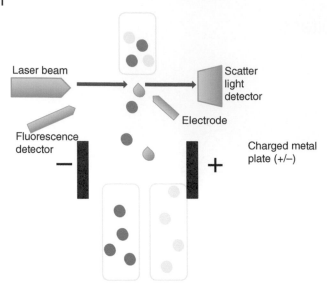

Figure 11.7 Schematic representation of fluorescence-activated flow cytometry. The cell mixture (e.g. blood sample) is treated with a label, that labels target cells. The cells are passed single file through a laser beam. Forward scattered light is detected by a scatter light detector. The excited labelled cells emit a fluorescence signal that is detected by the fluorescence detector. The labelled cells are then given a charge to sort them into a separate test tube. In this application cell sorting is achieved. Other systems can count different cells types or examine their physical and chemical characteristics.

step, none will be available and the cells will not be lysed. If the antigen was not present in the sample, complement will still be available to lyse the erythrocytes in the detection step.

Fluorescent Antibodies

This test uses antibodies conjugated with a fluorescent marker to detect microorganisms or other antigens. Direct fluorescence involves incubating tissues with fluorescent antigen-specific antibodies. Antigen-specific binding occurs and excess antibodies are washed away with a buffer solution. Similar methods are used for histopathogical sections, ELISA-type serum assays, cytology samples and blood samples. The bound fluorescent labelled antibodies can then be detected either by fluorescence-activated flow cytometry (Figure 11.7), with a fluorescence plate reader or fluorescence microscope (see also Chapter 9).

In indirect fluorescence (indirect fluorescent antibody [IFA or IFAT]) testing the patient's serum is incubated with antigen. A wash step removes excess antibodies before the fluorescent antibodies, specific for the patient's antibodies (e.g. anti-dog IgG antibodies), are added. A further wash step removes unbound anti-patient antibodies and fluorescence can then be detected with the methods described above. Examples include antinuclear antibody (ANA) tests and some pathogen-specific serology tests. Indirect fluorescence testing on histopathogical sections is similar except that the patient's serum is incubated on a specific tissue substrate (see Chapter 9).

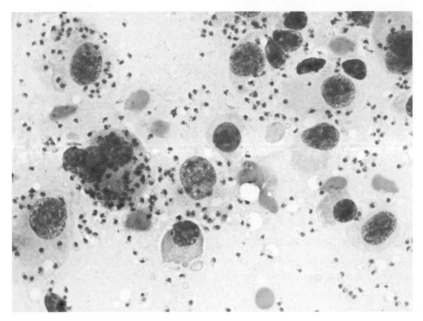

Figure 11.8 Photomicrograph showing numerous *Leishmania infantum* organisms and macrophages on cytology. *Source:* Courtesy of F. Albanese.

Diagnosis of Infectious Diseases

Leishmania

With more and more pets travelling, diseases such as leishmaniasis are diagnosed in non-endemic areas with increasing frequency. Leishmaniasis can cause a variety of skin changes and has often been called 'the great impersonator'. Various cutaneous signs, including alopecia, ulcerative and exfoliative dermatitis, nodules, depigmentation, ulcerated nodules, onychogryphosis and pustular dermatitis, have been reported.

Several different methods are useful in the diagnosis of this disease.

- Demonstration of *Leishmania infantum* organisms on cytology (Figure 11.8) or histopathology. Direct impression smears from lesional skin and fine-needle aspirates or biopsy specimens from bone marrow, lymph node, spleen or joint fluid are suitable samples, particularly if the tissue shows signs of clinical disease (e.g. pyogranulomatous inflammation). Bone marrow samples can be obtained from the humerus, iliac crest or ribs. The technique for obtaining a good quality sample is described in the next paragraph.
- Serology demonstrating *Leishmania* IgG in the patient's serum by ELISA or immunofluorescence techniques is a useful method, particularly in dogs in non-endemic areas with a history of travel to an endemic area and compatible clinical signs. The incubation period is long and seroconversion takes a few months. High titres in dogs with compatible clinical signs are therefore likely to be due to clinical leishmaniasis, whereas low titres warrant careful monitoring, repeat sampling or alternative laboratory techniques (e.g. PCR).

- Real-time qPCR amplifies and quantifies *Leishmania* kinetoplast DNA (kDNA), which can be used for diagnosis and monitoring of therapy. High kDNA levels are consistent with severe clinical disease. Suitable tissues are the same as for demonstration of the organisms. In addition conjunctival swabs have proven to deliver encouraging results with a high sensitivity and specificity. However, as PCR indicates infection but not clinical disease and negative PCR does not necessarily rule out leishmaniasis, the combination of both serology and PCR is very useful in the investigation of this disease.

Bone Marrow Samples

Bone marrow samples are not necessarily routinely performed in first-opinion practice but are a useful tool in the diagnosis of many blood disorders. Not many contra-indications exist, but if bleeding disorders with prolonged coagulation times are present, sampling should be delayed until the coagulopathy is under control. The risk of bone fracture is low unless the needle size is inappropriate for the patient to be sampled. Just as cytology and histology examine different aspects, bone marrow core biopsy and bone marrow aspirates also yield different types of information and are therefore comple-mentary techniques. Core samples allow for evaluation of the overall cellularity, the presence of myelofibrosis, myelonecrosis and architectural relationships of the cells. Aspirates allow for better characterisation of the individual cell morphology, which is needed to determine cell morphology abnormalities, identify the cell lineage and calculate cell ratios (e.g. myeloid to erythroid ratios and maturation ratios).

Special bone marrow aspiration needles and bone marrow core biopsy needles are available. For bone marrow core biopsies a Jamshidi bone biopsy needle is used; for most dogs a 13-gauge needle is suitable, but for smaller dogs and cats use a 14-gauge, and for larger dogs use 8–12-gauge needles. Bone marrow aspiration is carried out using a Klima or Rosenthal needle with an interlocking stylet; size 14 gauge will be suitable for most dogs and size 16 or 18 for small dogs and cats. Haematopoiesis is most active in the flat bones (e.g. the skull and ribs), however, bone marrow samples are more commonly obtained from the pelvis or femur due to ease and safe accessibility. Potential collection sites include the dorsal iliac crest, the femoral shaft (via the intertrochanteric fossa), humeral shaft (via the lateral aspect of the greater tubercle), the costochondral junction (through the cartilage and into the rib marrow cavity) or the sternum.

Depending on the patient's temperament, heavy sedation or general anaesthetic are required to provide analgesia and keep the patient still. For bone marrow biopsies and for cats (even for bone marrow aspirates) a general anaesthetic is preferred. Local anaes-thesia with 1 or 2% lidocaine is used to block the cutaneous, subcutaneous and periosteal nerves. However, the endosteal nerves remain intact and there will be some pain on sampling. If needed, post-procedure analgesia can be provided with non-steroidal anti-inflammatory agents or other means. The chosen site is clipped and surgically prepared to prevent infection. The surgical field is maintained with sterile drapes and sterile gloves need to be worn. A small incision above the collection site is made into the skin.

The sample needle is inserted through the soft tissues with the stylet in place until the bone is reached. For aspiration, the Klima or Rosenthal needle is placed securely in the bone marrow cavity. This is best achieved by securely holding the needle in a modified pencil grip with the end of the needle lodged again the palm of the hand or first metacarpophalangeal joint of the operator's hand to keep the stylet in place and generate the force needed to enter the bone. The other hand compresses the skin and soft tissue to provide more control. The needle is steadily pushed and rotated into the bone perpendicular to the cortex and then the bone marrow. The decrease in resistance may be hard to perceive. Correct placement is achieved when the needle has no give and will move with the humerus or femur.

Before aspiration, the barrel of a 10-mL syringe can be rinsed with 4% disodium- or dipotassium-EDTA to reduce clotting during collection. Once the stylet has been removed from the aspiration needle, the syringe is attached and full suction is applied until some blood is seen. The vacuum is released immediately to prevent haemodilution. The syringe can now be removed and some of the sample transferred onto a slide and some into an EDTA tube.

The sample on the slide needs to be processed immediately, ideally by a second person. The slide should be tilted to allow excess blood to run off. A second, clean slide is placed perpendicularly to the first one and used to squash to marrow particles across the first slide to ensure that the sample is not too thick to interpret. Ideally, one of the two slides should be stained with a rapid stain (e.g. a modified Romanovsky-type stain such as RapiDiff® or DiffQuik® – see Chapter 1) and examined to ensure that there is sufficient cellularity. If the sample is poorly cellular, a second aspirate should be attempted before recovery. If a sufficiently cellular slide cannot be obtained, a bone marrow biopsy should be performed. The bone marrow aspirate needs to be interpreted alongside a peripheral blood sample, which should ideally be submitted at the same time. Additional unstained slides should be submitted in case special stains (e.g. Prussian blue for iron or immunohistochemistry for leukaemia lineages) are required.

Any clotted aspirate can be submitted in formalin and processed like a biopsy. However, care needs to be taken to separate the formalin sample from the slides, as formalin vapours may fix the slides, rendering them unstainable. A very small core biopsy sample can be obtained by advancing the aspiration needle a further 10–20 mm into the marrow cavity without the stylet in place. The needle is then rotated vigorously and subsequently removed. The core sample is removed from the needle with a blunt probe or the stylet. However, the sample size is not always adequate and sampling with a Jamshidi needle is more likely to reveal a diagnostic sample.

Poor-quality and/or low-cellularity samples can be caused by poor technique, including improper seating of the needle, excessive aspiration leading to haemodilution, and sample clotting. Pathological conditions leading to poor samples include myelofibrosis with increased collagen and reticulin fibres and sampling of patients with aplastic anaemia, which usually yields fat tissue rather than haematopoietic spicules. Bone marrow biopsies are indicated in these patients.

The same bone can be used for aspiration and biopsy, but the bone needs to be entered a few millimetres away from the first sampling site. The technique for bone marrow biopsy is similar to that for aspiration. After performing a skin incision with a scalpel blade in the shaved and surgically prepared area, the needle is inserted through the soft tissues perpendicular to the bone cortex until the bone has been reached. Once the needle has reached the cortex, the needle is advanced by about 1 cm (depending on patient size) to obtain the biopsy core sample. Then needle is then rocked vigorously to section the sample at the base. Slight retraction, redirection and re-advancement can also help cut the core. The biopsy needle is subsequently gently removed from the biopsy site by continuously slowly twisting the needle on retraction. The biopsy sample is removed by carefully inserting a blunt probe into the cutting end and retrograde pushing the sample out of the needle. The sample is placed into a formalin collection pot. Good samples have a visually white (cortex) and red (marrow) end, and are longer than 1 cm. If desired, the sample can be very gently rolled over a slide prior to formalin fixation, to obtain a sample similar to an impression smear.

A technique for sternal bone marrow aspiration in dogs has recently been described by Paparcone et al. (2013), and appears safe and relatively easy to perform. The patients received butorphanol intramuscularly for analgesia 10–15 minutes prior to sampling, but sedation was only rarely required and most samples were obtained conscious. The dogs were positioned in right lateral recumbency with the right foreleg forward and the left foreleg backward, but parallel to the body axis. The skin over the second, third or fourth sternebra (Figure 11.9) was clipped and surgically prepared. An 18-gauge needle was inserted through the skin and pushed into the sternebra's wall in a rotating fashion. A distinct reduction in resistance was observed on entering the bone marrow. A vacuum of about 5 mL was applied with an attached 10-mL syringe for 5–10 seconds (Figure 11.10). Incorrect insertion or bone splinters leading to failure to obtain an adequate sample occurred in about 5% of cases. In those cases, a second attempt was performed in the same manner using a fresh needle.

The samples were prepared and stained with Giemsa or DiffQuik® to evaluate cellularity, differential cells counts, myeloid to erythroid ratios and parasite examination. *Leishmania* amastigotes were found either in macrophages or free in the extracellular environment in cases of macrophage membrane destruction. Samples from the patients were also submitted for *Leishmania* nested PCR examination. The author reported that no significant accidents occurred due to the technical procedure; some of the patients enrolled were sampled more than four times a year. As examination of bone marrow aspirates has an increased sensitivity due to a high density of *Leishmania* amastigotes in

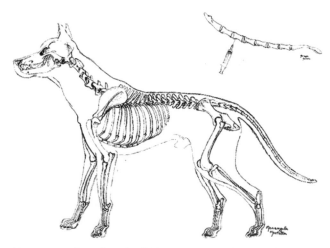

Figure 11.9 Sampling site for bone marrow aspiration from the sternebrae. *Source:* Paparcone et al., http://www.hindawi.com/journals/jvm/2013/217314/. Used under CC-BY 3.0 http://creativecommons. org/licenses/by/3.0/.

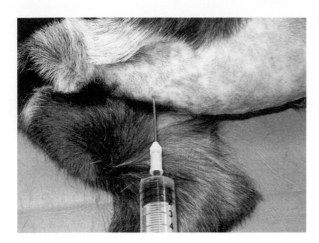

Figure 11.10 Bone marrow aspiration in process from the sternebrae with syringe *in situ*. *Source:* Paparcone et al., http://www.hindawi.com/journals/jvm/2013/217314/. Used under CC-BY 3.0 http://creativecommons.org/licenses/by/3.0/.

bone marrow, spleen and lymph node tissue, this technique provides a direct method (cytology and/or PCR) for diagnosis, rather than an indirect method such as serology, which may be less useful in endemic areas (where almost all dogs can be seropositive).

Borrelia

Tick-borne Lyme disease or Lyme borreliosisis is diagnosed in patients with compatible clinical signs and positive serology. Polyarthritis and lameness is the most common presentation in dogs infected with *Borrelia burgdorferii*. In humans a typical target-like rash – *erythema chronica migrans* – is commonly seen, but this is uncommon in canine patients. Dogs may also develop azotaemia, hypoalbuminaemia and proteinuria. A specific C5-based assay is available, which is not influenced by whole cell vaccines unlike some ELISA and IFA tests. Therefore, this is considered a good initial screening test. Suitable samples include EDTA blood and synovial fluid in EDTA tubes. *Borrelia* culture, direct microscopy and PCR are less reliable and less readily available. Western blot analysis can identify the exact proteins that the patient's serum binds to – this can distinguish dogs that have been vaccinated, dogs that are infected and dogs that are vaccinated and infected.

Bartonella

The presence of this flea-borne organism can be confirmed by serology, immuno-histochemical analysis of tissue samples or PCR (native samples or after culture). Serology with IFAT is the most commonly available technique, although some patients remain seronegative despite infection. Cross-reactivity with *Coxiella* and *Chlamydia* is also possible, leading to false-positive results. PCR of native samples can fail to identify the organisms due to the low-grade bacteraemia. More recently *Bartonella* culture using a *Bartonella*/alpha-*Proteobacteria* growth medium (BAPGM) followed by PCR has been developed, and seems to be the most sensitive method thus far. Suitable samples include EDTA blood, tissue aspirates in EDTA tubes and fresh tissue biopsy material.

Babesia

Babesiosis is a tick-borne disease caused by a haemoprotozoan parasite that mainly causes anaemia. Skin lesions apart from petechial and ecchymotic haemorrhage are rare but vasculitis, oedema, ulceration and necrosis of the axillae, pinnae, limbs, groin and scrotum have been reported. Infection can be diagnosed by serology or PCR on EDTA blood or tissue samples (lymph node, bone marrow or splenic aspirates).

Ehrlichia

Ehrlichiosis is caused by a Gram-negative, obligate intracellular bacterial agent. The predominant clinical signs are those of systemic disease, e.g. pyrexia, lethargy, weight loss and anorexia. However, vasculitis and (rarely) skin lesions involving a crusting facial dermatitis and papulocrustous or pustular lesions have been reported. Infection with *Ehrlichia canis* is another tick-bone blood disease and can be diagnosed by demonstrating the organism in white blood cells in a blood smear or by PCR on peripheral blood or a splenic aspirate. Although serological testing is available, cross-reactivity between *Ehrlichia canis* and other ehrlichial species is common and therefore serology is not reliable.

Treponema

Treponema paraluiscuniculi (rabbit syphilis) can be diagnosed by observing the characteristic spirochaete bacteria in material from smears or scrapes using dark-field microscopy. They can also be demonstrated using silver stains on histopathology. It may also be possible to use human serological tests.

PCR for Dermatophytes

The internal transcribed spacer of ribosomal DNA (ITS) is the genome fragment targeted in most veterinary tests.

- Advantages: rapid and sensitive. The current diagnosis of dermatophytosis can be problematic given the low sensitivity of Wood's lamp and direct microscopy techniques, and the length of time needed for culture.
- Disadvantages: dermatophyte PCR tests are still in their infancy. In veterinary medicine the major problem we have is the extremely high sensitivity of the PCR test. As dermatophyte DNA can also be found in gardens, how does one interpret a positive PCR test in an animal with no associated dermatophyte spores on hair shafts and/or in an animal with no clinical lesions? Difficult situations include a kitten in a household where a child has developed ringworm, screening rescue animals, monitoring the response to treatment and in alopecia from other causes. The cat or dog may have picked up a small fragment of dermatophyte DNA from the environment and the coat could only be transiently contaminated.

The results of PCRs for dermatophytosis must be interpreted very carefully in light of the history, clinical signs and differential diagnoses. The results should be confirmed by direct microscopy or culture before making a diagnosis of dermatophytosis. For other ways to diagnose dermatophytosis, see Chapter 6.

Virology Techniques

Virus Isolation

As viruses are oligate intracellular parasites and require living cells for replication, they need to be cultured on cell cultures, embryonated eggs or laboratory animals. Due to ethical considerations, cell cultures are becoming the most frequently used culture media. Different types of cell cultures exist.

- Primary cells prepared from directly from tissue samples. These can only be sub-cultured once or twice.
- Semi-continuous diploid cells derived from foetal tissue can be subcultured 20–50 times before they undergo culture senescence and cannot be transferred any longer.
- Continuous cells derived from tumours. These cells are immortalised and have an unlimited life span but retain contact inhibition.

Cell cultures are prepared by dissociating tissue using collagenase or trypsin and incubating the resulting cell suspension in a flat-bottomed plastic or glass container with a culture medium to ensure optimum growth. The cells attach to the bottom, spread and divide to form the primary culture. As the cells need continual nutrition, the supernatant has to be changed on a regular basis. After several cycles of cell division, the container may become too crowded and require division into secondary cultures. EDTA or trypsin is added to the primary culture to detach the cells and aliquots can be used to set up new cultures. Different viruses require different cell lines to replicate. Therefore, unless a specific virus is suspected, patient samples may need to be incubated with different types of cell lines to reach a diagnosis. Slow rotation in a low-speed centrifuge can speed up the infection/replication process for some viruses and may lead to a faster diagnosis. The cultures should be examined daily for evidence of viral damage to the cells. During virus incubation the culture medium must be changed when needed to keep the cultured cells alive. Detection of specific viral antigens may be possible after staining with monoclonal antibodies.

Electron Microscopy

Electron microscopy (EM) can be used to visualise virus particles *in situ* (e.g. on tissue samples) in order to identify the virus based on its specific morphology. The advantage is that specimens can be processed rapidly and there is no requirement for a preconceived diagnosis, as no virus-specific probe or tissue for culture is needed. However, EM requires highly skilled personnel, is expensive and is only successful if a minimum number of virus particles are present in the examined tissue. Direct and immunoelectron microscopy techniques are also available. Special fixative is required, and is usually supplied by the laboratory on request.

Diagnosing Viral Diseases

Poxvirus

Feline cowpox infection usually occurs through transmission from a rodent, which is the natural reservoir species. Cat-to-cat, cat-to-human and cat-to-dog transmission is also possible but very rare. A wound sustained during hunting leads to a single ulcerated nodule (typically on a foreleg, the head or neck). There is then a 7–10-day viraemic phase, which may be asymptomatic or manifest with mild malaise and pyrexia. The multiple epidermal papules and nodules then develop, and these ulcerate to form characteristic craters and ulcers ('pocks'). Systemic signs can develop and administration of glucocorticoids or other immunosuppressive agents can lead to a fatal pneumonia. Several methods are useful to make a diagnosis of pox virus in cases with compatible clinical signs. These include histopathology of biopsy material, virus isolation, serology and electron microscopy of crusts. Material for virus isolation should be submitted in plain or virus transport medium (VTM) pots. Similar techniques can be used for orthopoxvirus infection in Guinea pigs.

Herpesvirus

Feline herpesvirus infections lead primarily to respiratory signs but can also cause oral and facial ulceration. The virus can be detected in oropharyngeal or conjunctival swabs by virus isolation or PCR. VTM swabs can be submitted for PCR and virus isolation. Biopsy specimens of affected skin show ulceration, necrosis and often eosinophilic inflammation. Intranuclear viral inclusion bodies can be found in the keratinocytes in some cases.

Papillomavirus

This is most commonly a problem in young dogs with an immature immune system. Biopsy and histopathology can be used to distinguish oral or other viral papillomas and pigmented plaques from neoplastic conditions as there can be some overlap in clinical presentation. Histopathological findings include epidermal hyperplasia, ballooning degeneration (koilocytosis) of the keratinocytes with clumped, enlarged and pleomorphic keratohyalin granules. Intranuclear basophilic inclusion bodies can also occur. PCR can be used to identify different papillomaviruses in tissue samples, although the tests are not widely available.

Calicivirus

Feline calicivirus (FCV) is another primarily respiratory disease, although calicivirus infection can also cause cutaneous oedema, ulcerative dermatitis and oropharyngeal and conjunctival ulceration if the patient is affected by FCV-associated virulent systemic disease (VSD). The diagnosis is by virus isolation from oral or conjunctival swabs in cats with compatible clinical signs. However, a small proportion of infected cats shed virus beyond the usual 30-day period and remain carriers, so a positive virus isolation test does not always mean that the virus is involved in the pathogenesis.

Feline Immunodeficiency Virus (FIV)

FIV infection can lead to a chronic immunosuppressive disease. Common clinical signs include chronic gingivitis, stomatitis and periodontal disease, chronic or relapsing abscesses, pyoderma, dermatophytosis and demodicosis. Although ELISA testing exists and various easy in-house rapid ELISA test versions are commercially available, testing for FIV is not straightforward. This is because kittens born to affected mothers receive passive immunity and, more importantly, vaccination results in antibodies indistinguishable from those occurring during infection. In-house rapid ELISA tests are, however, useful as a first screening test, particularly prior to vaccination and to screen cats that may have been exposed to the virus (Figure 11.11). A positive result has to be interpreted with caution and follow-up tests should be performed, for example Western blot analysis of positive serum samples or PCR analysis. Unfortunately, even some commercially available PCR tests seem to be affected by vaccination, which causes a major diagnostic dilemma.

The American Association of Feline Practitioners (AAFP) recommends testing all at-risk and sick cats as well as kittens. However, most vaccinated cats will test positive on in-house rapid ELISA tests and Western blots, making a diagnosis in a vaccinated cat very difficult. Cats should therefore be tested before vaccination to check whether they are already infected.

In an in-house rapid ELISA test, antibodies can be detected from 60 days post exposure. In a sick cat, with compatible history and clinical examination, an in-house rapid ELISA test is recommended. If this proves negative, this is likely to be a true result and other differential diagnoses should be pursued. If the test is positive, a Western blot

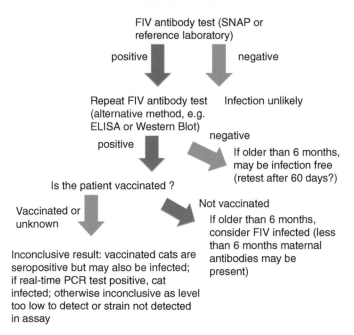

Figure 11.11 Decision algorithm for FIV testing, based on the Feline Retrovirus Management Guidelines from the American Association of Feline Practitioners.

should be performed to confirm the diagnosis. If there is a discrepancy with a positive in-house rapid ELISA test and a negative Western blot, both tests should be repeated 60 days later. If both repeat tests prove positive, FIV infection is likely but if any doubt persists, real-time qPCR may be useful. If both tests are negative, the patient is likely to not be FIV infected. If there is again a discrepancy, the tests should be repeated.

Feline Leukaemia Virus (FeLV)

FeLV is another common feline infectious disease that leads to a variety of different presentations. Cutaneous disorders that have been associated with FeLV infection include exfoliative dermatitis, cutaneous lymphosarcoma, giant cell dermatosis, epidermal horns, epidermal vasculitis, plasma cell stomatitis, plasma cell pododermatitis and plasma cell chondritis. Unlike FIV, however, vaccination does not lead to false-positive results in diagnostic tests.

ELISA testing for the so-called p27 antigen can be performed in most body fluids, including tears, saliva, blood, plasma and serum, with serum giving the most reliable results. Rapid in-house diagnostic ELISA tests are widely used, often in combination with FIV testing, although false-positive results can be seen where the virus is relatively rare in the test population (i.e. false-positives outnumber true-positives giving a low positive predictive value). Virus isolation, PCR and IFA can be used to confirm the diagnosis and stage the disease.

Other Viruses

PCR tests are available for avian feather disorders including psittacine beak and feather disease (PBFD; circovirus) and polyomavirus.

12

Diagnostic Imaging

Diagnostic imaging is routinely carried out in general practice with many surgeries well equipped with radiography and an ultrasound machine. More advanced imaging techniques, such as computed tomography (CT) and magnetic resonance imaging (MRI), are mostly restricted to bigger centres, universities and private referral clinics but are becoming more easily available to most patients and more affordable. Cases of otitis, in particular, can benefit from diagnostic imaging, but it can also be useful in patients with endocrine disease and suspected paraneoplastic conditions.

Imaging for Patients with Ear Disease

The main purpose of using imaging for cases of otitis is to examine the extent of the disease, which will in turn determine the prognosis and if the problem can be approached medically or if surgical intervention is needed. Distinguishing otitis externa from otitis media and/or interna is important. Up to 50% of patients with chronic otitis externa suffer from otitis media as well and, if left untreated, otitis media can progress to otitis interna or even a brain abscess. Most cases of otitis media are an extension of chronic or severe otitis externa, with stenosis of the horizontal canal and Gram-negative infections particular risk factors. Primary otitis media is less common in dogs, although primary secretory otitis media is becoming more commonly recognised in Cavalier King Charles Spaniels and other brachycephalic breeds. Nasopharyngeal inflammatory polyps in cats are an extension of upper respiratory diseases extending into the middle ear, although these can arise in the middle ear and base of the horizontal ear canal.

Dogs with otitis externa can show a number of clinical signs (Box 12.1). In mild cases owners may be unaware of the problem, particularly as the outside of the ear might look unremarkable. However, severe changes can be present in the horizontal canal, which will only become apparent on otoscopic examination. Otitis media can be missed, as the signs may be mild initially and/or masked by the otitis externa. Subtle signs can include head shaking, resistance to handling of the head and decreased activity. More severe signs include neurological signs, such as ipsilateral keratoconjunctivitis sicca, ipsilateral dry nose, Horner's syndrome, head tilt, deafness, vestibular signs with inner ear involvement, pain on palpation of the base of the ear, and pain on opening the mouth and dysphagia (Box 12.2). Neurological signs should be treated as an emergency–prompt treatment is needed to avoid permanent deficits.

Diagnostic Techniques in Veterinary Dermatology, First Edition. Ariane Neuber and Tim Nuttall.
© 2017 Ariane Neuber and Tim Nuttall. Published 2017 by John Wiley & Sons, Ltd.

Box 12.1 Clinical signs of otitis externa.

Head shaking
Scratching ear
Hot spot at base of ear
Otic discharge
Head tilt (particularly if unilateral disease present)
Malodour
Otic pain
Rubbing ear on objects
Otic erythema
Potential for muffled hearing/less responsive

Box 12.2 Clinical signs of otitis media.

Head shaking
Scratching ear
Hot spot at base of ear
Otic discharge (with concurrent rupture of the tympanic membrane and/or otitis externa)
Head tilt (particularly if unilateral disease present)
Malodour (with concurrent rupture of the tympanic membrane and/or otitis externa)
Otic pain
Rubbing ear on objects
Otic erythema (with concurrent otitis externa)
Potential for muffled hearing/less responsive
Aggression on examination of the ear (due to pain)
Hearing loss
Facial nerve paralysis
Horner's syndrome
Vestibular disease
Pain on chewing/avoiding hard food

Radiography

Radiography is very accessible and the findings are fairly specific. However, it is not the most sensitive form of imaging for patients with ear disease. Superimposition of other structures impede a clear picture of the tympanic bullae, making this technique difficult to interpret and not as sensitive as other imaging modalities. The ear canals can be better examined by direct visualisation with an otoscope or, even better, a video-otoscope. Due to a wide breed and individual variation, in-depth knowledge of the anatomy of the region in question and the influence of the head shape (Table 12.1) is very important and optimal positioning makes interpretation much easier.

To achieve accurate positioning, a general anaesthetic is required and several views need to be taken to optimise the result, making radiography a time-consuming

Table 12.1 Different head shapes.

Head shape	Features	Examples
Doliocephalic/ oligocephalic	Long, narrow head	Rough Collie, Saluki, Collie, Borzoi, Greyhound
Mesocephalic	Rounded head	Majority of breeds: Dobermann, Labrador Retriever, German Shepherd Dog, Bernese Mountain Dog
Brachycephalic	Short, wide head	English Bulldog, Pekinese, Pug, French Bulldog

diagnostic test. In patients with compromised upper airways (e.g. brachycephalic breeds), there is an increased anaesthetic risk. Lateral oblique views are taken to avoid superimposition over the bullae as seen on true lateral views. In order to allow for direct comparison between both bullae, positioning has to be very careful. Dorso-ventral and rostral open-mouth views are also used to compare both sides. Ideally, the endotracheal tube should be removed for these positions to avoid superimposition of the tube on the area of interest. Occasionally lateral and ventrodorsal views can add more information.

Radiography can detect changes such as calcification or ossification of the ear canals (Figure 12.1), changes to the bony tympanic bullae or soft tissue changes (Figure 12.2) (Table 12.2). However, mild changes to the bulla walls and soft tissues, and minimal fluid accumulations in the bulla pose a diagnostic challenge when radiography is used.

Dorsoventral View

The patient is placed in ventral recumbency, with the hard palate and the interpupillary line parallel to the cassette and the skull as close to the plate as possible. Support of the cervical spine and/or rostral mandible may be needed to stabilise this position and maintain symmetry. The radiographic beam should be centred through the expected position of the tympanic membranes (Figure 12.3). This is the most straightforward view to set up and may be done under sedation.

The ear canals should show a good air shadow with no calcification. The tympanic bullae should be seen as crisp, distinct, fine, smooth linear bony structures. However, the overlying petrous temporal bone and skull make it difficult to detect subtle soft tissue and bony changes in the middle ear.

Lateral Oblique View

The animal is placed in lateral recumbency (Figure 12.4). The bulla of interest is the one nearest to the film with the head parallel to the plate, which will minimise distortion and artefacts. The head is rotated around the long axis until the sagittal plane is approximately 20° to the horizontal with the mouth closed. Alternatively the nose can be elevated 15–20% to avoid the bullae superimposing each other. In order to ensure that the bulla of interest is clear of other structures, the beam should be centred around the base of the ear.

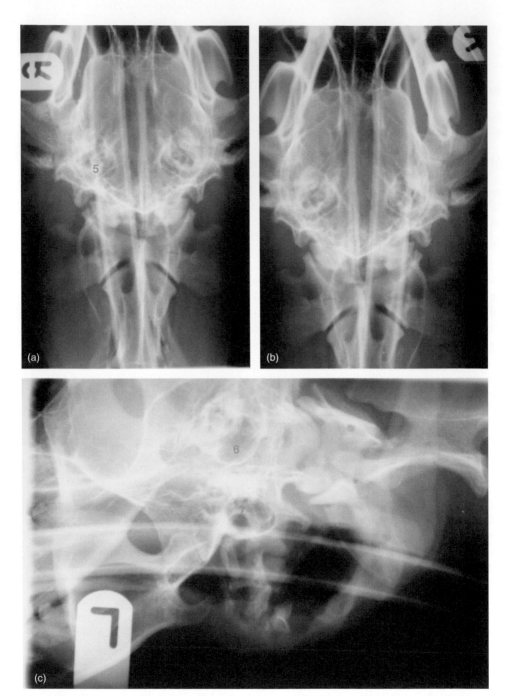

Figure 12.1 Bulla series of a 5-year-old male entire Hungarian Viszla with Pseudomonas otitis showing mineralisation of both ear canals consistent with chronic otitis externa. Slightly greater radio-opacity of the bullae is detected, requiring clarification with an advanced imaging modality to determine if otitis media is present. (a) Dorso-ventral (1 right mandible; 2 right temporo-mandibular joint; 3 narrowed lumen of the right ear canal; 4 mineralisation of the wall of the right ear canal; 5 right middle ear overlain by the petrous temporal bone, slightly more opaque than the left side). (b) Ventro-dorsal. (c) Left lateral oblique (6 right tympanic bulla, it is impossible to assess the opposite bulla in oblique views as it is obscured by the skull; 7 left tympanic bulla, there appears to be increased opacity and thickening of the bulla wall; 8 left mandible).

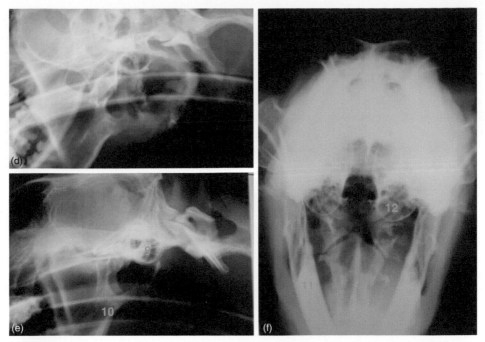

Figure 12.1 (Continued) (d) Same as 12.1(c) but right lateral oblique. (e) Lateral (9 tympanic bullae, it is possible to detect opacity and thickening in a lateral, but it is impossible to determine whether this is bilateral or unilateral, or which side is affected; 10 mandibles). (f) Rostro-caudal open mouth (11 mandibles; 12 tympanic bulla – the overlying hyoid bones and soft-tissues can make it difficult to detect subtle changes).

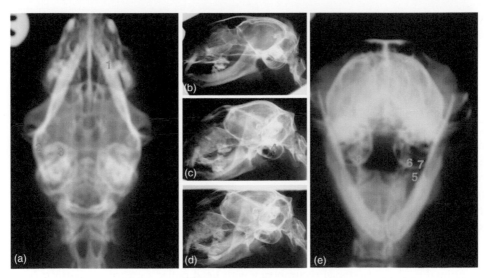

Figure 12.2 Bulla series of a 10-year-old female neutered cat showing obliteration of the left ear canal. There is diffusely increased soft tissue opacity in the left bulla. No obvious bony changes can be seen to affect the bullae. Note the internal bony shelf dividing the tympanic bulla into two compartments; this is only present in cats. The frontal sinus and visible parts of the nasal cavity are within normal limits. Multiple teeth are missing. (a) Dorso-ventral (1 left mandible; 2 air filled ear canal; 3 right tympanic bulla and petrous temporal bone). (b) Lateral. (c) Left lateral oblique (4 tympanic bulla). (d) Right lateral oblique. (e) Rostro-caudal open mouth (5 ventro-medial compartment; 6 dorso-lateral compartment; 7 internal bony shelf; 8 tympanic bulla).

Table 12.2 Radiographic features of ear canal and middle ear changes.

Radiographic change	Indicative of	Best radiographic view/s
Decreased air shadow in ear canal	Otitis externa/otic discharge	DV, VD, ROM, L
Calcification/ossification of the ear canal	Chronic otitis externa	DV, VD, ROM, L
Bilateral sclerosis and thickening of the tympanic bullae	Can be normal in elderly patients and some brachycephalic dogs Otitis media Bilateral inflammatory polyps Craniomandibular osteoarthropathy	ROM, LO, DV
Unilateral sclerosis and thickening of the tympanic bullae	Chronic unilateral otitis media Unilateral inflammatory polyp	ROM, LO, DV
Increased soft tissue opacity of the ear canal	Otitis externa/otic discharge	DV, VD, ROM, L
Lysis of the bulla wall	Chronic otitis media Middle ear neoplasia Osteomylelitis Chloesteatoma	ROM, LO, DV
Sclerosis of the petrous temporal bone	Otitis media Otitis media with osteomyelitis Middle ear neoplasia	ROM, LO, DV
Increased soft tissue opacity of the middle ear	Otitis media Inflammatory polyp	ROM, LO, DV

DV = dorsoventral view; L = lateral; LO = lateral oblique; ROM = rostrocaudal open-mouth view; VD = ventrodorsal view.

This view allows for good visualisation of the tympanic bullae and the petrous temporal bone. However, general anaesthesia is necessary and the positioning is difficult and not easily repeatable, making side-to-side comparisons difficult.

The ear canal (if visible) should show an air shadow with no calcification or ossification. The bullae should be air-filled, thin-walled, bony structures with smooth border and a crisp outline. Chronic inflammation or neoplasia may cause lytic changes in the petrous temporal bone and lytic changes in the bulla are most commonly caused by chronic inflammation. Expansion and lysis of the bulla is most commonly seen with a cholesteatoma. Lysis of the petrous temporal bone is a serious problem – this can be associated with cerebral infection and abscesses, and any ear flushing must be done with extreme care to avoid introducing material into the CNS.

Rostrocaudal Open-Mouth View

The animal is placed in dorsal recumbency with head pulled forward to align the hard palate vertical to the cassette (Figure 12.5). To avoid superimposition of the tongue, it is pulled out as far as possible and fixed to the mandible with a bandage. The interpupillary line is brought in parallel to the film. Positioning needs to take the shape of the head into account: in brachycephalic breeds the hard palate is angled by up to 20° away from the vertical. This helps to avoid superimposition of the wings of the atlas over the tympanic

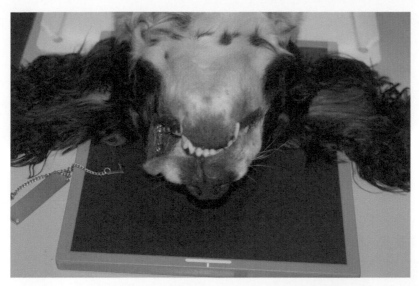

Figure 12.3 Positioning for bulla series: dorsoventral view. DV or VD positioning depends on the patient, for example deep-chested dogs are better imaged in VD position, brachycephalic and small-breed dogs and cats may be better imaged in a DV position. The skull needs to be as close as possible to the plate and positioned in a symmetrical fashion in sternal (DV) or dorsal (VD) recumbency; after positioning, place the L/R marker next to the head to avoid superimpositioning. Set the central beam to the level of the caudal zygomatic arch, just caudal to the eyes. The collimator should be opened to include C1/C2, the neurocranium, and the caudal portion of the nasal cavity to level of maxillary premolar 3.

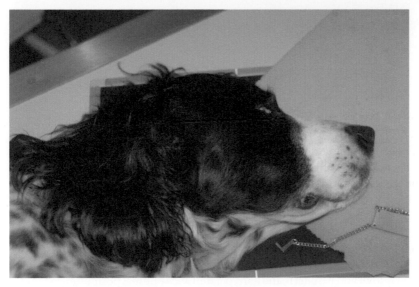

Figure 12.4 Positioning for bulla series: lateral oblique view. Both left and right lateral oblique views are needed; the patient is placed in a lateral recumbency with head and neck extended and a 30° angled foam sponge under the maxilla. The central beam is positioned ventral to the upper external auditory canal with the collimator to include the temporomandibular joint (TMJ) and tympanic bulla from C1/2 to the 3rd maxillary premolar. The marker is placed outside the soft tissue structures to avoid superimposition.

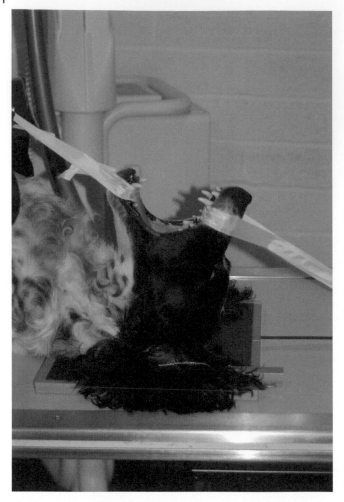

Figure 12.5 Positioning for bulla series: rostrocaudal open-mouth view. With the patient in dorsal recumbency the neck is flexed with the hard palate and mandibles perpendicular to the plate. The head needs to be fixed in this position with sponges or other positioning aids and tape or a tie is placed to fix the nose and the mandible to keep the mouth in an open position to avoid superimposition. The palate is angled at approximately 10° to the perpendicular plane of the body. Make sure the tube is not kinked while the patient is intubated and remove tube prior to taking the radiograph. Collimation is achieved by setting the central beam through the open mouth to the level of the soft palate with the cranium straight and free of rotation. C1 and the full tympanic bullae should be included.

bullae. Mesacephalic breeds require only slight angulation of the hard palate from the vertical (approximately 10°). In doliocephalic breeds the radiographic beam is centred through the open mouth and parallel to the hard palate. Once optimal positioning has been achieved, the endotracheal tube is temporarily removed during radiographic exposure, to avoid superimposition on the image, and replaced as soon as the image has been taken. This obviously poses an increased anaesthetic risk, particularly in brachycephalic breeds.

This view offers good visualisation of both tympanic bullae making it a good view to diagnose otitis media and compare both sides. However, it is difficult to avoid superimposition of soft tissue structures. These may give the impression of middle ear pathology, so any changes must be interpreted with caution.

Lateral View

The animal is placed in lateral recumbency with the head rotated to align in a true lateral. The sagittal plane should be parallel and the interpupillary line vertical to the plate. Padding may be needed to stabilise the position. The beam is centred between the eye and ear and the nasal pharynx, larynx and calvarium are included in the view.

There should be an air shadow in the ear canals and thickening may be appreciated if present. Similar to the other views, the bullae should be thin, crisp and smooth bony structures, however, superimposition of other structures in this view make their interpretation more difficult and the two sides cannot be compared.

Ventrodorsal View

The animal is placed in dorsal recumbency and aligned symmetrically with the hard palate parallel to the table. Support of the rostral mandible and/or the cervical spine can be helpful, and you can use a tie or tape positioned behind the canine and fixed to the table. The beam is centred between the expected position of the tympanic membranes.

This is a good view to detect changes consistent with otitis media, and may allow visualisation of changes in the bony septum in the middle ear. However, it is not suitable for brachycephalic breeds and subtle changes are difficult to detect due to super-imposition of the petrous temporal bone.

Canalography

This technique allows for better visualisation of the ear canal than plain radiography alone and helps determine the presence of tears in the tympanic membrane. The contrast medium used should be water soluble, iodine based and non-ionic and can be diluted 50:50 with sterile saline prior to instilling it into the ear canal to avoid ototoxicity. Contamination of the skin and outer ears (which will cause misleading shadows) can be avoided by using an appropriate volume of the contrast medium and a cotton wool plug in the outside of the ear canal orifice once the liquid has been instilled and massaged into the ear canal to ensure even distribution. Radiographs should ideally be taken in a rostrocaudal view but ventrodorsal images also allow interpretation of the ear canals. The ear canals can be evaluated for stenosis. Contrast medium entering the tympanic bulla can best be seen as opacification of the inner wall of the bulla on the rostrocaudal view and a tear in the tympanic membrane must be present to allow for this to happen. However, failure to detect contrast medium entering the middle ear does not rule out a ruptured tympanic membrane due to stenosis and/or material in the ear canal blocking the contrast medium. Otoscopy should be performed prior to contrast techniques to help rule out these factors. Advances in other imaging techniques, such as MRI and CT, have made contrast imaging largely obsolete.

Ultrasonography of the Middle Ear

Ultrasonography to diagnose fluid or soft tissue changes in the middle ears has been described. It has been reported to be very sensitive (between 80 and 100%) and specific (between 74 and 100%), but was evaluated in cadaver dogs rather than in clinical cases. Later reports comparing ultrasonography with other imaging modalities concluded that advanced imaging, such as CT and MRI, is far superior to both ultrasonography and radiography. Ultrasonography is particularly operator dependent and not easily reproducible. However, in the absence of access to advanced imaging, a combination of radiography and ultrasonography may be superior to one modality alone.

Advanced Imaging Techniques

Although false-positive findings are uncommon, radiography has an about 25–30% incidence of false-negative results compared to a surgical diagnosis of middle ear disease. Therefore, other techniques such as MRI and CT have been evaluated for their usefulness in the diagnosis of otitis media. In general, CT gives better resolution of the bony structures and MRI is more accurate in the evaluation of soft tissue structures.

MRI

MRI is an imaging technique that uses strong magnetic fields and radiowaves to record images of the body. This technique is widely used in veterinary referral hospitals and has the advantage of working without exposure to ionising radiation. Transportable MRI services are also available and can visit smaller practices. MRI relies on detecting a radiofrequency signal emitted by excited hydrogen atoms in the body using energy from an oscillating magnetic field applied at the appropriate resonant frequency. The orientation of the image is controlled by varying the main magnetic field using gradient coils. The coils are rapidly switched on and off, leading to the characteristic repetitive noises of an MRI scan. The contrast between different tissues is determined by the rate at which excited atoms return to the equilibrium state. Contrast agents may be given intravenously to enhance differences in tissues and help distinguish between soft tissue changes due to neoplasia or inflammation. Although the procedure is not painful, heavy sedation or a general anaesthetic is required to allow for optimal images without movement and ear protection for the patient is advised.

MRI is superior for the evaluation of soft tissue structures and therefore particularly useful for cases where otic neoplasia, inflammatory polyps or soft tissue changes of the external ear canal, bullae or inner ear are suspected (Figure 12.6). Referral is usually necessary for the patient to be able to undergo this investigation and the procedure is often combined with a video-otoscopic examination including a deep ear flush afterwards.

CT

CT images are created by a computer-calculated tomographic reconstruction of information obtained through a radiographic detector. CT produces a large volume of data that can be manipulated in order to demonstrate various bodily structures based on their ability to block the x-ray beam. Although, historically, the generated images were in the axial or transverse plane relative to the long axis of the body, modern scanners allow the data to be reformatted in various planes or even as volumetric (3D) representations of structures. Due to the tomographic images, superimposition is not relevant. Differentiation of soft tissues is possible due to the larger grey scale compared to radiography. Therefore, CT is far superior to radiography alone, particularly if changes to the tympanic bullae are suspected (Figure 12.7). It is often used to confirm the extent

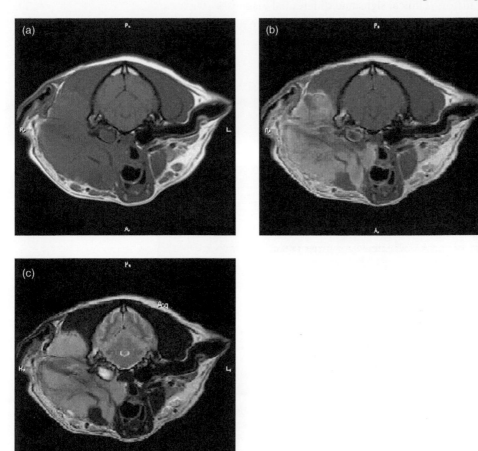

Figure 12.6 MRI series from a 6-year-old Beagle that presented with a history of unilateral right-sided otitis externa and facial paralysis. The images are (a) T1-weighted, (b) T1-weighted post-contrast and (c) T2-weighted slices. The left external ear canal and middle ear are normal and air-filled (black). In contrast, there is a large tumour in the soft tissues on the right side of the head that has obliterated the ear canal. There is also an otitis media with material in the tympanic bulla. This is especially obvious on the T1 post-contrast and T2 images. Compared to a CT scan (Figure 12.7), there is much better soft tissue delineation, but the bony structures around the ear cannot be visualised.

and location of changes, and is helpful in determining the best biopsy sites in suspected otic neoplasia and in planning any surgical treatments that may be necessary. However, false-positives can occur in about 11% of cases (this can be reduced with experience and combining CT with otoscopy) and false-negatives in about 17% of cases (compared to about 25–30% in radiography), making CT more sensitive but less specific than radiography. In particular, otoliths and pooled mucus can be seen in healthy middle ears, and there is individual and breed variation in the bulla wall. Brachycephalic dogs may show irregular thickening of the bulla wall. The lack of bony changes in early middle ear disease limits detection by radiography or CT unless there is a soft tissue accumulation in the bulla.

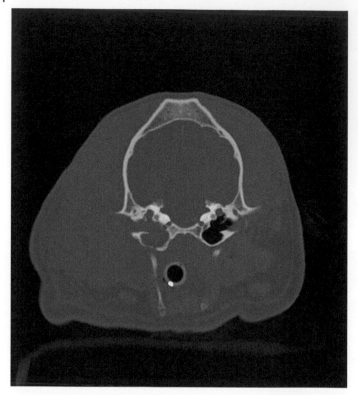

Figure 12.7 CT of a case of otitis media and paraural abscessation in a 10.5-year-old male neutered West Highland White Terrier. There is loss of the normal aerated appearance of the right tympanic bulla on this transverse image visualised on a bone window. There is mild expansion of the bulla, mild thickening of the bulla wall as well as focal areas of bone lysis affecting the ventral aspect of the wall. Marked soft tissue thickening or swelling is identified lateral to the affected bulla. The left bulla is normal. The tympanic membrane is intact, but the lumen of the ear canal is not visible (this would normally be air filled). *Source:* Courtesy of Francisco Llabres Diaz of Dick White Referrals.

CT is mostly confined to large veterinary referral institutions, although the cost is declining and it is becoming more widely available. Heavy sedation or general anaesthesia is required to obtain optimum images. Again, this procedure is usually combined with a subsequent video-otoscopic examination including a deep ear flush if indicated.

Imaging for Patients with Endocrine Disease

Hyperadrenocorticism

Diagnostic imaging of patients with suspected hyperadrenocorticism (HAC) can include imaging of the adrenal glands or pituitary gland, or tissues that show the effect of the metabolic changes. Radiography can detect the adrenals in severe cases with unilateral enlargement and calcification, but more sensitive techniques include ultrasonography, CT and MRI.

Ultrasonography

Abdominal ultrasonography in adrenal-dependent HAC should reveal one enlarged adrenal gland, with an atrophic to normal contralateral gland. Pituitary-dependent HAC patients usually have bilaterally enlarged adrenal glands, and they should both be atrophic to normal in iatrogenic HAC or hypoadrenocorticism. Finding the adrenal glands on ultrasonography requires a skilled operator and can be frustrating even for experienced ultrasonographers due to obesity, the deep and sometimes variable position of the glands, the small size of the glands, the interposition of visceral gas and lack of patient compliance.

The glands are less than 1 cm thick and are next to the aorta and vena cava, which can obscure the view of the gland. Using Doppler ultrasonography makes it easier to locate the glands as they can more easily be distinguished from the surrounding vessels with the Doppler feature. A high-frequency transducer (at least 7.5 MHz) should be used, occasionally a small transducer will be beneficial in some larger patients. The left adrenal is usually easier to find than the right as it is further caudal (Figure 12.8) and therefore less obscured by the ribs.

The patient should be placed in dorsal recumbency, although in some cases lateral recumbency for the non-dependent adrenal gland is useful. Sedation may be necessary. Considerable pressure is needed to displace overlying bowels, which would lead to gas artefact. The abdominal vessels can be used to help locate the adrenals. The left adrenal gland is located caudal to the coeliac and cranial mesenteric arteries, and cranial to the left renal artery. The phrenicoabdominal vein crosses the mid portion of the adrenal glands. The glands are small, elongated, hypoechoic structures that are surrounded by hyperechoic fat. The left adrenal gland is 'dumbbell' or 'peanut' shaped whereas the right

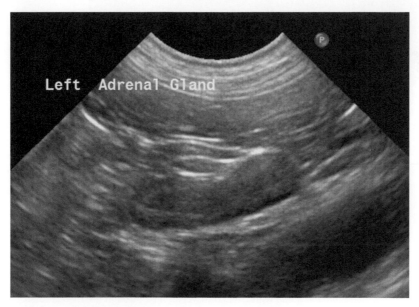

Figure 12.8 Enlarged left adrenal gland in a dog with HAC. The caudal pole shows a mildly washed out corticomedullary transition. The aorta can be seen at the right bottom of the image. *Source:* Courtesy of Karolin Kuehn.

adrenal gland is 'comma', 'wedge' or 'boomerang' shaped. It is often difficult to see the whole gland in one image and the poles of the glands are often asymmetric.

Rotation of the transducer enables the ultrasonographer to view and measure the whole adrenal gland in each plane and compare the dimensions. The transverse maximum diameter is considered to be the most sensitive and specific for adrenal gland enlargement and the upper limit is usually quoted as 7.4 mm, although this may need to be revised depending on the patient's body size. In patients with adrenal-dependent HAC, the size of the mass can be an indication of malignancy. Masses larger than 4 cm are usually malignant, between 2 and 4 cm are likely to be malignant and smaller than 2 cm are usually benign. In some normal cases, a distinct layering may be seen.

CT and MRI Imaging

The pituitary gland can be visualised by CT and MRI imaging. Large pituitary tumours with suprasellar expansion can usually be readily detected with conventional contrast-enhanced CT (Figure 12.9). Pituitary microadenomas can be localised with dynamic contrast-enhanced CT. Cisternography allows assessment of even small increases in the height of the pituitary gland. Assessment of the displacement and signal intensity of the posterior lobe of the pituitary on T1-weighted MRI images is useful for the diagnosis of pituitary adenoma.

Other Tissue Changes in HAC

Patients with HAC may show various radiological changes, although some of them may be incidental findings. Dystrophic mineralisation of various tissues, including the

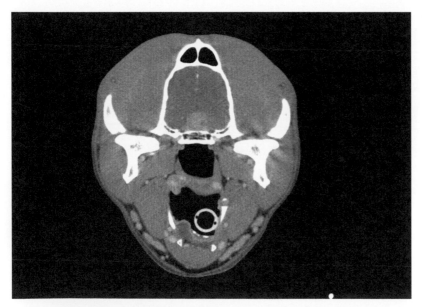

Figure 12.9 CT of a macroadenoma in a dog with HAC. Transversal slice through the medial fossa at the level of the TMJ, soft tissue window post contrast. There is a mildly heterogeneic, contrast-enhancing mass widely attached to the base of the skull. The hypophysis is not visible. *Source:* Courtesy of Karolin Kuehn.

tracheal rings and bronchial walls, kidneys, gastric mucosa, liver, skeletal muscle, branches of the abdominal aorta and skin (calcinosis cutis), can be seen. These changes are caused by the protein catabolism with protein damage leading to calcium and phosphorus deposition in the organic matrix of the abnormal protein, despite normal calcium and phosphorus concentrations in serum.

Thoracic radiographic features of canine HAC can also include a moderate to severe generalised interstitial lung pattern in some cases. Another important and commonly recognised feature is hepatomegaly, which is due to steroid hepatopathy. Cases of adrenal-dependent HAC show radiographically calcified adrenal masses in about a third to half of the cases. Those patients often show metastasis into the liver, vena cava or lungs, which can sometimes be detected radiographically as well. Osteoporosis is another radiographic feature of HAC and in most cases involves the vertebrae.

Thyroid Disease

Thyroid scintigraphy can provide valuable additional information and help in the diagnosis and management of patients with hyperthyroidism, hypothyroidism and thyroid neoplasia. Thyroid scintigraphy is performed by subcutaneous injection of a small amount of a radionuclide followed by a dorsoventral and/or lateral scan with a gamma camera. This will show uptake of the radionuclide by active thyroid tissue. The nuclides of choice are isotopes of iodine (principally ^{123}I and ^{131}I) or technetium as pertechnetate (^{99m}TcO4-), depending on financial restraints and the purpose of the scan. Radioactive iodine and pertechnetate ions are actively concentrated in the thyroid gland. However, unlike pertechnetate, iodine is subsequently incorporated into thyroglobulin (organification). Pertechnetate is also concentrated in the salivary glands and gastric mucosa. The half-life of pertechnetate is much shorter (6 hours) than the cheaper ^{131}I, but it is technically much superior. Images can be taken about 20 minutes after administration of pertechnetate and, due to short scanning time, sedation can be avoided in most patients.

In cats with hyperthyroidism scintigraphy will show ectopic thyroid tissue as well as large displaced thyroid tumours in the thoracic cavity. In dogs with hypothyroidism, scintigraphy is the most helpful imaging modality to distinguish hypothyroid patients from euthyroid sick animals. Scintigraphy can also help plan treatment for dogs with thyroid carcinomas by determining the size of the tumour and detecting metastasis in most cases. Ultrasonography can also be used, but scintigraphy seems to be the more sensitive technique.

Imaging for Patients with Paraneoplastic Associated Skin Disease

A variety of paraneoplastic and other syndromes have been described with skin disease associated with systemic neoplasia and other conditions, e.g. hepatocutaneous syndrome, feline lung digit syndrome, feline paraneoplastic alopecia, feline thymoma-associated exfoliative dermatitis and nodular dermatofibrosis. Hyperadrenocorticism is also a paraneoplastic disease in the strictest sense of the word. Other specific skin diseases can be triggered or induced by systemic neoplasia, for example pemphigus foliaceus, pemphigus vulgaris, vasculitis and sterile pyogranulomatous dermatitis. A 'tumour hunt' may be indicated to rule out or diagnose neoplasia. This could include CT, MRI, thoracic radiography and abdominal ultrasonography and/or radiography.

Hepatocutaneous Syndrome

Hepatocutaneous syndrome is also known as necrolytic migratory erythema, metabolic epidermal necrosis or superficial necrolytic dermatitis. This condition can be caused by glucogonomas in the pancreas and elsewhere, but it is most commonly associated with hepatic disease. The exact pathogenesis of the skin lesions is unknown but may be related to low serum amino acid levels. Abdominal ultrasonography often reveals diffuse liver disease (so-called 'honeycomb pattern') (Figure 12.10) or neoplasia in the pancreas or elsewhere. The most diagnostic test is dermatohistopathology, which reveals a 'red, white and blue' pattern consisting of a severe parakeratosis, upper epidermal pallor with oedema, and a superficial dermal infiltrate of mononuclear cells. Haematology shows non-regenerative or mildly regenerative anaemia. Biochemistry reveals an increased alanine aminotransferase (ALT), aspartate aminotransferase (AST) and alkaline phosphatase (ALP), hyperglycaemia without ketoacidosis, hypoalbuminaemia, severe hypoaminoacidaemia and elevated bile acids. Hepatic cytology consists of severe, vacuolar degeneration of hepatocytes.

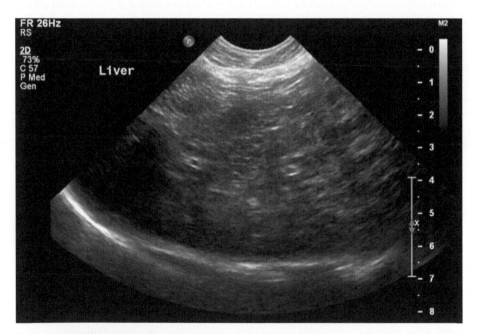

Figure 12.10 Ultrasonographic image of the multinodular appearance of the liver ('honeycomb pattern') in an 8-year-old male neutered Husky with hepatocutaneous syndrome. *Source:* Courtesy of Francisco Llabres Diaz of Dick White Referrals.

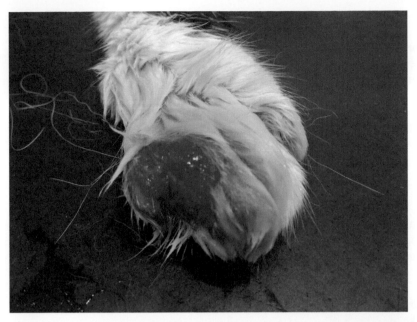

Figure 12.11 Lung digit syndrome in a cat. Pedal lesions in a cat shortly prior to euthanasia due to breathing problems. *Source:* Courtesy of Sarah Hatton.

Feline Lung Digit Syndrome

Feline lung digit syndrome is a rare condition of older cats with a guarded prognosis (mean survival time at presentation is only 58 days). A primary lung tumour, particularly bronchial and bronchoalveolar adenocarcinomas, metastasise to the digits (Figure 12.11) with the weight-bearing digits most commonly affected. Radiography of the distal extremities often shows extensive bony lysis of the distal phalanx, which can be transarticular to the second phalanx. Metastasis can also occur to other organs, including the skeletal muscle and bone in other regions, multiple thoracic and abdominal organs, skin and eyes. Thoracic radiography should be performed in suspicious cases.

Feline Paraneoplastic Alopecia

Feline paraneoplastic alopecia is a rare paraneoplastic disorder characterised by a ventral abdominal alopecia with a shiny, smooth and glistening appearance. It is usually associated with a pancreatic adenocarcinoma, which can be detected on abdominal ultrasonography. Rarely, this can be associated with a thymoma. At the time of diagnosis, metastasis to the liver and lungs has usually already occurred. Histopathology usualy shows an absent stratum corneum or, if the stratum corneum is present, it is parakeratotic and lifts away from the living epidermis. There is moderate to severe acanthosis. The hair follicles are usually diffusely miniaturised and in telogen. Dermal inflammation is commonly absent unless there is ulceration present.

Feline thymoma-associated exfoliative dermatitis is another rare feline paraneoplastic disease. Coughing and dyspnoea may occur, and advanced cases can show lethargy and anorexia, although the dermatological lesions usually precede the systemic clinical signs. The histopathology is characterised by epidermal and follicular apoptosis and hyperkeratosis, interface dermatitis extending to the superficial hair follicles to the level of the isthmus and a striking mononuclear follicular interface inflammation with scattered basal cell apoptosis. Finding a thymic mass radiographically or on CT is diagnostic.

Nodular Dermatofibrosis

Nodular dermatofibrosis is a rare hereditary condition in dogs (most commonly German Shepherd Dogs) that is characterised by multiple dermal nodules associated with internal malignancy (Figure 12.12, Figure 12.13, Figure 12.14). Affected organs include the kidneys (multifocal renal cystadenocarcinoma) or uterus (uterine leiomyomas).

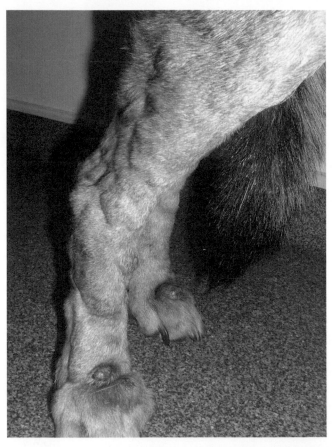

Figure 12.12 Nodular dermatofibrosis. Nodular lesions affecting the skin on the hind legs. *Source:* Courtesy of Jonathan Wray.

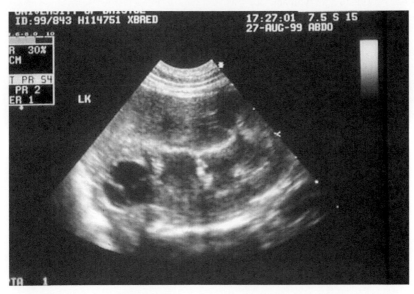

Figure 12.13 Nodular dermatofibrosis. Ultrasonographic image of the cycstic lesions of the kidney. *Source:* Courtesy of Jonathan Wray.

Ultrasonography and CT can be useful in finding the kidney or uterine lesions. Ultrasound-guided biopsies can be performed for diagnosis. Genetic mapping for the FLCN mutation, which is inherited in an autosomal dominant fashion, can be performed for a definitive diagnosis. This will also distinguish carriers from healthy dogs.

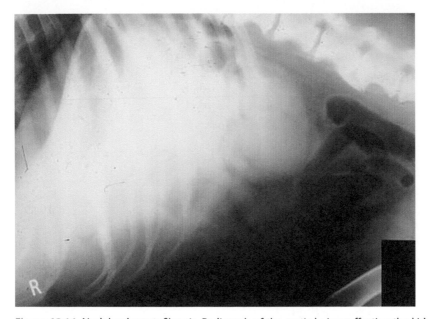

Figure 12.14 Nodular dermatofibrosis. Radigraph of the cystic lesions affecting the kidneys. *Source:* Courtesy of Jonathan Wray.

Other Uses for Imaging

Radiography and CT can be used to detect foreign bodies in draining sinus tracts, and musculoskeletal lesions that may be triggering self-trauma and/or leading to altered weight-bearing and pododermatitis. Similarly, MRI can be helpful in animals showing neurological signs consistent with central vestibular disease or a neuropathy. Finally, ultrasonography can be used to help determine the nature of some subcutaneous masses, abscesses and draining sinus tracts.

13

Otoscopy and Examination of the Ear

Ear disease is very common in small animal practice and can have serious implications for the quality of life of the patient and the owner. Owners who have in the past suffered from ear disease themselves can often better understand the pain associated with this condition and are often more motivated to fully evaluate the patient and ensure adequate analgesia during the course of the investigation and therapy. Accurate diagnosis and successful management include treating the acute symptoms but also finding the primary underlying disease in these cases. As with all dermatological diseases, a thorough history and clinical examination are very important. The various diagnostic tests are used afterwards used to help formulate a list of differential diagnoses and come up with a management plan. Ear disease is very complex and needs to be addressed from several angles. The infection needs to be treated, secondary (perpetuating) changes, such as glandular hyperplasia, stenosis, mineralisation of the cartilage and overproduction of ceruminous material or purulent discharge, need to be reversed or removed if possible, predisposing factors addressed where possible, and the primary disease needs to be diagnosed and treated.

Examination of a patient with otitis has to include a general examination, including an oral examination, palpation of the lymph nodes, chest auscultation, abdominal and testicular palpation as well as inspection of the remaining mucous membranes prior to a thorough examination of all of the structures of the ear. Examination of the respiratory system, soft palate and pharynx is indicated in animals where otitis media is suspected. A neurological examination should be carried out in all patients that present with ataxia, head tilt, nystagmus and/or Horner's syndrome.

Examination of the Pinnae, Ear Canal and Tympanic Membrane

After the general and dermatological examination, a more specific otological examination is indicated. Inspection of the pinnae (Figure 13.1, Figure 13.2, Figure 13.3, Figure 13.4) can give important clues, so both the medial and lateral aspects should be evaluated. A positive pinnal–pedal reflex, which involves rubbing the edge of the pinna between fingers and thumb and watching for a scratch reflex from the ipsilateral hind limb, can be associated with scabies. Mueller reported a good sensitivity and specificity for this test. However, other pruritic dermatoses such as atopic dermatitis, *Malassezia*

Diagnostic Techniques in Veterinary Dermatology, First Edition. Ariane Neuber and Tim Nuttall.
© 2017 Ariane Neuber and Tim Nuttall. Published 2017 by John Wiley & Sons, Ltd.

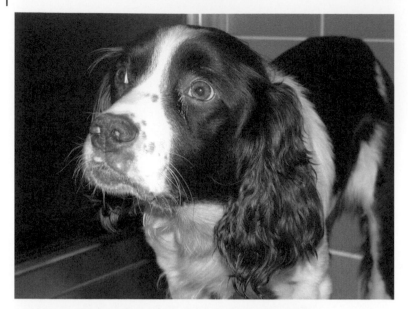

Figure 13.1 English Springer Spaniel with hanging pinnae restricting air flow to the ear canal.

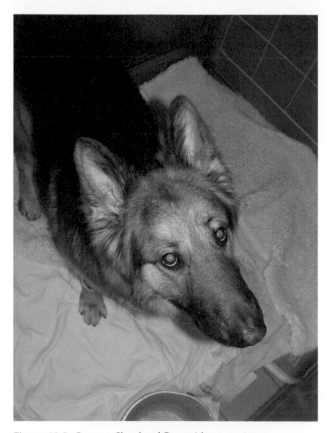

Figure 13.2 German Shepherd Dog with erect pinnae.

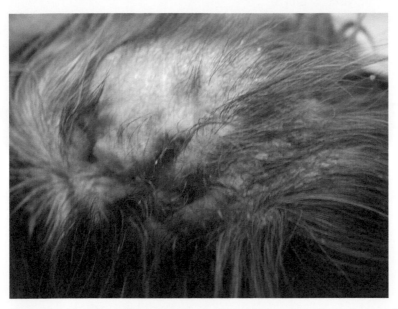

Figure 13.3 Severely erythematous pinna with crusting in a dog with atopic dermatitis and a secondary *Malassezia* otitis.

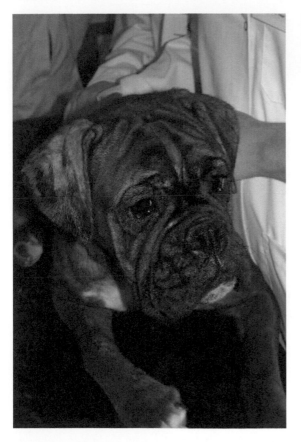

Figure 13.4 A young Boxer dog with intense pruritus due to atopic dermatitis. Self-trauma is leading to alopecia on the concave aspects of the pinnae.

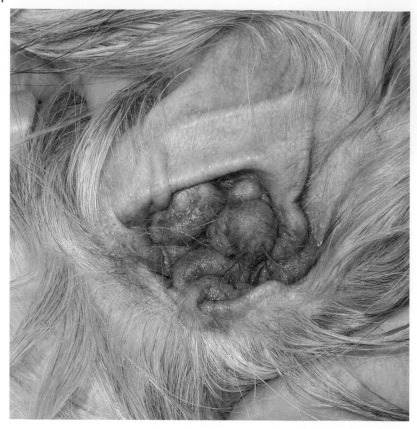

Figure 13.5 Erythema on the pinna of a dog with atopic dermatitis with no sign of otic discharge.

dermatitis and otitis, other ectoparasites and other inflammatory diseases involving this region, can also lead to a positive reflex. Diffuse erythema of the inner pinnae is commonly found in patients with allergic skin disease (Figure 13.5). In contrast erythema of the outer pinnae, particularly in white-haired animals and on the distal parts, is suggestive of sun damage or actinic dermatitis. Alopecia on the pinnae may be due to self-trauma caused by pruritus and therefore related to scabies, otitis externa with secondary infection, allergic otitis (Figure 13.5), *Otodectes*, other ectoparasites affecting the ears or dermatophytosis. Primary alopecia can occur on the pinnae in cases of endocrinopathy or in pattern baldness. Clearly defined ulcerations on the outer pinnae of a feline patient can be indicative of feline cowpox infection, whereas the same lesions on the inner pinnae of a dog can be seen in cases of vasculitis. Scaling and crusting on the pinnal margins can be associated with sarcoptic mange, pediculosis, hormonal disease, fly bite/mosquito hypersensitivity, zinc deficiency, sebaceous adenitis, and other corni-fication defects and vasculitis. Pustular lesions, vesicles and crusts can be caused by pemphigus foliaceus (Figure 13.6a), and less commonly by pyoderma and dermatophy-tosis. Curling pinnae in cats can be due to relapsing auricular chondritis and can be seen

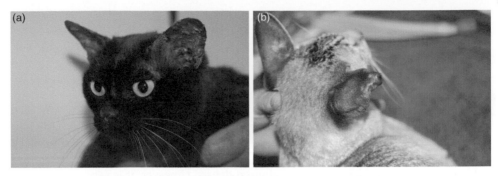

Figure 13.6 (a) Concave aspect of the pinna of a cat with pemphigus foliaceus. (b) Convex aspect pinna of a cat with curling pinna due to glucocorticoid use.

as a side effect of glucocorticoid therapy (Figure 13.6b). Polyps and comedone-like lesions on the pinna and in the opening of the ear canals can be associated with feline cystadenomatosis.

Inspecting the visible ear canal by lifting the pinnae and palpating the vertical and horizontal ear canals also gives valuable information about the degree of changes, the nature and quantity of the discharge, signs of pain or pruritus, and the range of mobility and pliability (which reflect the degree of stenosis, fibrosis or even mineralisation). The amount of hair should be noted (Figure 13.7) and this may need to be clipped at some stage if it traps the otic discharge and interferes with aeration of the ear canal. Infections of the ear canal are commonly associated with an unpleasant odour, particularly if Gram-negative organisms are involved.

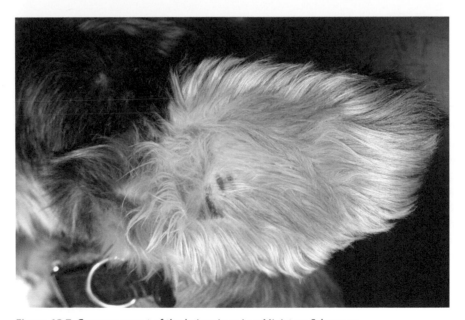

Figure 13.7 Concave aspect of the hairy pinna in a Miniature Schnauzer.

Nature of the Discharge

The nature of the debris can be indicative of the type of infection, but this should not replace cytological examination of the material. *Otodectes* spp. infestation tends to produce a characteristic brown coffee-ground-like discharge. Pale yellow and waxy debris is often associated with coccal infection, yeast overgrowth or *Demodex* spp. infestation. However, infection with cocci and *Malassezia* spp. overgrowth can also cause a pale brown waxy otic discharge. Gram-negative infections, in particular *Pseudomonas* spp., can lead to purulent yellow to green malodorous material or black fucoid–watery discharge. Biofilms are thick, slimy and green to black. Cornification defects can result in thick chocolate-coloured debris. However, it is very important to remember that visual assessment of the otic discharge cannot under any circumstances replace cytology and/or culture and sensitivity testing.

The nature of the discharge will also determine how cytological preparations are fixed and choice of ear cleaner. It may be useful to heat fix or use the one-stain method (see Chapter 1) with very waxy samples as these may be dissolved in the alcohol fixative. Seborrhoeic and purulent material can usually be air dried and alcohol fixed, although using a hair-dryer to ensure thorough drying can be helpful.

Thick, waxy and tightly adherent ear discharge will need to be broken down with a cleaner that provides very good ceruminosolvent and ceruminolytic activity. Seborrhoeic and purulent material is better removed with a cleaner with a high water content and a detergent, which will break down the mucoid and purulent discharge more efficiently. Acidic and alcohol-containing ear cleaners can be painful in ulcerated ears. Take great care with oil- and detergent-based ear cleaners if the tympanic membrane is ruptured. Some cats present with excessive cerumen as an apparently normal finding – if there are no associated clinical signs this does not need treatment.

Otoscopy and Cytology

Otoscopy and cytology are probably the most important ways to collect information about ear disease. However, otitis is often very painful and some dogs become head shy or even aggressive if they have a long history of recurring ear disease, making them resistant to examination. Postmortem studies on stray dogs euthanased for aggression found about 30% had signs of chronic ear disease, suggesting this is under-recognised, and that the chronic pain may be associated with behavioural changes.

In many cases, even when the patient is compliant, visualisation of the tympanic membrane is difficult or impossible due to changes in the ear canal (e.g. the amount of debris or stenosis). A good light source is essential in increasing the chances of visualisation of the deeper structures (Figure 13.8). A wall-mounted mains-operated system may have a more reliable power supply. Patient compliance is often better if the ear cone is warmed up prior to inserting it into the ear canal, for example by holding it in the hand for a while, and if the animal is allowed to see and smell the otoscope before insertion.

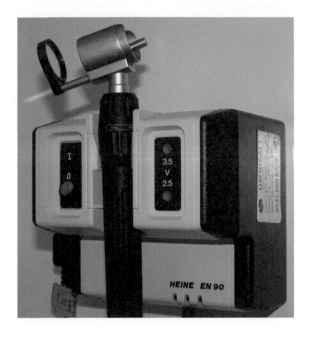

Figure 13.8 Wall-mounted mains-operated otoscope.

How to Use the Otoscope

1) The patient should be carefully restrained – firmly enough to keep them still but not overly so to cause distress. A second handler may be needed to keep the head still and level (Figure 13.9).

2) Choose an appropriate size cone – this must be able to pass into the ear canal without force. In practice, most animals will not accept cones larger than 5–6 mm.

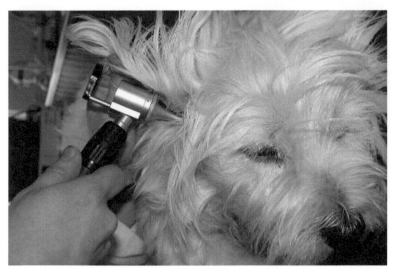

Figure 13.9 Otoscopy is performed in this West Highland White Terrier by lifting the pinna, gently inserting the warmed otoscopy cone into the ear canal and examining the ear canal.

3) Locate the most ventral notch among the cartilage folds at the opening of the vertical ear canal. Inserting the cone here will automatically lead it between the cartilage folds and into the vertical canal.

4) As you insert the cone pull the pinna downwards and towards you – this straightens the ear canal and flattens the dorsal ridge at the junction of the horizontal and vertical ear canals allowing you to pass the otoscope cone into the horizontal ear canal without force (Figure 13.9).

5) In some larger dogs (depending on their ear canal anatomy) it may be easier to pull the pinna upwards as you insert the otoscope. In most animals though, this accentuates the dorsal ridge making it harder to get into the horizontal ear canal.

Otoscopy is a skill that takes time to master. Practising on compliant, sedated or anaesthetised dogs with healthy ears reinforces the technique and helps you understand the anatomy of the ears canals and tympanic membrane (Figure 13.10).

Some patients benefit from a short course of glucocorticoids for a few days prior to otoscopic examination to reduce the inflammation, which will 'open up' the ear canal and make the patient more amenable to the examination. Some patients are too painful to examine conscious or due to their temperament or long-standing history of ear disease resulting in reluctance to be examined. Do not use force on these patients, as this will make the situation worse – use appropriate sedation or a general anaesthetic to perform a thorough, safe and non-traumatic examination. Thorough ear cleaning or an ear flush is usually useful if you sedate or anaesthetise a patient.

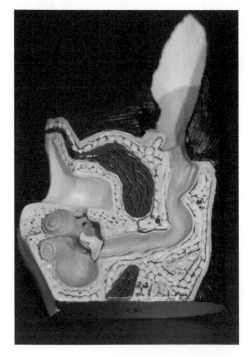

Figure 13.10 Ear anatomy of the dog.

Types of Otoscope

Different types of otoscope are available, which have different advantages and disadvantages.

- An open or surgical otoscope allows good access (e.g. to remove foreign bodies or flush ears) but has a more limited field of vision. This is probably the most commonly used type in small animal practice.
- A closed otoscope offers a good view and allows for tympanometry (see later in this chapter), but gives limited access for foreign body removal, ear flushing or obtaining material from the deeper ear canal (e.g. for cytology or culture).
- A video-otoscope is an endoscopic camera with a specialised attachment. This offers far better visualisation of the ear canal and deeper structures. Most models have a working channel, enabling the operator to remove foreign bodies, flush the ear canals and middle ear, perform biopsy of masses, and perform myringotomy and laser surgery. Most will record videos and still images, which are very useful for the clinical record, to monitor progress and for client education.

Normal Otoscopy Findings

The normal ear canal lining is smooth, with or without hairs, pale pink and, depending on the breed, usually offers enough space to advance the otoscope far enough to visualise the tympanic membrane (TM). The healthy TM (Figure 13.11) is shiny, translucent and

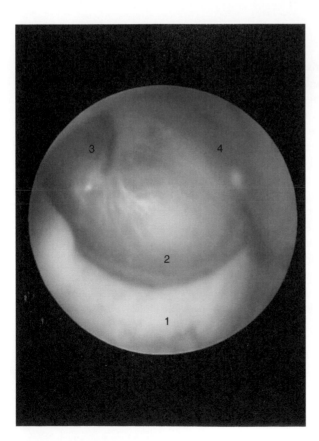

Figure 13.11 Video-otoscopic image of the tympanic membrane of the left ear of a cat. (1 Ventral wall of the ear canal; 2 pars tensa; 3 attachment of the malleus; 4 pars flaccida.)

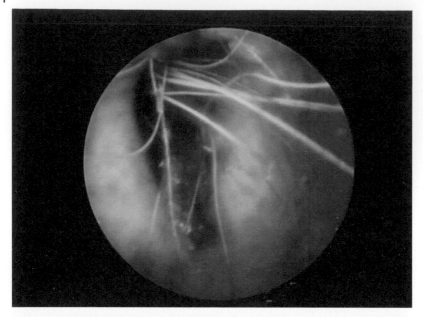

Figure 13.12 Video-otoscopic image of an erythematous ear canal with hairs growing in the ear canal with some brown waxy discharge attached.

taut in the region of the pars tensa and at times bulging in the dorsal pars flacida. The manubrium of the malleus should be visible as a rostral and dorsal white C-shaped structure. The pars tensa is slightly concave, slopes away from you (i.e. medially) ventrally, and has fine striations radiating out from the malleus. You may be able to see the bony wall of the middle ear and the darker caudoventral opening to the tympanic bulla in some dogs. However, even in normal ears the TM cannot be visualised in about 25% of cases. There are two good landmarks for the tympanic membrane. Firstly, there are always a few hairs that arise from the ventral insertion of the membrane. Secondly, it sits just inside a bony prominence on the skull (the external acoustic meatus), and if you feel this with the otoscope you are very close to the membrane. The external acoustic meatus may be narrow in some healthy dogs (particularly brachycephalic breeds), making it very hard to see the tympanic membrane.

A small amount of pale yellow or brown otic discharge is generally normal. Hairs can be seen in the ear canals of many dogs (Figure 13.12), and some breeds are particularly prone to hairy ears, e.g. Poodles, Cocker Spaniels, Schnauzers, Airedale and other terriers. This may be extensive enough to block the ear canal and prevent effective otoscopy.

Abnormal Findings
Some primary diseases, such as *Otodectes* spp. infestation, *Otobius megnini* (spinose ear tick), foreign bodies (FB) and masses can be easily identified and either removed (FB), have biopsies performed (masses) or be diagnosed and have specific treatment prescribed (ear mites). However, ear mites cannot always be visualised on otoscopy and a preparation of ear wax mixed with liquid paraffin may need to be examined

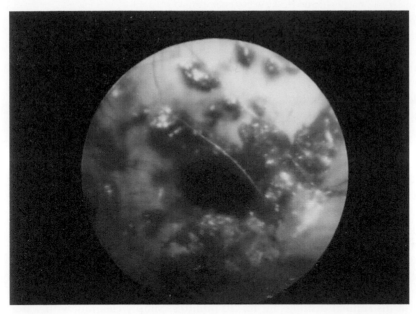

Figure 13.13 Video-otoscopic image of brown waxy debris in the ear canal of a dog with *Malassezia* otitis.

microscopically for a better chance of achieving a diagnosis. In very suspicious cases, trial therapy may be indicated to rule out *Otodectes* spp.

Any changes in the lining of the ear canal, such as ceruminous gland hyperplasia, stenosis, debris (Figure 13.13), erythema, and changes to the TM such as opacity, ruptures (Figure 13.14) or absence of the structure altogether can be appreciated, noted

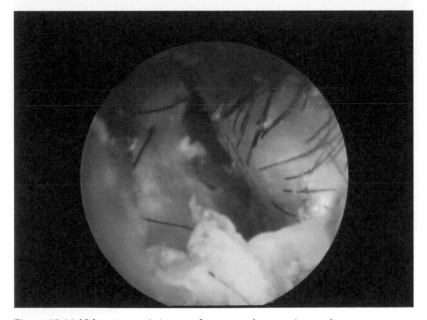

Figure 13.14 Video-otoscopic image of a ruptured tympanic membrane.

and interpreted. Sebaceous hyperplasia results in a characteristic 'cobblestone' appearance to the ear canal lining, and is one of the first signs that the dog has started to develop chronic pathological changes in the ears. In some instances, the TM cannot be seen without performing an ear flush. Severe stenosis of the horizontal ear canal can make it impossible to see the TM even after ear cleaning. Changes to the lining of the ear canal often occur along the whole length of both the horizontal and vertical canal but can also be localised to either one of them. Therefore, even if the ear looks normal from the outside, it is possible for significant changes to be present in the deeper portions of the ear canal and vice versa.

Cleaning the Otoscope and Ear Cones

A clean cone should be used for each ear, and otoscopes and ear cones must be cleaned and disinfected between patients. Otoscopes can be wiped down with antiseptic wipes if visibly clean, but any debris or other material must be removed before disinfecting. This should be done carefully as most otoscopes cannot be immersed in water. Debris can be removed from ear cones using cotton buds, tissue paper or cleaning brushes. They can then be disinfected by soaking in 20% chlorhexidine gluconate solution, Cetylcide®, Medistel® or other high-level broad-spectrum instrument disinfectant for 20 minutes. Simply cleaning with water and a cotton bud or with an alcohol wipe does not reliably remove contamination with bacteria such as *Pseudomonas aeruginosa*.

Techniques to Assess the Integrity of the TM

Prior to choosing ear drops and cleaners, it is important to establish whether the integrity of the TM is compromised. Damage to the TM will allow liquids to enter the tympanic bulla and ototoxicity can occur. If TM integrity is compromised or cannot be established, agents with high safety should be used and the owners be made aware of the risk. There is no product available that is licensed to be used in the middle ear and toxicity can always occur, either due to the physical presence of material (including water or saline) or to the disease process itself. Essentially anything that enters the middle ear cavity can potentially damage the inner ear.

It can be very difficult to assess the integrity of the TM in inflamed ears with a handheld otoscope, as the TM may be obscure and it is impossible to see small tears. The high-quality magnified image from a video-otoscope is much more sensitive to small TM lesions.

In an anaesthetised patient the ear can be filled with saline – large bubbles emerging from the bottom of the ear canal are likely to represent air escaping from the bulla, indicating rupture of the TM. Fluid appearing from a nostril or the mouth during the procedure is also indicative of a ruptured TM. Sedated or conscious dogs may cough or gag during ear cleaning if fluid gets into the pharynx.

Griffin has described inserting a soft rubber feeding tube through an otoscope towards the TM. The tube bounces back if the TM is intact, but passes out of view if there is false middle ear (distended TM with accumulated debris bulging into the bulla) or a ruptured TM. However, this technique may not detect a small tear in the TM as the tube may bounce off the intact part of the TM.

Contrast canalography is another way to determine to integrity of the TM (see Chapter 12), although failure of the contrast material to flow into the middle ear does not rule out otitis media or a rupture of the TM.

CT and MRI studies can also give an indication of the integrity of the TM as debris often accumulates near the TM. If there appears to be a separation between the ear canal and the tympanic bulla with debris in the ear canal and not the bulla, it is likely that the TM is intact. It is also possible to see the outline of the TM on high-quality CT images. However, CT and MRI are usually only available in referral institutions and may not be widely accessible.

Tympanometry is a routine audiometric test in human patients. It is not a hearing test, and it assesses energy transmission through the TM and middle ear. It relies on measuring changes in compliance of the TM to different pressures in the external ear canal and is a non-invasive, objective and reliable method in human ears. It is used to assess the integrity of the TM and pressure in the middle ear. However, it is difficult to align the equipment (which has to be modified from human use) and get a reliable seal between the probe and the lining of the ear canal due to the anatomical differences. This test is not routinely used in practice but may be available in some referral institutions.

Sample Collection for Cytology

Material for cytology should be collected from all cases with otitis externa. Even in cases, which are not amenable to otoscopy, a cytology sample can usually be obtained. In most cases this can be done by carefully inserting a cotton bud into the ear canal, ideally as far as the base of the vertical ear canal (see Chapter 5). Material can be obtained with a gentle swabbing action from the lining of the ear canal. The cotton bud is then gently rolled on the surface of a glass slide and the sample prepared for cytology. If the patient is not cooperative, a gloved finger can gently be inserted into the ear canal to collect some material from the opening of the vertical ear canal. This is successful in even reluctant patients if it is done carefully and the ear canal massaged first to gain the patient's trust. However, it is important to follow basic safety precautions, such as firm constraint and the use of a muzzle if indicated.

The rolled out, unstained sample from a patient without ear disease is translucent and barely perceptible due to its high lipid and low cellular content. The more inflammatory cells and organisms are present the more opaque the sample is, even unstained and to the naked eye.

Cytological preparations are can be air dried (seborrhoeic or purulent) or heat fixed (if very waxy), although opinions about the necessity for heat fixing are divided amongst dermatologists – see Chapter 1. The slide is subsequently stained with a modified Romanowsky type stain (e.g. DiffQuik® or RapiDiff®) using a two-stain or one-stain method (see Chapter 1). This is sufficient to demonstrate inflammatory cells and/or microorganisms. Commercial laboratories will often use Gram stains instead as this allows classification of Gram-positive and Gram-negative organisms as well as a morphological description (cocci and rods), which is not possible with the rapid stains. However, these are more time consuming and complex, and rapid staining techniques are preferred in practice.

A separate sample should be obtained from each ear as the nature of the inflammation and/or infection can vary between ears in the same patient. Some authors even advocate obtaining shielded samples from the different portions of the ear canal (vertical and horizontal canal) by inserting a cotton bud (or sterile swab for samples for culture) through a sterile otoscope cone into the deeper portion of the ear canal and the middle ear if the TM is ruptured or otitis media is present or suspected.

Interpretation of Otic Cytology

See also Chapter 5.

Some microorganisms can be present in a normal ear canal, however, if clinical signs are present any inflammatory cells or microorganisms are likely to be relevant for the disease process and antimicrobial therapy is indicated. Some studies have shown cytology is more sensitive in detecting bacterial and yeast infections than culture and sensitivity testing.

The stained sample should be inspected with the naked eye first. If a large proportion of the sample has taken up the purple stain, a high number of inflammatory cells and/or microorganisms is likely to be present.

Low numbers of anucleate keratinocytes are present in samples from patients without significant ear disease (Figure 13.15). Inflammatory changes in the ear canal lead to an increase in the cell turnover and an increase in the number of anucleate keratinocytes. Parakeratotic keratinocytes, which possess a retained nucleus as the normal apoptotic process has not been completed as usual, can also be seen.

Microbial overgrowth without a significant inflammatory cell exudate is present in most cases of erythroceruminous otitis, and it is of utmost importance to characterise the nature of the organisms (Figures 13.16, 13.17, 13.18, 13.19, 13.20, 13.21, 13.22, 13.23). Yeast infections (usually *Malassezia* spp.) are most common, closely followed by coccoid

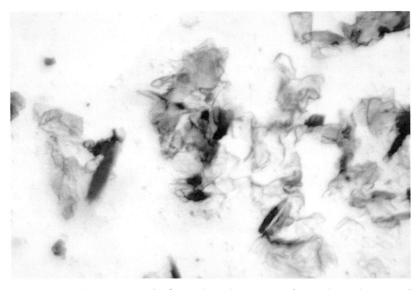

Figure 13.15 Photomicrograph of a cytological preparation from a dog without significant ear disease. There are keratinocytes but no inflammatory cells or microorganisms.

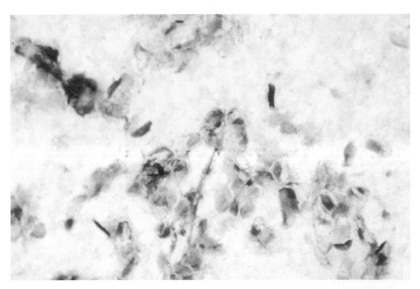

Figure 13.16 Photomicrograph under low-power magnification of a cytological preparation of bacterial overgrowth from an ear. Note the increased basophilic staining, which is probably associated with inflammatory cells and microorganisms.

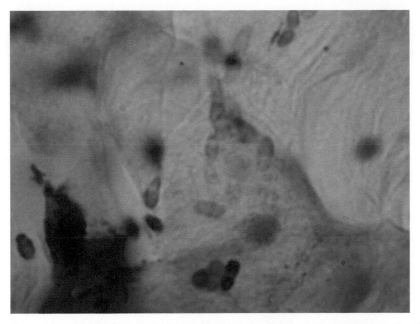

Figure 13.17 Photomicrograph of a cytological preparation from the ear of a dog with *Malassezia* otitis. Note that some yeast organisms seem to take up the stain better than others.

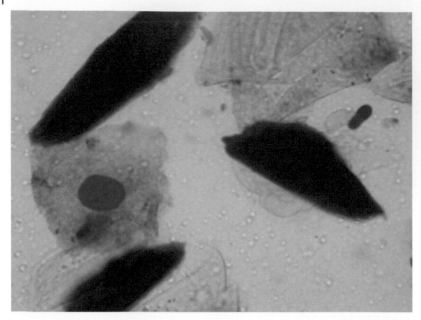

Figure 13.18 Photomicrograph of a cytological preparation showing parakeratotic keratinocytes caused by *Malassezia* otitis.

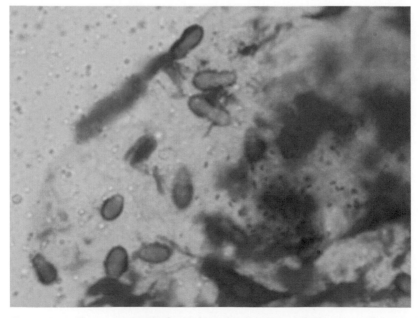

Figure 13.19 Photomicrograph of a cytological preparation under high magnification of *Malassezia* spp. in a dog with otitis. Some brown piment granules are also visible.

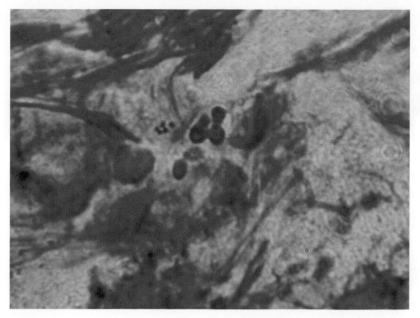

Figure 13.20 Photomicrograph of a cytological preparation from a dog with mixed ear infection with cocci and yeast. Degenerate neutrophils and nuclear strands can also be seen.

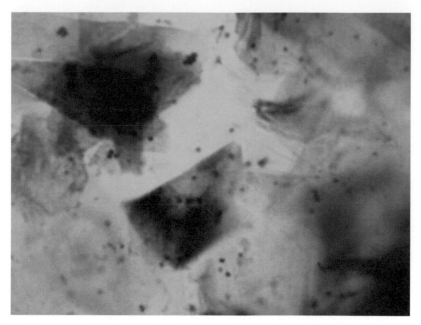

Figure 13.21 Photomicrograph of a cytological preparation showing keratinocytes and numerous cocci in the absence of inflammatory cells characteristic for bacterial overgrowth.

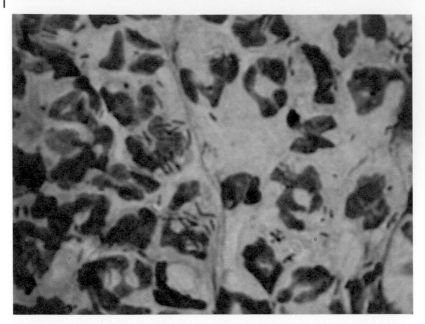

Figure 13.22 Photomicrograph of a cytological preparation showing numerous degenerate neutrophils and intracellular rods in a cytological preparation from a dog with *Pseudomonas* otitis.

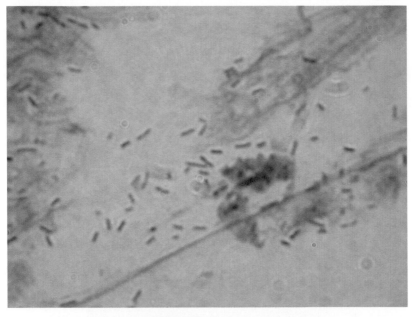

Figure 13.23 Photomicrograph of a cytological preparation showing nuclear strands and rods in a sample from a dog with *Pseudomonas* otitis.

bacteria (usually *Staphylococcus pseudintermedius*), and, less commonly, rod bacteria. However, mixed overgrowths are common. It is important to be able to distinguish coccoid bacteria from other small round structures such as melanin granules, debris in the stain or droplets of the stain. The former will change colour to yellow or brown on changing the focus very slightly. Debris and stain precipitates can be avoided by changing or filtering the stain solutions on a regular basis. They are also irregular in size, shape and staining, while bacteria are usually perfectly round or rod-shaped, usually of similar size (or sizes if a mixed infection is present) and will always be dark blue to purple, even if the level of focus is changed. Stain precipitates also form finely granular washes over large areas of the slide.

Suppurative otitis will involve a neutrophilic or pyogranulomatous (usually in more chronic cases) exudate. This is most commonly associated with Gram-negative infections (e.g. *Pseudomonas* spp., *Escherichia coli* and *Proteus* spp.), but can also be seen with staphylococci and, rarely, in some cases of *Malassezia* otitis. In a severe infection the inflammatory cells usually show signs of cell degeneration, e.g. loss of their ability to control water retention.

Reviewing the cytology in chronic and relapsing cases of otitis is important. In some cases the organism is the same, suggesting failure to manage primary and other factors or, less commonly, resistance. However, a change (for example from *Malassezia* to a Gram-negative population such as *Pseudomonas* spp.) can be quickly detected and the patient moved onto more appropriate therapy. Cytology is therefore a very important tool in the follow-up of ear cases during treatment.

Pemphigus foliaceus can lead to the presence of acantholytic cells (exfoliated keratinocytes from deeper layers of the living epidermis) in the ear canal. These will be surrounded by neutrophils, which can be non-degenerative; this is called a positive Tzanck test. Neoplastic cells are rarely encountered on cytology from otic exudate, but may be seen with sebaceous adenomas or adenocarcinomas. However, it is difficult to evaluate these for signs of malignancy reliably as the context of the tissue structure is required to be able to draw useful conclusion. Needle cores or aspirates taken from lesions under otoscopic guidance can be more useful. Eosinophils may been seen in cats with eosinophilic granuloma complex affecting the ear canals.

Bacterial Culture and Antimicrobial Sensitivity Testing

This is much less useful than cytology. The main reason is that culture results are poorly predictive of the response to topical therapy (see Chapter 6). The main benefit is to precisely identify the organisms to give a guide to appropriate antimicrobial therapy. This is more important with Gram-negative organisms – for example, *Pseudomonas* show inherent resistance to many antimicrobials but will usually be sensitive to aminoglycosides and fluoroquinolones given topically at high concentrations. Culture may therefore be useful if rod bacteria are seen on cytology. Other indications for culture include a failure to respond to appropriate cleaning and treatment despite good compliance, and where systemic therapy is considered (e.g. if topical therapy is not feasible or there is an otitis media).

Concurrent antibacterial therapy may interfere with the culture results, and ideally the patient should be off antimicrobial therapy for a few days prior to obtaining a sample.

The sample for culture should ideally be taken before obtaining a sample for cytology to avoid contamination. If a sample can only be obtained with the gloved hand, sterile gloves need to be used and some material transferred onto a transport swab. Otherwise, much in the same way as a sample is obtained for cytology, a sterile transport swab is inserted deep into the ear canal and the sample submitted to the laboratory in a suitable transport medium (see Chapter 6).

Myringotomy and Evaluation of the Middle Ear

Myringotomy means the deliberate rupture of the TM to gain access to the middle ear. This is mostly performed in cases where middle ear disease behind an intact TM has been diagnosed, for example in cases of primary secretory otitis media of brachyce-phalics, where middle ear changes are seen on imaging and/or where an abnormal TM is seen on otoscopy.

A good myringotomy is difficult to perform without the use of a video-otoscope and needs to be done by an experienced clinician. It can be performed in dogs and cats but is easier on larger-breed dogs due to the smaller diameter of the ear canal in small-breed dogs and cats. However, due to the length of the ear canal, it can be more difficult in giant breeds.

The procedure needs to be performed under general anaesthetic with good analgesia. The patient needs to be intubated with a close fitting or cuffed endotracheal tube to avoid aspiration pneumonia and is placed in lateral recumbency with the affected ear up. Steps need to be taken to avoid contamination of the face and surrounding area by placing towels, incontinence pads or similar absorbent materials over the face and around the opening of the ear canal to soak up fluid that flows back from inside the ear canal. Ideally this procedure should be done with a video-otoscope.

The ear canal needs to be flushed to remove any debris and to assess the integrity of the TM. If it is intact but there is a high index of suspicion for middle ear disease, myringotomy may be indicated. If the TM is ruptured or missing, the ear canal and middle ear can be flushed using solutions that are safe in the middle ear, such as a warmed saline solution. The myringotomy incision should be made in the caudoventral quadrant of the pars tensa. If the manubrium can be visualised this should be avoided. If visualisation of the manubrum is impossible due to opacity of the TM or masses or fluid in the middle ear cavity, the rostral and dorsal area of the TM should be avoided. To determine the correct place for the myringotomy incision the pars flaccida should ideally be in the dorsal position at 12 o'clock. In the left eardrum, the pars tensa is incised at the 5 o'clock position opposite to the manubrium of the malleus; for the right ear, the incision is made in the pars tensa at the 7 o'clock position opposite and ventral to the manubrium of the malleus. Correct positioning is important to avoid damage to the ossicles and the round window in the bulla and to preserve the blood supply to the TM. If a tear in the TM can be seen but is present in a different part of the TM, flushing is best done through a new myringotomy to avoid damage to structures in the middle ear. The actual incision of the TM can be done with a rigid sterile catheter or feeding tube with the tip cut off at an approximately 45–60° angle to leave a sharp point, a sterile spinal needle, a Buck curette, the tip of a laser, a small cotton-tipped applicator or a myringotomy blade. The instrument of choice should be poked through the myringot-omy site in one firm motion to create a small hole.

A sterile tube can be used to collect any material from the middle ear cavity for culture and cytology. If no fluid is present, 0.5–1 mL of sterile saline can be infused and re-aspirated. The middle ear cavity is then flushed with copious amounts of sterile saline until no more opaque fluid and debris can be seen. Often, fluid will be seen coming out of the patient's nose or mouth, indicating that the Eustachian tube is patent. Suitable antimicrobial and/or corticosteroid medication can be instilled directly into the bulla. Post-procedure neurological signs, such as head tilt, Horner's syndrome, deafness, facial nerve paralysis or vestibular signs, can occur but are rare with a careful technique. These complications are more commonly seen in cats than in dogs and are usually reversible. Suitable analgesia after a myringotomy includes non-steroidal anti-inflammatory drugs (NSAIDs) (not with glucocorticoids), paracetamol (not in cats), tramadol or gabapentin. Glucocorticoids are often administered to treat the otitis, and their anti-inflammatory effect will reduce pain; however, they are not analgesics and specific pain relief for a few days is always indicated.

Small myringotomy incisions usually heal within 3–4 weeks if infection and inflammation are controlled. However, if the incision is made in an incorrect place, is too large and/or there is ongoing infection and inflammation, the healing process will take longer.

BAER Testing

Brainstem auditory evoked response (BAER) testing is a quick and non-invasive test to assess deafness in dogs and cats. BAER testing requires specialised equipment and is usually done in referral institutions. It involves positioning recording electrodes on the head and ears of a patient. Headphones are used to pass a series of clicks at varying decibel levels into one ear at a time and the electrical brain response is recorded. Puppies can usually be tested for congenital hearing defects conscious, but cats and older dogs may require sedation for the procedure. BAER testing has been used to investigate the potential for ototoxicity of agents used in ear medication for research purposes and to monitor the response to therapy in clinical patients (e.g. if conductive deafness is suspected).

Deafness can be classified as follows.

- Conductive deafness due to interference in the transmission of sound waves to the inner ear (e.g. a foreign body, obstruction in the ear canal, rupture of the ear drum or infection in the middle ear).
- Sensorineural deafness resulting from damage or defect in any part of the auditory (hearing) pathway from the cochlea in the inner ear, via the auditory nerve to the auditory cortex of the brain. This can be a result of ototoxicity following the use of topical or systemic medication or due to the aging process.
  - Congenital deafness is present at birth.
  - Inherited deafness is passed down through one or both parents, and is usually congenital.
  - Late-onset deafness occurs later in life, and includes hearing loss associated with old age.
  - Acquired deafness is due to external factors such as ototoxic medication, injury or disease.

Biopsy

Biopsy of the ear canal may be useful if a mass is identified, in order to plan surgery and give a more accurate prognosis. Other than this biopsies are rarely performed in the evaluation of otic disease. Other indications include severe changes in the lining of the ear canal when the clinician would like to assess the severity and likely outcome (e.g. fibrosis and mineralisation are not readily reversible, whereas hyperplasia can usually be reduced with glucocorticoid therapy) or if ulceration is present, particularly in the absence of severe purulent *Malassezia* or Gram-negative infection.

Performing a biopsy requires general anaesthetic with good analgesia and, depending on the location of the lesion, a 4-mm punch can be used, a shave biopsy (particularly if the pinna is sampled), or an excisional biopsy specimen from a mass can be obtained. It is difficult to get meaningful biopsy specimens from the deeper ear canals as the biopsy forceps designed for endoscopes struggle to adequately grip and cut the epidermis.

14

Which Test to Choose When

Introduction

The aim of this book is to explain the diagnostic tests used in veterinary dermatology. This chapter focuses on which test is useful in which clinical situation, to help clinicians choose the appropriate test.

Ectoparasites are a major cause of skin problems, particularly pruritus, alopecia and scaling. They are important differentials that should be confirmed or eliminated early in the investigation of virtually all animals presenting with skin problems. In chronic cases, ectoparasites can act as flare factors (particularly fleas and *Sarcoptes* spp.) or complications of therapy (*Demodex* spp. in dogs on long-term glucocorticoids). Techniques used to detect ectoparasites and/or immunological reactions to them are therefore useful in most patients with skin disease. These include: visual inspection, coat combing, tape-strips, skin scrapes, faecal examination, intradermal tests and/or serology, and trial therapy. All of these approaches have their advantages and disadvantages. The sensitivity and specificity, furthermore, varies both between tests and the ectoparasites they are used to detect. Interpretation can, therefore, be difficult for the inexperienced clinician and this chapter aims to give guidance on when to perform which test in a symptom-based manner for the most common dermatological complaints seen in practice. Obviously, the tests need to be chosen after having taken a detailed history and having performed a very thorough clinical examination – both general and dermatological. The most common conditions are: pruritus, otitis, alopecia, scaling and crusting, papular and pustular diseases, pigmentary changes, erosive/ulcerative diseases, draining tracts and cutaneous/subcutaneous masses. The most appropriate tests for these conditions will be discussed.

Pruritus

Pruritus is one of the most commonly encountered complaints in small animal general practice. It can have a devastating effect on the quality of life of both the patient and the owner. The majority of cases are due to an allergic skin disease, an ectoparasite infestation or a secondary infection. Rare diseases, such as epitheliotropic lymphoma, syringohydromelia or pemphigus foliaceus, can also cause pruritus. In cats, pruritus is usually found in the form of one of the following cutaneous reaction patterns: miliary

Diagnostic Techniques in Veterinary Dermatology, First Edition. Ariane Neuber and Tim Nuttall.

dermatitis, head and neck pruritus, symmetrical alopecia or eosinophilic granuloma complex. These are explained in more detail later on.

Differential Diagnoses for Pruritus in the Dog

Pruritic diseases in dogs tend to have a characteristic lesion distribution (Figure 14.1), although certain breeds seem to have variations in the areas affected, particularly in

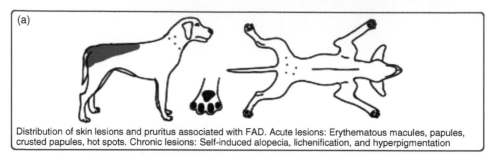

(a)

Distribution of skin lesions and pruritus associated with FAD. Acute lesions: Erythematous macules, papules, crusted papules, hot spots. Chronic lesions: Self-induced alopecia, lichenification, and hyperpigmentation

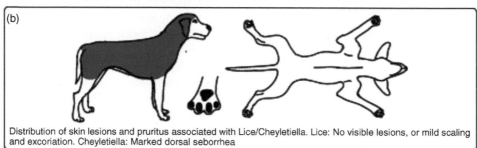

(b)

Distribution of skin lesions and pruritus associated with Lice/Cheyletiella. Lice: No visible lesions, or mild scaling and excoriation. Cheyletiella: Marked dorsal seborrhea

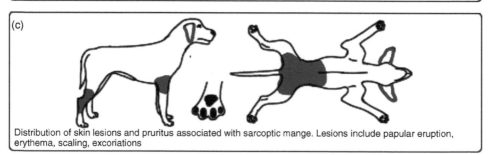

(c)

Distribution of skin lesions and pruritus associated with sarcoptic mange. Lesions include papular eruption, erythema, scaling, excoriations

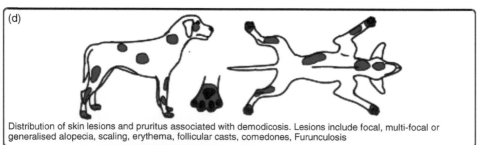

(d)

Distribution of skin lesions and pruritus associated with demodicosis. Lesions include focal, multi-focal or generalised alopecia, scaling, erythema, follicular casts, comedones, Furunculosis

Figure 14.1 Lesion distribution for pruritic skin conditions in dogs. *Source:* Hensel et al. (2015), http://bmcvetres.biomedcentral.com/articles/10.1186/s12917-015-0515-5. Used under CC-BY 4.0 http://creativecommons.org/licenses/by/4.0/

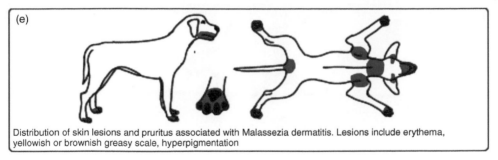

Distribution of skin lesions and pruritus associated with Malassezia dermatitis. Lesions include erythema, yellowish or brownish greasy scale, hyperpigmentation

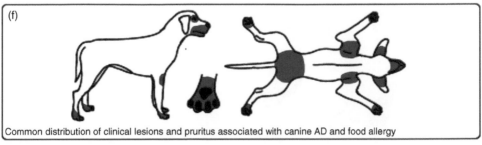

Common distribution of clinical lesions and pruritus associated with canine AD and food allergy

Figure 14.1 (Continued)

atopic dermatitis (Figure 14.2). It is important to consider all the possible differential diagnoses for your patient. The classical lesion distribution is as follows:

- facial pruritus is usually due to atopic dermatitis (which may be associated with food and/or environmental allergens), lip fold or facial fold intertrigo, otitis, secondary infections, dermatophytosis, or behavioural or neuropathic problems, or (rarely) Aujesky's disease;
- pruritus affecting the neck and shoulder is most commonly associated with flea allergic dermatitis or syringohydromelia;
- very localised pruritus (e.g. individual digits, single joints, single lesions etc.) can be associated with pyotraumatic dermatitis, acral lick granuloma, behavioural problems, neuropathies and/or musculoskeletal disorders;
- irritation of the limbs but sparing the paws can be due to a peripheral neuropathy or a behavioural problem;
- pedal pruritus is most commonly due to interdigital foreign bodies, atopic dermatitis (food or environmentally induced), *Malassezia* dermatitis, interdigital furuncles, harvest mite infestations and dermatophytosis, or hookworm or hepatocutaneous syndrome (footpads);
- pruritus affecting the tail base is commonly due to flea allergic dermatitis, whereas tail tip irritation can be associated with behavioural issues and neuropathies;
- dorsal and particularly caudal dorsal pruritus is often due to flea allergic dermatitis, *Cheyletiella*, lice or back pain (disc protrusion);
- flea allergic dermatitis, atopic dermatitis (food or environment) and behavioural problems can cause flank irritation;
- pruritus on the ventral abdomen is most commonly associated with atopic dermatitis, flea allergic dermatitis or cystitis.

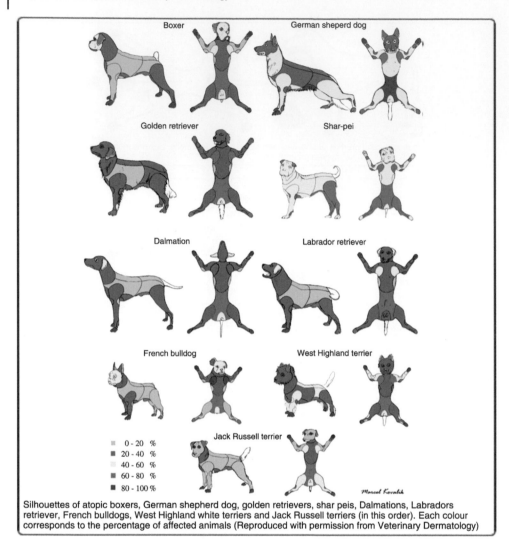

Silhouettes of atopic boxers, German shepherd dog, golden retrievers, shar peis, Dalmations, Labradors retriever, French bulldogs, West Highland white terriers and Jack Russell terriers (in this order). Each colour corresponds to the percentage of affected animals (Reproduced with permission from Veterinary Dermatology)

Figure 14.2 Breed-specific distribution of skin lesions in canine atopic dermatitis. *Source:* Hensel et al. (2015), http://bmcvetres.biomedcentral.com/articles/10.1186/s12917-015-0515-5. Used under CC-BY 4.0 http://creativecommons.org/licenses/by/4.0/

A logical approach, taking into consideration the history and clinical findings (understanding the importance of the primary lesions and lesion distribution) will then lead to a problem list and subsequently a list of differential diagnoses.

Minimum Database for Pruritus in the Dog

As parasitic skin diseases are common, the minimum database needs to take this into consideration. Figure 14.3 summarises the diagnostic approach to the pruritic dog. For all cases a flea combing, surface cytology, and deep and superficial skin scrapings, as well as cytology to investigate the possibility of a microbial overgrowth or infection, should be

Approach to pruritus

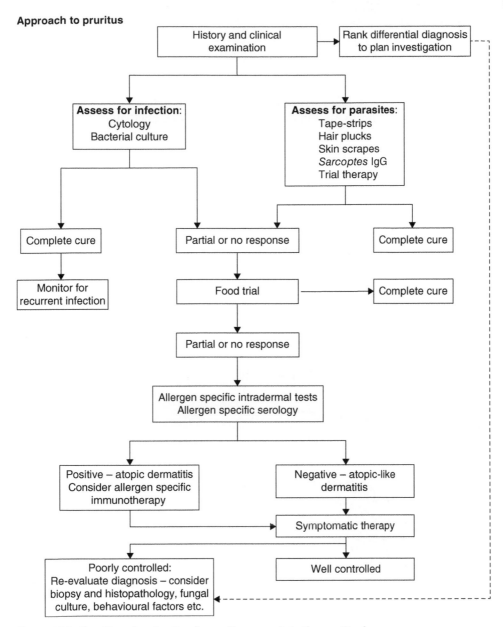

Figure 14.3 Algorithm showing the diagnostic approach to the pruritic dog.

performed. An ectoparasite control trial (to include fleas and mites) and, if required, *Sarcoptes* IgG, should also be performed if relevant for the geographical location and presentation. Microbial infection or overgrowths need to be treated. Although allergic skin disease is common, other differential diagnoses need to be ruled out first and therefore allergy testing should only be considered after a thorough work-up has been performed.

Differential Diagnoses for Pruritus in the Cat

Pruritic skin diseases in cats may not be recognised by the owner, as cats may retreat to overgroom, lick and scratch. They may therefore be presented for alopecia, eosinophilic lesions or other problems secondary to the pruritus and inflammation. A careful history will reveal the pruritus in many cases, and a trichogram will demonstrate anagen hairs with broken tips (Figure 14.4). If in doubt, you can fit an Elizabethan collar to prevent self-trauma and demonstrate regrowth of hair or healing of lesions (although many cats dislike collars intensely).

Unfortunately, the history, clinical signs and lesion distribution are not as helpful as in dogs to determine the most likely differential diagnosis (Figure 14.5). Cats present with well-defined cutaneous reaction patterns including the eosinophilic granuloma complex (indolent ulcers, eosinophilic plaques and/or eosinophilic granulomas, bilaterally symmetrical [self-induced] alopecia, head and neck pruritus, and miliary dermatitis). These can be associated with multiple and overlapping differential diagnoses. All of these

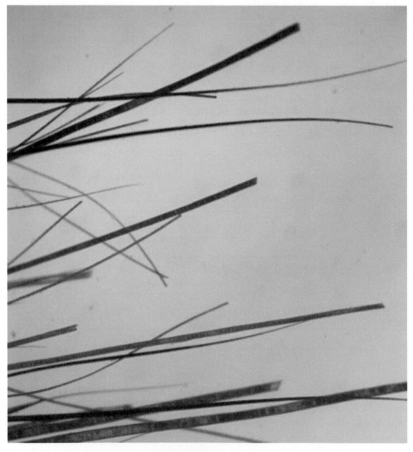

Figure 14.4 Broken, blunt and split hair tips seen in a trichogram, indicating pruritus in this cat. *Source:* Courtesy of J. Declercq.

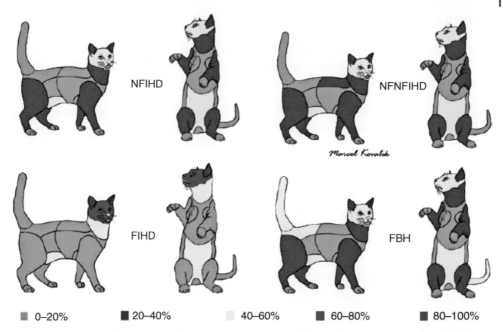

Figure 14.5 The distribution of skin lesions in cats with different hypersensitivity dermatoses (NFIHD = non-food induced hypersensitivity dermatitis; NFNFIHD = non-flea non-food-induced hypersensitivity dermatitis; FIHD = food-induced hypersensitivity dermatitis; and FBH = flea bite hypersensitivity). *Source:* Hobi et al. 2011. Reproduced with permission of John Wiley & Sons, Inc.

reaction patterns can be caused by flea allergic dermatitis, food allergy and feline atopic dermatitis. Other differential diagnoses include bacterial pyoderma, *Malassezia* dermatitis, dermatophytosis, herpesvirus dermatitis, mosquito bite hypersensitivity, *Demodex* spp., *Neotrombicula (Trombicula) autumnalis, Notoedres cati, Otodectes* spp., pemphigus foliaceus, cystitis, paraneoplastic pruritus, disc protrusion and psychogenic dermatosis. Therefore, in cats it is even more important to carefully demonstrate or rule out all of the possible differential diagnoses in each case.

Minimum Database for Pruritus in the Cat

The minimum database for pruritic cats includes superficial and deep skin scrapings, cytology, a dermatophyte culture (additional Wood's lamp examination is optional), a thorough flea control trial and, later on in the process, an exclusion diet. Food trials are more difficult to perform in feline patients due to their indoor–outdoor lifestyle, fussy eating behaviour and the potential for hepatic lipidosis (see Chapter 8).

Depending on geographical location and the likelihood of *Demodex gatoi*, a faecal flotation and a treatment trial for *Demodex* might also be useful. Similarly to canine patients with pruritus, all other differentials need to be ruled out before considering allergy testing. Allergy testing in the cat is more difficult as reactions on intradermal allergy testing tend to be less pronounced and fleeting and serum allergy testing is more controversial than in the dog (see Chapter 8).

Otitis

Otitis is also a very common clinical presentation and can be a very complex condition, especially in dogs. In cats, otitis is much less common and more often associated with ear mites or inflammatory polyps. Most cases in dogs tend to be chronic and relapsing (unless they are caused by an easily cured problem such as ear mites or a foreign body), and the changes caused by each episode of otitis make the ear more susceptible to future episodes of otitis. Many factors are involved and a classification system for the contributing factors has been created by August and recently modified by Griffin.

Primary diseases are those that actually trigger the inflammation in the ears. These include atopic dermatitis and/or adverse food reactions (Figure 14.6), contact dermatitis (to topical ear medications), foreign bodies, ear mites, cornification defects, hormonal diseases (e.g. hypothyroidism or hyperadrenocorticism), autoimmune disease and neoplasia.

Predisposing factors are those that rarely cause the inflammation, but make otitis more likely to occur or more likely to be severe in animal with a primary condition. These

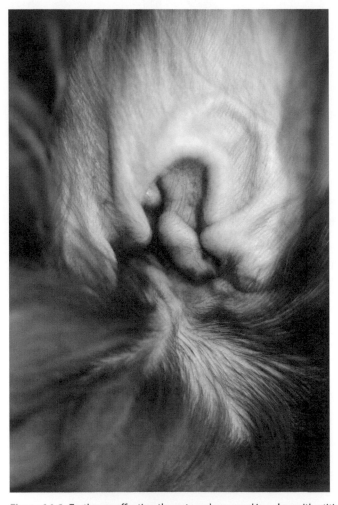

Figure 14.6 Erythema affecting the external ear canal in a dog with otitis externa due to atopic dermatitis.

include conformation of the pinna (e.g. pendulous and hairy), opening of the ear canal (e.g. very narrow as in Shar-peis) and anatomy of the ear canal (e.g. narrow and hairy), and life style choices such as frequent swimming, the use of cotton ear buds and the frequent use of harsh cleaners.

Perpetuating factors prevent resolution of the otitis and involve secondary changes following repeated bouts of inflammation and infection. These include stenosis due to swelling of the lining of the ear canal, otitis media, ceruminous gland hyperplasia, increased humidity, excessive discharge, dysfunction of epithelial migration, calcification of the ear canals, dilated or ruptured tympanic membrane, debris in the middle ear, cholesteatoma and otitis media.

Griffin modified the original classification and considered infections as secondary factors. It is important to realise that almost all ear infections are secondary to a series of underlying causes.

It is important to address all the contributing factors to achieve not just resolution of the current episode of otitis but to avoid recurrence of the problem in the future. This is a particular challenge as the perpetuating factors that occur in response to the current disease make it more likely for the disease to persist or relapse in the future. Due to the complicated nature of otitis it is important to be systematic and to identify and rectify, if possible, all the different factors involved.

Minimum Database for Patients with Otitis

The minimum database for cases of otitis includes otoscopy, ear cytology and examining the discharge for ear mites. However, otoscopy may not be possible at the first presentation due to the severe pain and/or stenosis. Culture and sensitivity testing may be indicated where rods have been identified on cytology or where the otitis cannot be resolved (see Chapter 13). Advanced imaging is useful for chronic or severe cases of otitis to determine the extent of the disease. Further tests depend on other possible clinical signs that may give a clue as to the primary disease, e.g. allergy testing, endocrine tests or biopsies.

Alopecia

Alopecia is another common clinical presentation (Figure 14.7). It is important to distinguish between primary or secondary (self-induced) alopecia, particularly in cats. Cases of secondary alopecia should be worked up like any other pruritic disease. This section deals with primary, non-pruritic, spontaneous alopecia. It is important to recognise whether the alopecia is focal or multifocal (patchy, moth eaten), or symmetrical to diffuse alopecia, as this influences the likely differential diagnoses and approach to diagnosis. A good history and thorough clinical examination is important to detect other clinical signs that help with the differential diagnosis (Table 14.1, Table 14.2, Table 14.3).

Minimum Database for Patients with Alopecia

The minimum database is slightly different for the different presentations of alopecia, and the history and clinical signs should be taken into account in each case.

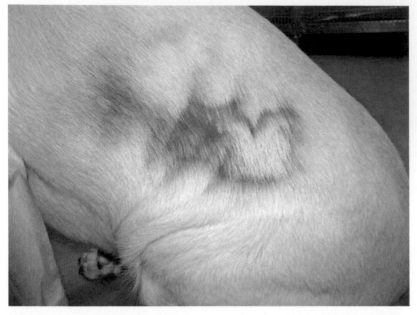

Figure 14.7 A yellow Labrador Retriever showing classical features of seasonal flank alopecia.

Table 14.1 History and clinical findings in patients with alopecia.

Useful pointers from the history

Age	Young animal	Demodicosis
		Dermatophytosis
		Congenital alopecia
	Middle-aged	Endocrine alopecia
	Old	Epitheliotropic lymphoma
		Paraneoplastic alopecia
Sex	Intact male	Sertoli cell tumour
		Hyperandrogenism
	Intact female	Hyperoestrogenism
Breed		Breed-related problems
Systemic signs	Polyuria/polydypsia	Hyperadrenocorticism
	Lethargy, weight gain	Hypothyroidism
	Vomiting, weight loss	Paraneoplastic alopecia
Seasonality		Cyclical flank alopecia
Travel abroad		Leishmaniasis
Prior illness		Telogen/anagen defluxion
Injections		Vaccine-associated vasculitis
		Steroid injection site alopecia
Contagion		Dermatophytosis

Table 14.1 *(Continued)*

Useful clinical findings

Inflammatory lesions (papules, pustules, crusts)	Pyoderma
	Dermatophytosis
	Demodicosis
	Leishmaniasis
Scaling	Sebaceous adenitis
	Follicular dysplasias
	Keratinisation defects
	Hypothyroidism
	Sertoli cell tumour
Thickened skin	Hypothyroidism
Atrophic skin (+/− comedomes)	Hyperadrenocorticism
	Steroid injection site alopecia
	Paraneoplastic alopecia
Normal skin	Congenital alopecia
	Endocrine alopecia
	Cyclical flank alopecia
	Pattern baldness
	Telogen effluvium/anagen defluxion
Pot belly and calcinosis cutis	Hyperadrenocorticism
Abdominal mass	Sertoli cell tumour
	Hyperoestrogenism
Pyrexia and lymphadenopathy	Leishmaniasis
Muscle atrophy	Dermatomyositis
Gynaecomastia, oestrus	Hyperoestrogenism
Linear preputial erythema	Sertoli cell tumour

Table 14.2 Clinical features of focal to multifocal and symmetrical diffuse alopecia.

	Focal or multifocal alopecia	Symmetrical or diffuse alopecia
Lesion distribution	Focal Multifocal and non-symmetrical	Symmetrical across the sagittal plane
Hair loss	Usually complete	Usually partial and diffuse May be complete in centre of lesions
Margin of hair loss	Well demarcated	Poorly demarcated and diffuse
Hairs	Anagen; may be broken	Telogen; usually intact
Skin	Inflamed (erythema, lichenification, scaling, follicular casts, comedones, hyperpigmentation) May be normal	Normal to atrophic May see comedones (hyperadrenocorticism), hyperpigmentation (endocrine) and thickening (hypothyroidism)
Rest of coat	Normal	Dull, dry, scaling

Table 14.3 Differential diagnoses for focal to multifocal and symmetrical diffuse alopecia.

Focal to multifocal alopecia	Symmetrical or diffuse alopecia
Infectious/parasitic	
Staphylococcal pyoderma	
Demodex	
Dermatophytosis	
Leishmania	
Immune-mediated	
Dermatomyositis	
Alopecia areata	
Pseudopelade	
Vasculitis	
Vaccine-associated vasculitis	
Lymphocytic mural folliculitis (cats)	Lymphocytic mural folliculitis (cats)
Endocrine/metabolic	
Steroid injection site	Hyperadrenocorticism
	Hypothyroidism
	Sex hormone dermatoses
	Telogen effluvium
	Anagen defluxion
	Paraneoplastic alopecia
	Pituitary dwarfism
Neoplasia	
Epitheliotropic cutaneous T-cell lymphoma	Epitheliotropic cutaneous T-cell lymphoma
Congenital/hereditary	
Keratinisation defects	
Sebaceous adenitis	
Follicular dysplasias (including colour-dilute and black-hair follicular dysplasia)	Follicular dysplasias (including colour-dilute and black-hair follicular dysplasia)
Congenital alopecias	Congenital alopecias
Pattern baldness	Pattern baldness
Miscellaneous	
Post-clipping alopecia (idiopathic or associated with underlying conditions)	Cyclical flank alopecia
Scars	Alopecia X
Traction alopecia (e.g. rubber bands, ties etc.)	

The approach to focal and multifocal alopecia can include hair plucks, tape-strips, deep skin scrapings, cytology, Wood's lamp examination, trichography and dermatophyte cultures. If these tests fail to yield a positive result, a biopsy is indicated.

Symmetrical alopecia has a wider range of potential differential diagnoses and may require a more involved work-up of endocrine and metabolic conditions (see

Chapter 10). A hair pluck and trichogram is always indicated to determine hair growth cycles and shaft abnormalities. Haematology, biochemistry and urinalysis are screening tests for potential endocrine or metabolic disease, and further tests may be indicated according to the results. Other tests may include diagnostic imaging. Biopsies are indicated to investigate the less common differential diagnoses and/or where screening or endocrine tests fail to achieve a diagnosis.

Scaling and Crusting Dermatoses

Excessive scaling (seborrhoea) and crusting are commonly mentioned as if they were synonymous but they are fundamentally different primary lesions. Scaling describes abnormal shedding of superficial epidermis, the stratum corneum, which forms visible dandruff. This can be due to increased cellular turnover and/or abnormal desquamation. Orthokeratotic hyperkeratosis (orthokeratosis) is an increase in normal keratinocytes, which is common in inflammatory diseases and keratinisation disorders. Parakeratotic hyperkeratosis (parakeratosis) is a thickened stratum corneum with nucleated keratinocytes, which is more specific for *Malassezia* dermatitis, zinc-responsive dermatosis and superficial necrolytic dermatitis. Crusting, in contrast, is the accumulation of skin cells and dried exudates, secretions, inflammatory cells or medications. However, scaling and crusting may occur together.

Scaling and crusting diseases can be primary or (more commonly) secondary to other skin diseases (Table 14.4). If pruritus is present, the reason for the pruritus needs to be investigated first. Ichthyosis and other hereditary disorders are usually seen in young patients (Figure 14.8).

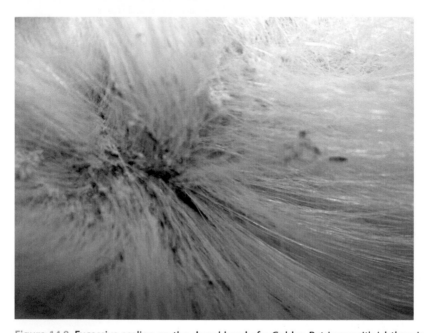

Figure 14.8 Excessive scaling on the dorsal head of a Golden Retriever with ichthyosis.

Table 14.4 Differential diagnosis of scaling.

Causes of secondary scaling	
Pruritic	
Ectoparasites	Fleas
	Sarcoptes
	Cheyletiella
Infections	Pyoderma
	Malassezia
Hypersensitivities	Atopic dermatitis
	Adverse food reactions
Immune-mediated	Drug reactions
Neoplasia	Cutaneous epitheliotropic lymphoma
Non-pruritic	
Infections	*Demodex*
	Dermatophytosis
	Leishmania
Metabolic	Endocrinopathies
	Superficial necrolytic dermatitis
	Lymphocytic mural folliculitis
	Thymoma-associated exfoliative dermatitis
	Zinc-responsive dermatosis
	Essential fatty acid deficiency
	Malabsorption diseases
	Severe systemic diseases
Immune-mediated	Pemphigus foliaceus
	Exfoliative cutaneous lupus erythematosus
	Drug reactions
Environmental	Low humidity, dry heat
	Hard surfaces – calluses

Primary scaling diseases: keratinisation disorders	
Nasodigital hyperkeratosis	Common
Idiopathic keratinisation disorders ('idiopathic seborrhoea')	Relatively common
Sebaceous adenitis	Relatively common
Schnauzer comedo syndrome	Uncommon
Ear margin dermatosis	Uncommon
Ichthyosis	Rare
Lethal acrodermatitis	Rare

The minimum database for scaling and crusting disorders entails cytology, skin scrapings and hair plucks/trichograms for all patients. Over and above these tests, the choice depends on the history and clinical examination, which determines the list of differential diagnoses. Biopsies are required to diagnose primary scaling disorders and can be helpful in many cases with secondary scaling and crusts.

Pigmentary Changes

Changes in the skin pigmentation can be caused by too much (hyperpigmentation) or too little pigment in the skin (hypopigmentation). Hyperpigmentation is most commonly an expression of post-inflammatory changes in the skin or hormonal disease, such as hypothyroidism, hyperadrenocorticism, or adrenal or gonadal sex hormone imbalances. Some congenital disorders can also cause increased pigmentation. Post-inflammatory hyperpigmentation is usually associated with other presenting signs, such as pruritus or alopecia, and tests appropriate for those conditions should be conducted. It usually forms a lace-like pattern of pigmentation on affected skin. Macular melanosis is more common with endocrinopathies. It can occur on the anus, scrotum, prepuce and ventral proximal tail in association with testicular tumours. An abdominal ultrasound scan should be conducted to check for metastasis, and castration is often curative. Lentigo is a congenital condition that can occur in dogs and ginger cats, which present with sharply demarcated hyperpigmented macules. Acanthosis nigricans is a condition seen in Dachshunds that develop pigmentation and lichenification in the axillae. It is often associated with *Malassezia* dermatitis. It is a paraneoplastic condition in humans, but this appears to be rare in animals. Some breeds of cats naturally have darker hair at the extremities and coat darkening can occur after clipping the hair, for example when spaying female cats. Melanomas, melanocytic naevi or basal cell tumours can be hyperpigmented and a biopsy is necessary to diagnose these conditions.

Hypopigmentation is rarer. It is usually either congenital, or due to a specific autoimmune attack on the melanocytes, diseases that affect the dermo-epidermal junction or epitheliotrophic lymphoma. Some syndromes, such as Chediak–Higashi or Waardenburg syndrome cause diffuse hypopigmentation from birth. Acquired hypopigmentation can be associated with autoimmune diseases (uveodermatological syndrome, vitiligo and discoid lupus erythematosus), neoplasia (epitheliotropic lymphoma), environmental factors (rubber toxicity, burn, trauma, cold or chemical or physical injury) or idiopathic changes (snow nose, Dudley nose and age-associated or idiopathic leucotrichia). In some cases a clinical diagnosis can be made. Most cases will require a biopsy.

Macules, Papules and Pustules

Macules are small (<1 cm diameter), circular, flat areas of skin discolouration, whereas papules and pustules are small elevated lesions – papules are solid and pustules contain pus. If any other clinical sign is present, such as pruritus, this should be pursued first. Diseases that can cause erythematous macules include staphylococcal pyoderma, flea

Table 14.5 Differentiating exfoliative staphylococcal pyoderma from pemphigus foliaceus.

Clinical signs	Pemphigus foliaceus	Pyoderma
Symmetrical facial and periocular lesions	+	−
Medial pinna affected	+	−
Footpads affected	+	−
Trunk initially affected	+/−	+
Irregular, polycyclic or annular pustules	+	−
Coalescing pustules	+	−
Non-follicular pustules	+	+/−
Flaccid pustules	+	+/−
Turgid pustules	−	+/−
Epidermal collarettes	−	+
Expanding collaretes and lesions	−	+
Pallisading crusts	+	−
Moist erosions	+	−

allergic dermatitis (FAD), fly bite hypersensitivity, contact dermatitis and erythema multiforme (often associated with specific target lesion macules). Bleeding into the skin can lead to haemorrhagic macules, which can be caused by vasculitis or coagulopathies.

Papules are commonly seen in patients with staphylococcal pyoderma, FAD, fly bite hypersensitivity, sarcoptic mange, atopic dermatitis, contact dermatitis, feline cowpox and miliary dermatitis. Diseases that can cause pustules include pemphigus foliaceus, pemphigus erythematosus, bullous impetigo, sterile eosinophilic pustulosis, subcorneal pustular dermatosis and linear IgA disease.

Minimum Database for Macular, Papular and Pustular Diseases

The minimum database for these conditions incudes cytology, skin scrapings, coat brushings, dermatophyte culture and ectoparasiticidal trial therapy. If sarcoptic mange is suspected, *Sarcoptes* IgG serology can be performed. The clinical signs should be carefully evaluated to help differentiate exfoliative staphylococcal pyoderma and pemphigus foliaceus (Table 14.5). In many cases a biopsy is required to make a final diagnosis, unless in-house tests have already yielded a diagnosis. For macules, diascopy is useful – erythema will blanch on pressure but haemorrhagic lesions will not. Dermoscopy (see Chapter 4) can be useful to distinguish the nature of pigmented, macular, papular and pustular lesions.

Ulcers and Erosions

As with many other clinical signs, it is important to establish if any other clinical signs, such as alopecia or pruritus are present. These should be worked up first. Once pruritic, alopecic, pustular, depigmenting, nodular and scaling and crusting diseases have been excluded, you should consider trauma (thermal, chemical and physical), neoplasia (various, including squamous cell carcinoma), infections (herpesvirus, calicivirus, poxvirus, mucocutaneous pyoderma, deep pyoderma and *Candida*) and autoimmune diseases (cutaneous and systemic lupus erythematosus, erythema multiforme/toxic epidermal necrolysis, pemphigus vulgaris, epidermolysis bullosa acquisita and other autoimmune subepidermal blistering diseases, and vasculitis).

Often these cases are severely ill and some of these conditions can be life threatening. A swift diagnosis and treatment are therefore vital, and in some cases decisions need to be made before the results from histopathology and cultures are available. Careful evaluation of the history, signalment and clinical signs can help in the differential diagnosis (Table 14.6). Nikolskiy's sign is useful, but should be performed and interpreted carefully (Table 14.7). Erythema multiforme, Stevens–Johnson

Table 14.6 Features of the signalment and history useful in cases with erosions and ulcers.

(a) Predisposed breeds.

Condition	Predisposed breeds
Pemphigus foliaceus (PF) Insecticide-trigger contact PF (ITC-PF)	Spaniels, Akita, Chow Large-breed dogs (72% >20 kg)
Epidermolysis bullosa acquisita (EBA)	Great Dane
Mucous membrane pemphigoid (MMP)	German Shepherd Dog
Classical discoid lupus erythematosus (CDLE)	Shetland Sheepdog, Rough Collie, German Shepherd Dog, Siberian Husky
Generalised DLE (GDLE)	Chinese crested dog?
Vesicular cutaneous lupus erythematosus (VCLE)	Rough Collie, Border Collie, Shetland Sheepdog
Exfoliative CLE (ECLE)	German Short-Haired Pointer
Mucocutaneous lupus erythematosus (MCLE)	German Shepherd Dog
Systemic lupus erythematosus (SLE)	German Shepherd Dog, Rough Collie, Shetland Sheepdog, Beagle, Afghan Hound, Old English Sheepdog, Poodles, Irish Setter
Alopecia areata (AA)	Dachshund?
Mural isthmic folliculitis	Lundehund
Anal furunculosis, metatarsal fistula and German Shepherd Dog pyoderma	German Shepherd Dog
Injection site vasculitis	Bichon Frise, Poodles, Yorkshire/Silky Terriers
Proliferative arteritis of the nasal philtrum	St Bernard
Cutaneous and renal glomerular vasculopathy (CRGV/Alabama rot)	Greyhound (although many breeds have been affected in the UK)
Idiopathic ear margin vasculitis	Dachshund
Dermatomyositis	Rough Collie, Shetland Sheepdog, Beauceron
Familial cutaneous vasculopathy	German Shepherd Dog
Adverse drug reaction (sulphonamides)	Dobermann
Uveodermatological syndrome	Akita

Table 14.6 *(Continued)*

(b) Clinical significance of skin lesions.

Clinical lesion	Significance	Examples
Crusts	Exudation, discharge, haemorrhage	Common and non-specific
Scale	Exfoliation; chronic disease	ECLE, PF, pemphigus vegetans (Pveg), sebaceous adenitis (SA), GDLE, ADRs
Lichenification	Chronic disease	GDLE
Erosions	Superficial disease above basement membrane; acute/subacute disease	PF, ECLE, CDLE, GDLE
Ulcers that move with the skin	Deep disease affects whole epidermis, basement membrane and upper dermis; acute/subacute disease	SLE, VCLE, CDLE, MCLE, MMP, EBA, pemphigus vulgaris (PV)
Skin moves over ulcers	Full-thickness necrosis	Vasculitis, Stevens–Johnson syndrome (SJS), toxic epidermal necrolysis (TEN), anal furunculosis, GSD pyoderma
Cutaneous atrophy and scarring	Vasculopathy and hypoxia	Vasculitis, SLE, dermatomyositis
Alopecia	Targets follicles	AA, pseudopelade, mural isthmic folliculitis, feline mural folliculitis (degenerative mucinotic or lymphocytic), dermatomyositis (+ other vasculopathies), SLE
Nail loss	Specific for SLO; with other clinical signs in other conditions	Symmetrical lupoid onychodystrophy (SLO), vasculitis, DLE
Draining sinus tracts	Lesions affect subcutaneous tissues	Vasculitis, panniculitis, SLE, anal furunculosis, GSD pyoderma
Mucosal	Mucosa; mucocutaneous junctions	MCLE, MMP, EBA, PV, SJS, TEN
Affects footpads		EBA, vasculitis
Target lesions		Erythema multiforme (EM)
Purpura, petechiae, ecchymoses	Vascular lesions	Vasculitis
Extremities		Vasculitis
Muscle atrophy		Dermatomyositis
Loss of pigment		Vitiligo, DLE, uveodermatological syndrome
Ocular signs		Uveodermatological syndrome

Table 14.6   (*Continued*)

(c) Autoimmune subepidermal blistering diseases (AISBDs).

AISBD	Frequency	Breed	Clinical features	Predominant lesion distribution
MMP	50%	GSD	Heal by scarring; symmetrical lesions	Oral cavity; mucocutaneous junctions; pinnae
EBA	25%	Great Dane	Symmetrical lesions	Mucosal surfaces; mucocutaneous junctions; skin; pinnae; footpads
Junctional EBA	Rare			
BP	10%			Skin (frictional sites)
Mixed AISBD	Rare			Oral cavity; mucocutaneous junctions
Linear IgA dermatosis	Rare			Oral cavity; footpads
Pemphigoid of gestation	Rare		Pregnancy	Oral cavity
Bullous SLE	Rare			Oral cavity; footpads; skin (frictional sites)

(d) Types of vesicle in blistering diseases.

Type of vesicle	Disease
Flaccid vesicle	PV; EM/SJS; VCLE
Turgid vesicle	AISBDs
Haemorrhagic vesicle	AISBDs
Erythematous margin	AISBDs; EM/SJS; VCLE

syndrome and toxic epidermal necrolysis cannot be reliably differentiated on histopathology alone, and the clinical signs must be carefully evaluated to make the diagnosis (Table 14.8).

If there is a history of trauma, supportive care and wound care should be given. Cases typical of intertrigo, lick granuloma, acral lick dermatitis or feline eosinophilic granuloma complex should be subjected to skin scrapings and cytology. Any severe

Table 14.7   Nikolskiy's sign. Nikolskiy's sign is the ability to split the epidermis forming an erosion or ulcer with digital or blunt force. There are a number of clinical variants.

Nikolskiy's sign	Description	Examples
Direct	Normal skin splits distant from primary lesions	PV
Marginal	Normal perilesional skin splits	PV
Pseudo	Erythematous perilesional skin splits	EM/SJS; VCLE
False	Bulla expands with digital pressure	AISBDs

Table 14.8   Clinical differentiation of erythema multiforme complex conditions.

	EM minor	EM major	SJS	SJS–TEN	TEN
Flat or raised, erythematous polycyclic to target lesions	Y	Y	N	N	N
Mucosal surfaces involved	N (or 1)	>1	>1	>1	>1
Erythematous or purpuric macules/patches (% body surface area)	<50%	<50%	>50%	>50%	>50%
Epidermal ulceration (% body surface area)	<10%	<10%	<10%	10–30%	>30%

undiagnosed diseases after skin scraping and cytology will need a biopsy and in some cases additional tests, such as ANA testing, routine haematology, biochemistry and urinalysis, bacterial culture and antibiotic sensitivity testing, fungal culture and virus isolation/serology, may be indicated.

Importance of Making the Correct Diagnosis and Specialist Referral

More and more effective drugs for many skin conditions in animals and humans have been developed and are available for use in practice. This can greatly improve the quality of life for many patients with skin disease. Symptomatic therapy for pruritus, in particular, has had many advances recently. Due to the efficacy of these drugs for pruritus and other lesions, regardless of the diagnosis, it can be tempting to treat symptomatically rather than making a diagnosis. This is often initially successful, but this approach is flawed as it can lead to missing patients with pruritic and non-allergic skin disease, such as cases of sarcoptic mange or epitheliotropic lymphoma, and mask underlying problems and infections. A failure to achieve a diagnosis may also prevent an accurate prognosis for the owner and consideration of more appropriate treatments. A delayed diagnosis can also significantly impact the clinical outcome.

Although the vast majority of mild cutaneous diseases can be successfully managed in general practice, many patients will benefit from referral to a dermatology specialist. The cost per disease ratio is often favourable as the expertise of the specialist means that more specific and relevant tests are performed, leading to a quicker diagnosis, enabling discussion of the prognosis and appropriate treatment options with the owners. Resources are therefore used more efficiently, despite the perceived higher consultation fees. In addition, rare conditions, such as autoimmune diseases, may require therapy with drugs that are rarely used in first-opinion practice and can have severe side effects if not monitored appropriately. Chronic cases, including atopic dermatitis, pododermatitis and otitis, can also greatly benefit from specialist input, particularly if the disease cannot be controlled easily. It is therefore prudent to offer this option to owners of patients with more complicated skin disease.

15

Genetic Tests for Skin Diseases

Many skin diseases have a genetic basis, and there are clear breed and familial risk factors for developing many conditions. However, relatively few common conditions involve a single gene and gene defect with a clear pattern of inheritance. Most involve multiple genes (i.e. they are polygenic) with the disease outcome dependent both on the underlying genotype and environmental influences. These may or may not actually involve a 'gene defect' as such, as the overall pattern of interactions within the genotype is most important. The terminology used in genetics can be confusing – please refer to the glossary (see Table 15.7) for more information about the terms used in this chapter.

Patterns of Inheritance

In autosomal recessive disorders each of the offspring inherit one allele of the affected gene from each parent (Figure 15.1). Animals that are homozygous for the abnormal allele will develop the condition, but animals that are heterozygous with one normal allele and one abnormal allele will be clinically unaffected carriers of the condition. It does not matter whether the affected or carrier parent is male or female. Note that the percentages in Tables 15.1, 15.2, 15.3 and 15.4 are averages over a population; it is impossible to predict the exact frequency of affected, unaffected and carrier animals in any one mating.

In autosomal dominant disorders each of the offspring inherit one allele of the affected gene from each parent. Animals will develop the condition whether they inherit one (heterozygous) or two (homozygous) abnormal alleles (Figure 15.2). Clinically unaffected carriers of the condition are not seen as the phenotype is governed by the dominant abnormal allele. It does not matter whether the affected or normal parent is male or female.

In sex-linked recessive disorders all the male offspring inherit their X-chromosome and X-associated allele from their mother, but the female offspring inherit one X-chromosome from their mother and one from their father. Female offspring that are homozygous for the abnormal allele will develop the condition, but animals that are heterozygous with one normal allele and one abnormal allele will be clinically unaffected carriers of the condition (Figure 15.3). However, males only have one X-chromosome

Diagnostic Techniques in Veterinary Dermatology, First Edition. Ariane Neuber and Tim Nuttall.
© 2017 Ariane Neuber and Tim Nuttall. Published 2017 by John Wiley & Sons, Ltd.

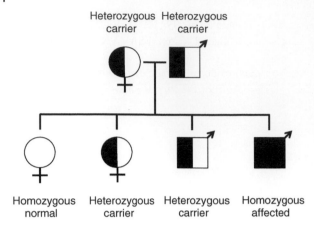

Figure 15.1 Autosomal recessive inheritance.

Table 15.1   Autosomal recessive patterns of inheritance.

Parents	Offspring
unaffected × unaffected	100% unaffected
unaffected × carrier	50% unaffected 50% carriers
unaffected × affected	100% carriers
carrier × carrier	25% unaffected 25% affected 50% carriers
carrier × affected	50% carriers 50% affected
affected × affected	100% affected

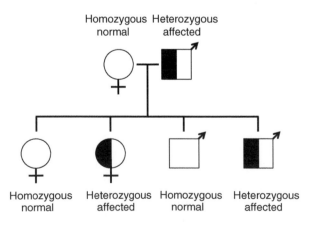

Figure 15.2 Autosomal dominant inheritance.

Table 15.2 Autosomal dominant patterns of inheritance.

Parents	Offspring
unaffected × unaffected	100% unaffected
unaffected × affected (heterozygous)	50% unaffected 50% affected (heterozygous)
unaffected × affected (homozygous)	100% affected (heterozygous)
affected × affected (heterozygous) (heterozygous)	25% unaffected 25% affected (homozygous) 50% affected (heterozygous)
affected × affected (homozygous) (heterozygous)	50% affected (homozygous) 50% affected (heterozygous)

and therefore will either develop the condition or not depending on whether they inherit an abnormal or normal allele from their mother. Clinically unaffected male carriers of the condition are not seen. The percentages in Table 15.3 are averages over a population; it is impossible to predict the exact frequency of affected, unaffected and carrier animals in any one mating.

In sex-linked dominant disorders all the male offspring inherit their X-chromosome and X-associated allele from their mother, but the female offspring inherit one X-chromosome from their mother and one from their father (Figure 15.4). Female offspring that inherit either one (heterozygous) or two (homozygous) abnormal alleles will develop the condition. However, males only have one X-chromosome and therefore will either develop the condition or not depending on whether they inherit an abnormal or normal allele from their mother. Neither female nor male clinically unaffected carriers of the condition are seen.

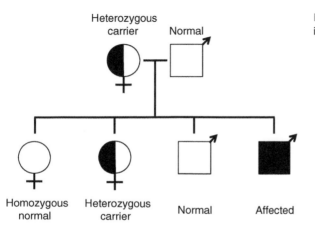

Heterozygous
carrier   Normal

Homozygous   Heterozygous   Normal   Affected
normal   carrier

Figure 15.3 Sex (X)-linked recessive inheritance.

Table 15.3 Sex-linked recessive patterns of inheritance.

Parents		Offspring	
Male	**Female**	**Male**	**Female**
unaffected	unaffected	100% unaffected	100% unaffected
unaffected	carrier	50% unaffected 50% affected	50% unaffected 50% carriers
unaffected	affected	100% affected	100% carriers
affected	unaffected	100% unaffected	100% carriers
affected	carrier	50% unaffected 50% affected	50% unaffected 50% carriers
affected	affected	100% affected	100% affected

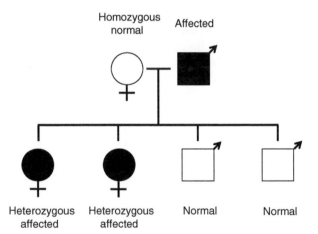

Figure 15.4 Sex (X)-linked dominant inheritance.

Genetic Tests

Genetic conditions that may be relevant in skin diseases are listed in Table 15.5. This table also indicates whether or not genetic tests are available for each condition.

More complete and up-to-date lists of available genetic tests can be found at Online Mendelian Inheritance in Animals (OMIA; http://omia.angis.org.au/home/home), Inherited Diseases in Dogs (IDID; http://idid.vet.cam.ac.uk/search.php) and WSAVA Testing Laboratories for DNA-based and other Genetic Tests (http://research.vet .upenn.edu/DNAGeneticsTestingLaboratorySearch/tabid/7620/Default.aspx).

Submitting Samples for Genetic Tests

Genetic tests can be run on DNA isolated from whole blood submitted in EDTA, from buccal swabs, dried blood collected on swabs, hairs, claws and other tissue samples. Most tests are performed on whole blood in EDTA or buccal swabs in DNA

Table 15.4 Sex-linked dominant patterns of inheritance.

Parents		Offspring	
Male	Female	Male	Female
unaffected	unaffected	100% unaffected	100% unaffected
unaffected	affected (heterozygous)	50% unaffected 50% affected	50% unaffected 50% affected (heterozygous)
unaffected	affected (homozygous)	100% affected	100% affected (heterozygous)
affected	unaffected	100% unaffected	100% affected (heterozygous)
affected	affected (heterozygous)	50% unaffected 50% affected	50% affected (heterozygous) 50% affected (homozygous)
affected	affected (homozygous)	100% affected	100% affected (homozygous)

collection media, but it is important to discuss the appropriate collection method for each test with the laboratory before submitting the sample. Home test kits for owners are also available for some tests. It is very important to avoid any contamination with DNA from other animals during collection, and that the samples are labelled correctly.

Laboratories that offer a range of genetic tests include University of California Davis (https://www.vgl.ucdavis.edu/), North Carolina State University (http://www.ncstatevets.org/genetics/), Texas A&M University (http://vetmed.tamu.edu/vibs/service-labs), the Animal Health Trust (http://www.aht.org.uk/cms-display/genetics_cares.html), Anatgene (http://www.antagene.com), Laboklin (http://www.laboklin.co.uk/laboklin/index.jsp), Veterinary Genetics Services (https://www.vetgen.com/), Paw Print Genetics (https://www.pawprintgenetics.com), Animal Genetics (http://www.animalgenetics.eu/), The Vet DNA Center (https://vetdnacenter.com/) and Optigen (http://www.optigen.com/).

Results

Most diseases that are tested for are single-gene autosomal recessive defects with high penetrance. The results may be reported in a number of similar ways:

- clear or unaffected (N/N, +/+, homozygous normal or homozygous wildtype);
- carrier (N/n, N/JEB [gene name – e.g. junction epidermolysis bullosa], +/- or heterozygous);

Table 15.5   Genetic conditions that may be relevant in skin diseases.

Condition	Breed	Inheritance	Test available
Ichthyosis	American Bulldog	Autosomal recessive	Yes
	Golden Retriever	Autosomal recessive	Yes
	Great Dane	Autosomal recessive	Yes
Ichthyosis/epidermolytic hyperkeratosis (EHK)	Norfolk Terrier	Autosomal recessive	Yes
Footpad hyperkeratosis	Irish Terriers Kromfohrländer Dogue de Bordeaux	Autosomal recessive	Yes
Hereditary nasal parakeratosis	Labrador Retriever	Autosomal recessive	Yes
Congenital keratoconjunctivitis sicca and ichthyosiform dermatosis (CKSID; dry eye and curly coat syndrome)	Cavalier King Charles Spaniels	Autosomal recessive	Yes
Lethal acrodermatitis	Bull Terriers	Autosomal recessive	No
Ectodermal dysplasia – skin fragility syndrome (ED-SFS)	Chesapeake Bay Retriever	Autosomal recessive	Yes
Dystrophic epidermolysis bullosa	Golden Retriever	Autosomal recessive	Yes
Junctional epidermolysis bullosa	German Short-Haired Pointer	Autosomal recessive	Yes
Herlitz junctional epidermolysis bullosa (H-JEB)	Belgian Horses French Draft Horse	Autosomal recessive	Yes
Hereditary equine regional dermal asthenia (HERDA)	Paint Horse Quarter Horse Appaloosas	Autosomal recessive	Yes
Warmblood fragile foal syndrome	Warmblood horses	Autosomal recessive	Yes
Alopecia	American Hairless Terrier	Autosomal recessive	Yes
Alopecia	Birman	Autosomal recessive	Yes
Smooth straight coat (improper coat)	Various	Autosomal recessive	Yes
Long coat	Various	Autosomal recessive	Yes
Colour point	Various (cats)	Autosomal recessive	Yes
Amber coat	Norwegian Forest Cat	Autosomal recessive	Yes

Table 15.5 (*Continued*)

Condition	Breed	Inheritance	Test available
Brown and yellow coat (coul mutations)	Various (dogs)	Autosomal recessive	Yes
Oculocutaneous albinism	Various	Autosomal recessive	Yes
Pituitary dwarfism	German Shepherd Dog Saarloos Wolfdog Czechoslovak Wolfdog	Autosomal recessive	Yes
Colour-dilution alopecia	Various	Autosomal recessive	Yes
Congenital hypothyroidism	French Bulldog Fox Terrier Spanish Water Dog Rat Terrier Tenterfield Terrier	Autosomal recessive	Yes
Ivermectin (multi-drug) sensitivity (MDR1 mutation; includes sensitivity to a range of related and other drugs using p-glycoprotein metabolism)	Australian Shepherd Collies Old English Sheepdog (bobtail) German Shepherd Dog Longhaired Whippet McNab Shepherd/Border Collie English Shepherd Dog Shetland Sheepdog Silken Windhound American White Shepherd Wäller Elo (and others)	Autosomal recessive	Yes
C3 deficiency	Brittany Spaniel	Autosomal reccssive	Yes
Leucocyte adhesion deficiency type III (LAD III)	German Shepherd Dog	Autosomal recessive	Yes
Canine leucocyte adhesion deficiency (CLAD)	Irish Setter	Autosomal recessive	Yes
Canine cyclic neutropenia (grey collie syndrome)	Rough and Smooth Collies	Autosomal recessive	Yes
Chediak–Higashi syndrome	Various	Autosomal recessive	
Trapped neutrophil syndrome	Border Collie	Autosomal recessive	Yes
Severe combined immunodeficiency (SCID)	Jack Russell Terrier Parson Russell Terrier Frisian Water Dog Arab horses	Autosomal recessive	Yes

(*continued*)

Table 15.5 (*Continued*)

Condition	Breed	Inheritance	Test available
X-linked severe combined immunodeficiency (X-SCID)	Bassett Hound Welsh Corgi	X-linked recessive	Yes
Lavender foal syndrome (LFS) or coat colour dilution lethal (CCDL)	Arab horses	Autosomal recessive	Yes
Lethal white foal syndrome	Paint Horse Pinto Horse Quarter Horse	Autosomal recessive	Yes
Renal cystadenocarcinoma and nodular dermatofibrosis	German Shepherd Dog	Autosomal dominant	Yes
Ligneous membranitis	Scottish Terrier	Autosomal recessive	No
Acral mutilation syndrome	Cocker Spaniel Brittany Spaniel English Springer Spaniel English Pointer German Short-Haired Pointer	Autosomal recessive	Yes
Connemara pony hoof wall separation disease	Connemara	Autosomal recessive	Yes

- affected or at risk (n/n, JEB/JEB, -/- or homozygous mutant); affected is normally used for animals that already exhibit the condition, whereas at risk is used for animals that are likely to develop the condition later in life;
- some laboratories will also give the actual DNA bases affected in each allele, e.g. A/A, A/G or G/G.

The format of the results may differ a little for dominant and sex-linked alleles. Testing for complex traits or alleles with lower penetrance is limited at present, but may become more frequent. The results for these tests are likely to be more nuanced, with less precise genetic data and more information about the genotype–phenotype correlation (e.g. there is a 70% chance that dogs with this genotype will develop atopic dermatitis before 3 years of age; there is 80% likelihood that dogs born to parents with this genotype will subsequently develop atopic dermatitis).

The results should also include the exact gene and alleles tested for, as some conditions may be associated with more than one allele and not all variants may have been tested (if indeed tests exist for all the variants). The evidence associating the condition with the tested gene should also be referenced. Finally, the laboratory should provide clear advice on the clinical and breeding significance of the results.

Using Genetic Tests to Confirm a Diagnosis

Genetic tests can be used to confirm a diagnosis, although it is important that the history and clinical signs are compatible with the diagnosis, and that, if appropriate, differential diagnoses have been ruled out. For example, nasal ulceration is most likely to be due to

Table 15.6   Relationship between genotype and clinical phenotype.

Genotype	Clinical phenotype	
	Dominant allele	Recessive allele
normal/normal	Unaffected	Unaffected
normal/abnormal	Affected	Unaffected carrier
abnormal/abnormal	Affected	Affected

hereditary nasal parakeratosis in a Labrador Retriever that is homozygous for the affected gene but this does not necessary **eliminate** other problems, such as discoid lupus erythematosus and squamous cell carcinoma.

In theory, genetic testing should have 100% specificity and 100% sensitivity. However, incorrect test results may be associated with poor sample collection (not enough DNA, DNA contamination and labelling errors), laboratory error (including DNA contamination) and poor correlation of the genotype with the condition (this is rare with most single-gene disorders with high penetrance, but may be significant if multiple-gene variants exist, with complex traits and with incomplete penetrance). A negative result does not therefore exclude all possible gene defects and cannot be used to absolutely rule out the condition. Different gene variants are a particular problem between different breeds, and it should not be assumed that a test validated in one breed will work in another breed even if the condition appears to the same.

In single-gene disorders showing classical or Mendelian inheritance, the genotype usually predicts the clinical phenotype (Table 15.6). However, the interpretation can complicated by non-Mendelian factors such as incomplete penetrance, incomplete or co-dominance, multiple alleles at a locus with a complex pattern of dominance, chromosome abnormalities, polygenic inheritance, and environmental triggers and factors. Some tests may therefore only predict the risk of the disease occurring in an individual. It is important to check the published information about the test for a condition and, if necessary, speak to the laboratory that performed the test.

Other Uses of Genetic Tests

A wide range of tests to predict coat colour, colour patterns, length and type are available. Breeders use these to predict and plan mating outcomes for desired traits. Identity and parentage tests using micro satellite marker analysis are also available. DNA profiling can also be used to determine assignment probabilities to particular breeds for any individual, assessing whether it is purebred, half-bred or the likely contributions of breeds in a cross-bred animal.

Breeding Advice

Breeding advice can be challenging and fraught with potential problems. Any advice must be evidence based, and you may need to discuss this with a specialist or the DNA

Table 15.7 Glossary of genetic terms

Autosomal	Inheritance through a non sex chromosome (i.e. not X or Y)
Allele	One of two or more forms of a gene or DNA sequence on a chromosome that may be associated with a phenotypic trait. Diploid organisms can be homozygous (i.e. two copies of the same allele) or heterozygous (i.e. two different alleles)
Dominant	A dominant allele will mask the phenotypic expression of a recessive allele at the same locus; phenotypic expression will occur with either one (heterozygous) or two (homozygous) dominant alleles
Exon	DNA sequences within a gene that make up the final RNA transcript; usually separated by one or more introns in a gene
Genotype	The specific genetic makeup of an individual. The genotype, epigenetic factors (i.e. changes in gene expression not associated with the DNA sequence) and environmental influences determine the phenotype
Haplotype	A combination of alleles at adjacent loci on the chromosome that are inherited together. Haplotype also refers to a set of SNPs on a single chromosome that are statistically associated
Intron	DNA sequences within a gene that are removed during transcription to produce the final RNA sequence
Linkage disequilibrium	Non-random association of alleles at two or more loci, which may be on the same or different chromosomes
Locus	Specific location of a gene or DNA sequence on a chromosome
Microsatellite markers	Polymorphic repeating sequences of two to six base pairs throughout the genome used in inheritance studies (simple sequence repeats [SSRs] or short tandem repeats [STRs])
Penetrance	The proportion of individuals with a particular genotype that develop the associated phenotype
Phenotype	An individual's observable characteristics or traits. These may include morphology, development, physiology, behaviour and/or disease states
Population stratification	Differences in allele frequencies between groups in a study population that are associated with ancestry (e.g. race, breed, geography, etc.) rather than a disease condition
Recessive	The effect on the phenotype of the recessive allele will be masked by a second allele at the same locus; phenotypic expression requires two recessive alleles at the same locus on each chromosome (i.e. homozygous)
Sex-linked	Inheritance through a sex chromosome (i.e. X or Y); often referred to as X-linked as Y-chromosomes carry very few genes Male offspring always inherit their X chromosome from their mother Female offspring always inherit one X chromosome from their father and one from their mother
Single nucleotide polymorphisms (SNPs)	A difference in single nucleotide (A, T, C or G) in a DNA sequence – for example AGC**C**TA and AGC**T**TA

testing laboratory. It is fairly straightforward to discuss conditions associated with single gene and allele defects as the patterns of inheritance are well understood, provided that the inheritance follows the classical or Mendelian genetic model. This pattern can be complicated by multiple alleles at a locus with complex patterns of dominance, co-dominance and incomplete penetrance, where traits can be said to 'not breed true'. In addition, many conditions involve multiple genes and/or the genotype may only increase the risk of the condition developing, which requires further triggers. Other complications include missing or duplicated chromosomes (e.g. XXY or XXYY). The outcome of breeding from an animal with a particular phenotype or genotype can therefore be unpredictable.

The frequency of the affected allele in a population can also cause a problem. For example, ichthyosis genotype frequencies in Swiss Golden Retrievers are 31% affected (abnormal/abnormal), 49% carriers (abnormal/normal), and only 20% unaffected (normal/normal) dogs. A strict approach would exclude 80% of the breeding population, severely restricting the available gene pool. This is a mild disease and producing some affected dogs may be preferable to extreme inbreeding that could spread other potentially more severe recessive traits in the breed. Therefore, a more sustainable approach could be mate to unaffected animals to carriers to limit the number of affected animals and more gradually lower the frequency of the abnormal allele within a population. Genetic counselling and advice should be discussed with specialists in each case.

Further Reading

General Reading and Guidance

Bexfield N, Lee K (2014) *BSAVA Guide to Procedures in Small Animal Practice* 2nd edn. BSAVA, Gloucester, UK.

Bilbrough G (2016) In-house versus external testing. In: *BSAVA Manual of Canine and Feline Clinical Pathology* 3rd edn. (eds E Villiers, J Ristic). BSAVA, Gloucester, UK. pp. 1–10.

Jackson H, Marsella R (2012) *BSAVA Manual of Canine and Feline Dermatology* 3rd edn. BSAVA, Gloucester, UK.

Mecklenburg L, Linek M, Tobin DJ (2009) *Hair Loss Disorders in Domestic Animals.* Wiley-Blackwell, Ames, IA.

Meredith A, Johnson-Delaney C (2010) *BSAVA Manual of Exotic Pets* 5th edn. BSAVA, Gloucester, UK.

Miller WH, Griffin CE, Campbell KL (2013) Diagnostic methods. In: *Muller and Kirk's Small Animal Dermatology*. Elsevier Mosby, St Louis, MO. pp. 57–107.

Monti P, Archer J (2016) Quality assurance and interpretation of laboratory data. In: *BSAVA Manual of Canine and Feline Clinical Pathology* 3rd edn. (eds E Villiers, J Ristic). BSAVA, Gloucester. pp. 11–26.

Nuttall TJ (2016) Laboratory evaluation of skin disease. In: *BSAVA Manual of Canine and Feline Clinical Pathology* 3rd edn. (eds E Villiers, J Ristic). BSAVA, Gloucester. pp. 492–510.

Palmeiro BS, Roberts H (2013) Clinical approach to dermatologic disease in exotic animals. *Veterinary Clinics of North America – Exotic Animal Practice* 16, 523–577.

Histopathology

Gross TL, Ihrke PJ, Walder EJ and others (2005) *Skin Diseases of the Dog and Cat* 2nd edn. Blackwell Publishing, Oxford.

Shearer DH (2012) Dermatopathology. In: *BSAVA Manual of Canine and Feline Dermatology* 3rd edn. (eds H Jackson, R Marsella). BSAVA, Gloucester, UK. pp. 31–36.

Yager JA (2014) Erythema multiforme, Stevens-Johnson syndrome and toxic epidermal necrolysis: a comparative review. *Veterinary Dermatology* 25, 406–413.

Cytology

Cowell RL, Tyler RD, Meinkoth JH (2008) *Diagnostic Cytology and Haematology of the Dog and Cat* 3rd edn. Elsevier-Mosby, St Louis, MO.

Mendelsohn C, Rosenkrantz WS, Griffin CE (2006) Practical cytology for inflammatory skin diseases. *Clinical Techniques in Small Animal Practice* 21, 117–127.

Monti P, Cian F (2016) Diagnostic cytology. In: *BSAVA Manual of Canine and Feline Clinical Pathology* 3rd edn. (eds E Villiers, J Ristic). BSAVA, Gloucester. pp. 398–434.

Paparcone R, Fiorentino E, Cappiello S and others (2013) Sternal aspiration of bone marrow in dogs: a practical approach for canine leishmaniasis diagnosis and monitoring. *Journal of Veterinary Medicine* Volume 2013, Article ID 217314, 4 pages, http://dx.doi.org/10.1155/2013/217314.

Raskin RE, Meyer DJ (2010) *Canine and Feline Cytology: a Colour Atlas and Interpretation Guide*. Saunders Elsevier, St Louis, MO.

Sharkey LC, Dial SM, Matz SE (2007) Maximising the diagnostic value of cytology in small animal practice. *Veterinary Clinics of North America – Small Animal Practice* 37, 351–372.

Ectoparasite

Fondati A, De Lucia M, Furiani N and others (2010) Prevalence of *Demodex canis* positive dogs at trichoscopic examination. *Veterinary Dermatology* 21, 146–151.

Lower KS, Medleau LM, Hnilica K and others (2001). Evaluation of an enzyme-linked immunosorbent assay (ELISA) for the serological diagnosis of sarcoptic mange in dogs. *Veterinary Dermatology* 12, 315–320.

Milley C, Dryden M, Rosenkrantz WS and others (2016) Comparison of parasitic mite retrieval methods in a population of community cats. *Journal of Feline Medicine and Surgery*. Online early publication. DOI: 10.1177/1098612X16650717.

Pereira AV, Pereira SA, Gremião ID and others (2012). Comparison of acetate tape impression with squeezing versus skin scraping for the diagnosis of canine demodicosis. *Australian Veterinary Journal* 90, 448–450.

Otitis

Griffin CE (2006) Otitis techniques to improve practice. *Clinical Techniques in Small Animal Practice* 21, 96–105.

Harvey RG, Paterson S (2014) *Otitis Externa: an Essential Guide to Diagnosis and Treatment*. CRC Press, Boca Raton, FL.

Kennis RA (2013) Feline otitis: diagnosis and treatment. *Veterinary Clinics of North America – Small Animal Practice* 43, 51–63.

Lehner G, Louis CS, Mueller RS (2010) Reproducibility of ear cytology in dogs with otitis externa. *Veterinary Record* 167, 23–26.

Newton HM, Rosenkrantz WS, Muse R and others (2006) Evaluation of otoscope cleaning and disinfection procedures commonly used in veterinary medical practices: a pilot study. *Veterinary Dermatology* 17, 147–150.

Paterson S, Tobias K (2013) *Atlas of Ear Diseases of the Dog and Cat*. Wiley Blackwell, Oxford, UK.

Radlinsky MAG (2016) Advances in otoscopy. *Veterinary Clinics of North America – Small Animal Practice* 46, 171–183.

Strain GM, Fernandes AJ (2015) Handheld tympanometer measurements in conscious dogs for the evaluation of the middle ear and auditory tube. *Veterinary Dermatology* 26, 193–197.

Toma S, Cornegliani L, Persico P and others (2006) Comparison of 4 fixation and staining methods for the cytologic evaluation of ear canals with clinical evidence of ceruminous otitis externa. *Veterinary Clinical Pathology* 35, 194–198.

Diagnosis of Pyoderma and Antimicrobial Susceptibility Testing

Beco L, Guaguère E, Lorente Mendez C, Noli C, Nuttall TJ, Vroom M (2013) Suggested guidelines for using systemic antimicrobials in bacterial skin infections: part one – diagnosis based on clinical presentation, cytology and culture. *Veterinary Record* 172, 72–78.

Beco L, Guaguère E, Lorente Mendez C, Noli C, Nuttall TJ, Vroom M (2013) Suggested guidelines for using systemic antimicrobials in bacterial skin infections: part two – antimicrobial choice, treatment regimens and compliance. *Veterinary Record* 172, 156–160.

Blondeau JM (2009) New concepts in antimicrobial susceptibility testing: the mutant prevention concentration and mutant selection window approach. *Veterinary Dermatology* 20, 383–396.

Brissot H, Cervantes S, Guardabassi L, Hibbert A, Lefebvre H, Mateus A, Noli C, Nuttall TJ, Pomba C, Schulz B (2016) *GRAM: Guidance for the Rational Use of Antimicrobials – Recommendations for Dogs and Cats* 2ⁿᵈ edn. Ceva Santé Animale, France.

Clinical and Laboratory Standards Institute (CLSI) (2015) *Performance Standards for Antimicrobial Disk and Dilution Susceptibility Tests for Bacteria Isolated from Animals* 3ʳᵈ edn. CLSI document Vet01-S. Wayne, PA.

Clinical and Laboratory Standards Institute (CLSI) (2016) *Performance Standards for Antimicrobial Susceptibility Testing* 26ᵗʰ edn. CLSI document M100-S. Wayne, PA.

Drlica K (2003) The mutant selection window and antimicrobial resistance. *Journal of Antimicrobial Chemotherapy* 52, 11–17.

Hillier A, Lloyd DH, Weese JS and others (2014) Guidelines for the diagnosis and antimicrobial therapy of canine superficial bacterial folliculitis (Antimicrobial Guidelines Working Group of the International Society for Companion Animal Infectious Diseases). *Veterinary Dermatology* 25, 163–175.

Nuttall TJ (2013) Choosing the best antimicrobial for the job. *Veterinary Record* 172, 12–13.

Rodrigues Hoffmann A, Patterson AP, Diesel A, Lawhon SD, Ly HJ and others (2014) *The Skin Microbiome in Healthy and Allergic Dogs*. PLoS ONE 9: e83197.

VetCAST (2015) Subcommittee of EUCAST (European Committee on Antimicrobial Susceptibility Testing) www.eucast.org/ast_of_veterinary_pathogens/(last accessed 13 Nov 2016).

Malassezia

Nuttall TJ, Halliwell RE (2001) Serum antibodies to *Malassezia* yeasts in canine atopic dermatitis. *Veterinary Dermatology* 12, 327–332.
Velegraki A, Cafarchia C, Gaitanis G and others (2015) *Malassezia* infections in humans and animals: pathophysiology, detection, and treatment. *PLoS Pathology* 11 e1004523.

Dermatophytosis

Chung TH, Park GB, Lim CY and others (2010) A rapid molecular method for diagnosing epidemic dermatophytosis in a racehorse facility. *Equine Veterinary Journal* 42, 73–78.
Moriella KA (2001) Diagnostic techniques for dermatophytosis. *Clinical Techniques in Small Animal Practice* 16, 219–224.

Other Bacterial, Mycobacterial, Fungal, Viral and Protozoal Infections

Allison RW, Little SE (2013) Diagnosis of rickettsial diseases in dogs and cats. *Veterinary Clinical Pathology* 42, 127–144.
García A, Martínez R, Benitez-Medina JM and others, (2013) Development of a real-time SYBR Green PCR assay for the rapid detection of *Dermatophilus congolensis*. *Journal of Veterinary Science* 14, 491–494.
Hegarty BC, Qurollo BA, Thomas B and others, (2015) Serological and molecular analysis of feline vector-borne anaplasmosis and ehrlichiosis using species-specific peptides and PCR. *Parasites and Vectors* 8, 320.
Jagger T (2016) Diagnosis of bacterial, fungal and mycobacterial diseases. In: *BSAVA Manual of Canine and Feline Clinical Pathology* 3rd edn. (eds E Villiers, J Ristic). BSAVA, Gloucester. pp. 511–532.
Krupa I, Straubinger RK (2010) Lyme borreliosis in dogs and cats: background, diagnosis, treatment and prevention of infections with *Borrelia burgdorferi* sensu stricto. *Veterinary Clinics of North America – Small Animal Practice* 40, 1103–1119.
Lappin MR (2010) Update on the diagnosis and management of *Toxoplasma gondii* infection in cats. *Topics in Companion Animal Medicine* 25, 136–141.
Paltrinieri S, Solano-Gallego L, Fondati A and others (2010) Guidelines for diagnosis and clinical classification of leishmaniosis in dogs. *Journal of the American Veterinary Medical Association* 236, 1184–1191.
Radford A, Dawson S (2016) Diagnosis of viral infections. In: *BSAVA Manual of Canine and Feline Clinical Pathology* 3rd edn. (eds E Villiers, J Ristic). BSAVA, Gloucester. pp. 533–540.

Shirian S, Oryan A, Hatam G-R and others (2014) Comparison of conventional, molecular, and immunohistochemical methods in diagnosis of typical and atypical cutaneous leishmaniasis. *Archives of Pathology and Laboratory Medicine* 138, 235–240.

Solano-Gallego L, Koutinas A, Miró G and others (2009) Directions for the diagnosis, clinical staging, treatment and prevention of canine leishmaniosis. *Veterinary Parasitology* 165, 1–18.

Solano-Gallego L, Miro G, Koutinas A and others (2011) LeishVet guidelines for the practical management of canine leishmaniosis. *Parasite Vectors* 4, 86.

Solano-Gallego L, Banetha G (2016) Diagnosis of protozoal and arthropod borne diseases. In: *BSAVA Manual of Canine and Feline Clinical Pathology* 3rd edn. (eds E Villiers, J Ristic). BSAVA, Gloucester. pp. 549–566.

Stillman BA, M Monn, J Liu and others (2014) Performance of a commercially available in-clinic ELISA for the detection of antibodies to *Anaplasma phagocytophilum, Anaplasma platys, Borrelia burgdorferi, Ehrlichia canis* and *Ehrlichia ewingii*, and *Dirofilaria immitis* antigen in dogs. *Journal of the American Veterinary Medical Association* 245, 80–86.

Yancey CB, Hegarty BC, Qurollo BA and others (2014) Regional seroreactivity and vector-borne disease co-exposures in dogs in the United States from 2004–2010: utility of canine surveillance. *Vector Borne Zoonotic Diseases* 14, 724–732.

Atopic Dermatitis, Food Trials and Allergy Testing

Baxter CG, Vogelnest LJ (2008) Determination of threshold concentrations of multiple allergenic extracts for equine intradermal testing using normal horses in three seasons. *Veterinary Dermatology* 19, 305–313.

Bethlehem S, Bexley J, Mueller RS (2012) Patch testing and allergen-specific serum IgE and IgG antibodies in the diagnosis of canine adverse food reactions. *Veterinary Immunology and Immunopathology* 145, 582–589.

Bexley J, Nuttall TJ, Hammerberg J and others (2013) Serum anti-*Staphylococcus pseudintermedius* IgE and IgG antibodies in dogs with atopic dermatitis. *Veterinary Dermatology* 24, 19–24.

Bexley J, Nuttall TJ, Hammerberg B and others (2016) Serological cross-reactivity between beef, lamb and cow's milk allergen extracts in dogs. *Veterinary Dermatology*. Online early publication. DOI: 10.1111/vde.12335.

Buckley L, Schmidt V, McEwan NA and others (2013) Cross-reaction or co-sensitisation among related allergens in canine intradermal tests. *Veterinary Dermatology* 24, 422–427.

Hardy JI, Hendricks A, Loeffler A and others (2014) Food specific serum IgE and IgG reactivity in dogs with and without skin disease: lack of correlation between laboratories. *Veterinary Dermatology* 25, 447–e70.

Fadok VA (2013) Update on equine allergies. *Veterinary Clinics of North America – Equine Practice* 29, 541–550.

Favrot C, Steffan J, Seewald W and others (2012) Establishment of diagnostic criteria for feline non flea induced hypersensitivity dermatitis. *Veterinary Dermatology* 23, 45–50.

Hensel P, Santoro D, Favrot C and others (2015) Canine atopic dermatitis: detailed guidelines for diagnosis and allergen identification. *BMC Veterinary Research* 11, 196.

Hobi S, Linek M, Marignac G and others (2011) Clinical characteristics and causes of pruritus in cats: a multicentre study on feline hypersensitivity-associated dermatoses. *Veterinary Dermatology* 22, 406–413.

Kunzle F, Gerber V, Van Der Haegen A and others (2007) IgE-bearing cells in bronchoalveolar lavage fluid and allergen-specific IgE levels in sera from RAO-affected horses. *Journal of Veterinary Medicine series A – Physiology, Pathology and Clinical Medicine* 54, 40–47.

Langner KF, Darpel KE, Drolet BS and others (2008) Comparison of cellular and humoral immunoassays for the assessment of summer eczema in horses. *Veterinary Immunology and Immunopathology* 122, 126–137.

Mueller RS, Thierry Olivry T, Prélaud P (2016) Critically appraised topic on adverse food reactions of companion animals (2): common food allergen sources in dogs and cats. *BMC Veterinary Research* 12, 9.

Noli C, Foster A, Rosenkrantz WS (2014) *Veterinary Allergy*. Wiley, Chichester, UK.

Olivry T, Mueller RS, Prélaud P and others (2015) Critically appraised topic on adverse food reactions of companion animals (1): duration of elimination diets. *BMC Veterinary Research* 11, 225.

Peeters LM, Janssens S, Goddeeris BM and others (2013) Evaluation of an IgE ELISA with *Culicoides* spp. extracts and recombinant salivary antigens for diagnosis of insect bite hypersensitivity in Warmblood horses. *Veterinary Journal* 198, 141–147.

Ricci R, Granato A, Vascellari M (2013) Identification of undeclared sources of animal origin in canine dry foods used in dietary elimination trials. *Journal of Animal Physiology and Animal Nutrition* 97, 32–38.

Rybnicek J, Lau-Gillard PJ, Harvey R and others (2010) Further validation of a pruritus severity scale for use in dogs. *Veterinary Dermatology* 20, 115–122.

Vogelnest LI, Cheng KY (2013) Cutaneous adverse food reactions in cats: retrospective evaluation of 17 cases in a dermatology referral population (2001–2011). *Australian Veterinary Journal* 91, 443–451.

White SD (2015) A diagnostic approach to the pruritic horse. *Equine Veterinary Education* 27, 156–166.

Wilhelm S, Kovalik M, Favrot C (2015) Breed-associated phenotypes in canine atopic dermatitis. *Veterinary Dermatology* 22, 143–149.

Genetic Testing

Grall A, Guaguère E, Planchais S and others (2012) PNPLA1 mutations cause autosomal recessive congenital ichthyosis in golden retriever dogs and humans. *Nature Genetics* 44, 140–147.

Nicholas FW (2009) *Introduction to Veterinary Genetics* 3rd edn. Wiley-Blackwell, Chichester, UK.

Nodtvedt A, Bergvall K, Sallander M and others (2007) A case-control study of risk factors for canine atopic dermatitis among boxer, bullterrier and West Highland white terrier dogs in Sweden. *Veterinary Dermatology* 18, 309–315.

Nuttall TJ (2014) The genomics revolution in canine atopic dermatitis. In: *Veterinary Allergy* (eds C Noli, AP Foster, WA Rosenkrantz). Wiley-Blackwell, Oxford. pp. 32–41.

Owczarek-Lipska M, Thomas A, André C and others (2011) Häufigkeit von Gendefekten in ausgewählten europäischen Retriever Populationen. *Schweizer Archive fur Tierheilkunder* 153, 418–420.

Shaw SC, Wood JLN, Freeman J and others (2004) Estimation of heritability of atopic dermatitis in Labrador and Golden Retrievers. *American Journal of Veterinary Research* 65 1014–1020.

Starkey MP, Scase TJ, Mellersh CS and others (2005) Dogs really are man's best friend – canine genomics has applications in veterinary and human medicine! *Briefings in Functional Genomics and Proteomics* 4, 112–128.

Wood SH, Ollier WE, Nuttall T (2010) Despite identifying some shared gene associations with human atopic dermatitis the use of multiple dog breeds from various locations limits detection of gene associations in canine atopic dermatitis. *Veterinary Immunology and Immunopathology* 138, 193–197.

Autoimmune and Immune-Mediated Diseases

Banovic F, Linder KE, Olivry T (2016) Clinical, microscopic and microbial characterization of exfoliative superficial pyoderma-associated epidermal collarettes in dogs. *Veterinary Dermatology*. Online early publication. DOI: 10.1111/vde.12352.

Hansson-Hamlin H, Lilliehook I, Trowald-Wigh G (2006) Subgroups of canine antinuclear antibodies in relation to laboratory and clinical findings in immune-mediated disease. *Veterinary Clinical Pathology* 35, 397–404.

Endocrine Testing

Behrend EN, Kooistra HS, Nelson R and others (2013) Diagnosis of spontaneous canine hyperadrenocorticism: 2012 ACVIM Consensus Statement (Small Animal). *Journal of Veterinary Internal Medicine* 27, 1292–1304.

Frank LA, Henry GA, Whittlemore JC and others (2015) Serum cortisol concentrations in dogs with pituitary dependent hyperadrenocorticism and atypical hyperadrenocorticism. *Journal of Veterinary Internal Medicine* 29, 193–199.

Graham PA, Mooney CT (2016) Laboratory evaluation of hypothyroidism and hyperthyroidism. In: *BSAVA Manual of Canine and Feline Clinical Pathology* 3rd edn. (eds E Villiers, J Ristic). BSAVA, Gloucester. pp. 333–352.

Hill KE, Scott-Moncrieff JC, Koshko MA and others (2005) Secretion of sex hormones in dogs with adrenal dysfunction. *Journal of the American Veterinary Medical Association* 226, 556–561.

Monroe WE, Panciera DL, Zimmerman KL (2012) Concentrations of non-cortisol adrenal steroids in response to ACTH in dogs with adrenal dependent hyperadrenocorticism, pituitary dependent hyperadrenocorticism and non-adrenal illness. *Journal of Veterinary Internal Medicine* 26, 945–952.

Mooney CT (2011) Canine hypothyroidism – a review of the aetiology and diagnosis. *New Zealand Veterinary Journal* 59, 105–114.

Ramsey I, Herrtage M (2016) Laboratory evaluation of adrenal diseases. In: *BSAVA Manual of Canine and Feline Clinical Pathology* 3rd edn. (eds E Villiers, J Ristic). BSAVA, Gloucester. pp. 353–372.

Sheil RE, Mooney CT (2007) Testing for hyperthyroidism in cats. *Veterinary Clinics of North America – Small Animal Practice* 37, 671–691.

Sheil RE, Sist M, Nachreiner RE and others (2010) Assessment of criteria used by veterinary practitioners to diagnose hypothyroidism in sighthounds and investigation of serum thyroid hormone concentrations in healthy salukis. *Journal of the American Veterinary Medical Association* 236, 302–308.

Zeugswetter FK, Bydzovsky N, Kampner D and others (2010) Tailored reference limits for urine cortisol:creatinine ratio in dogs to answer distinct clinical questions. *Veterinary Record* 167, 997–1001.

Dermoscopy

Dong C, Angus J, Scarampella F and others (2016) Evaluation of dermoscopy in the diagnosis of naturally occurring dermatophytosis in cats. *Veterinary Dermatology* 27, 275–e65.

Scarampella F, Zanna G, Peano A, Tosti A (2015) Dermoscopic features in 12 cats with dermatophytosis and in 12 cats with self-induced alopecia due to other causes: an observational descriptive study. *Veterinary Dermatology* 26, 282–e63.

Scarampella F, Zanna G (2015) Dermoscopy of canine and feline alopecia. In: *Dermoscopy of the Hair and Nails* 2nd edn. (ed. A Tosti). CRC Press, Boca Raton, FL. pp. 155–158.

Zanna G, Auriemma E, Arrighi S and others (2014) Dermoscopic evaluation of skin in healthy cats. *Veterinary Dermatology* 26, 14–e4.

Zanna G, Roccabianca P, Zini E and others (2016) The usefulness of dermoscopy in canine pattern alopecia: a descriptive study. *Veterinary Dermatology*. Online early publication. DOI: 10.1111/vde.12359.

Index

Note: page numbers in *italics* indicate figures and those in **bold** indicate tables.

acanthocytes   67
acantholytic cells
   cytology   65–67, *66*, 253
   histopathology   114, *114, 115*, **168**
acanthosis   112
acanthosis nigricans   269–271
acral mutilation syndrome   **284**
acromegaly   196
ACTH
   endogenous   192, *193*, 195
   stimulation test   186, 187–188,
      187–188, 194
Addison's disease   186, *188*
adhesive tape   *2*, 5
   avian skin biopsy   108, *109*
   fungal staining   14–15
   mounting coat brushings   24
   mounting hair plucks   29, 41
   skin sampling with *see* tape-strips
adrenal glands, ultrasonography   195,
      226–229, *227*
adrenal tumours   193
   biochemical tests   186, 187–188, 189,
      192
   imaging   192, 228, 229
adrenocorticotrophic hormone *see* ACTH
agglutination test   202, *202*
alanine aminotransferase (ALT)   179,
      180
albinism, oculocutaneous   **283**
alcohol   87, 89
algae   74
alkaline phosphatase (ALP)   179, 180

allergens
   environmental allergy
      testing   145–157
   extracts and mixes   146–148
   selection   146, **147–148**
   see also food allergens
allergen-specific immunotherapy
      (ASIT)   146, 156
allergen-specific (IgE) serology
      (ASIS)   146, 156
   drug withdrawal periods   148–149,
      149
   food allergens   145
allergy testing   125–157
   allergen extracts and mixes   146–148
   allergen selection   146, **147–148**
   drug withdrawal   148–149
   environmental allergens   145–157
   equipment   6, *8*
   food allergens   125–145
   food trials   125–144
      see also food trials
   indications   145–146
   intradermal *see* intradermal allergen
      tests
   Malassezia and staphylococci   156
   patch testing   145, 156–157, *157*
   serological *see* allergen-specific (IgE)
      serology
   skin prick testing   156
alopecia   *265*, 265–269
   clinical features   **266–267**
   colour-dilution   48–50, *49*, **283**

Diagnostic Techniques in Veterinary Dermatology, First Edition. Ariane Neuber and Tim Nuttall.
© 2017 Ariane Neuber and Tim Nuttall. Published 2017 by John Wiley & Sons, Ltd.

alopecia (*Continued*)
  cyclical (recurrent or seasonal)
      flank   44, *44*
  endocrine and metabolic
      diseases   173–174, 175–176
  feline paraneoplastic   231
  focal or multifocal   267, **267, 268**
  of follicular arrest   44, *45*
  hereditary   **282**
  histopathology   **117**
  hyperadrenocorticism   173–174, *177*
  hypothyroidism   173, *174–176*
  minimum database   267–269
  parasitic infections   21, *22*
  pinnal   *237*, 238
  steroid hormone assays   195
  symmetrical or diffuse   **267,** 267–269,
      268
  ulcers and erosions   **274**
alopecia areata (AA)   45, *46*, **168, 273**
alopecia X   44, *45*
  histopathology   *123*, 124
  steroid hormone testing   187, 195
amber coat colour mutation   **282**
amikacin   **96**
amino acid levels   196–197
amoxicillin(-clavulanate)   95, **96**
ampicillin   **96**
anaemia   178, 179
anagen defluxion   44, 45
anagen hairs   42, *43*, 44
anti-erythrocyte antibodies
      (AEABs)   170
antifungal susceptibility testing   104
antihistamines   149, **149**
antimicrobial resistance, suspected   84
antimicrobial sensitivity testing   89–97
  breakpoints   92, 93
  calculating drug doses   93, 94
  failed antibiotic therapy   83, *84*
  intermediate results   94
  Kirby-Bauer disc diffusion   90–92,
      91
  methods compared   90–92
  minimum inhibitory
      concentration   90–95, *91*
  mismatches with clinical response   95
  mutant prevention concentration   97,
      97
  otitis externa   92–93, *93*, 253
  predicting patterns   95–97, **96**
  predicting treatment response   92–94,
      93
  topical therapy and   94–95
anti-nuclear antibodies (ANA)   169
anti-platelet antibodies   170
apoptosis   115, *116*, **168**
arteritis of the nasal philtrum,
      proliferative   **273**
Arthroderma   101
aspartate aminotransferase (AST)   180
atopic dermatitis (AD)   125
  allergy testing   145, 146–157
      see also *allergy testing*
  diagnostic criteria   125, 126
  external ear   *237, 238, 264*
  food-induced see food-induced atopic
      dermatitis
  food trials   125–144
      see also *food trials*
  lesion distribution   **128–129,** 259, *260*
  skin microbiome   81, *82*
  vs. flea allergic dermatitis   37–38
atopic-like dermatitis (ALD)   125
atrophic pattern   122
autoimmune subepidermal blistering
      diseases (AISBDs)   121, 167, 168,
      168, 275
autosomal dominant disorders   277, *278*,
      279
autosomal recessive disorders   277, **278,**
      278
avian patients, biopsy   108, *109*

Babesia   210
bacilli (rod-shaped bacteria)   75, 83, *83*
bacteria
  antimicrobial sensitivity
      testing   89–97
      see also antimicrobial sensitivity
      testing
  commensal   81, *82*
  cytology   74–76
  detecting unusual   103–104

extracellular   71, 74–75
intracellular   71, 74
mimics   75–76
mucosal reservoirs   83
otic cytology   248–253, *249, 251–252*
transient   81
bacterial cultures   83–97
antibiotic-treated patients   85
common pitfalls   97
ear disease   253
indications   83–85
interpretation   89–97
sample collection   85–89
see also antimicrobial sensitivity testing
bacterial overgrowth syndrome   74
ballooning degeneration   114
BARF (biologically appropriate raw food or bones) diet   129–130
Bartonella   209
basket weave hyperkeratosis   112
basophils   69
berry bugs *see* harvest mites
biopsy   105–110
ear canal   255–256
equipment   5, *6*
immune-mediated diseases   160–169
indications   105
prior medical therapy   106
punch   107–108
site preparation   106–107
site selection   106
submission of samples   17, 109–110
technique   107–108, *109*
for tissue culture   89
wedge excision   108
Blastomyces   73
blood agar plate   *90*
blood samples, equipment   5, *7*
bone marrow samples   206–209, *208, 209*
Borrelia   209
brainstem auditory evoked responses (BAER)   255
breeding advice   285–287
brown and yellow coat   **283**
bulbitis   122
bullous dermatitis   121
bullous pemphigoid (BP)   **168, 275**

C3 deficiency   **283**
calcinosis cutis   174, *177*, 228–229
calcofluor-white   **16**
calicivirus, feline (FCV)   212
cameras, microscope   *3*, 8
canalography   223, 246
canine leucocyte adhesion deficiency   **283**
carcinomatous acanthosis   112
caseous necrosis   114
cefotaxime   **96**
cefoxitin   **96**
ceftazidime   93, *93*
cell cultures   211
cephalexin   **96**
Chediak–Higashi syndrome   271, **283**
Cheyletiella   36, *40*
coat brushings   24
eggs   50, *51*
tape-strips   28
visual inspection   23, *23, 27*
chiggers (*Eutrombicula* spp.)   22, 35
chloramphenicol   **96**
cholesterol, serum   179, 180
Chorioptes   23, 24
Civatte bodies   115
clefts
subepidermal   **168**
suprabasilar   **168**
clindamycin   95, **96**
clippers, electric   3
coagulative necrosis   115
coat brushings/combings
fungal cultures   *87*, 87–88
parasites   23, 24–25
coat colour dilution lethal   **284**
Coccidioides   73
coeliac disease   130
cold agglutinin titres   171
coliforms   75
colour-dilution alopecia   48–50, *49*, **283**
colour point   **282**
comedones   *22, 31*
comma-like hairs   55, 99
commensal organisms   81, *82*
compact hyperkeratosis   112
complement-fixation test   202–204, *203*

compliance, diet trials   142–143
computed tomography (CT)
   ear disease   224–225, *226*, 247
   endocrine disease   228, *228*
   other uses   233, 234
congenital keratoconjunctivitis sicca and ichthyosiform dermatosis (CKSID)   **282**
Congo red   **16**
Connemara pony hoof wall separation disease   **284**
cooked foods   129–130
Coomb's tests   169–170
cortisol, plasma
   ACTH stimulation test   187–188, *187–188*
   baseline   186
   see also dexamethasone suppression test
cortisol:creatinine ratio, urinary *see* urinary cortisol:creatinine ratio
corynebacteria   75
cotton buds   *2*, 5, *5*
   ear canal sampling   25, 62–63
   indirect impression smears   61
cover-slips   3, *4*, 11
cowpox, feline   212
creatine kinase (CK)   179
creatinine, plasma   180
crusts   111, *111*, **117,** 269, **274**
   minimum database   269
   pemphigus foliaceus   162, *163*
   pinnal margins   238
Cryptococcus   73
CT *see* computed tomography
Ctenocephalides felis felis   *39*
cultures, microbiological   83–97
   indications   83–85
   obtaining material for   85–89
   see also bacterial cultures; fungal cultures
Cushing's disease *see* hyperadrenocorticism
cutaneous adverse food reactions (CAFR)   125–145
   allergen testing   145
   food trials   125–144

cutaneous and renal glomerular vasculopathy   **273**
cutaneous lupus erythematosus (CLE)   162, *167*, 167–168
   exfoliative (ECLE)   **168, 274**
   vesicular (VCLE)   **168, 273, 274**
cyclic neutropenia, canine   **283**
cytology   57–80
   adhesive tape-strip   60
   algorithmic approach   78, *79*
   cell types   64–70
   common pitfalls and mistakes   78–80
   findings   64–78
   fine-needle aspirates   64
   immune-mediated diseases   159–160, **160,** *160–161*
   impression smears   60–61
   indications   57–60, 85, *85*
   inflammatory lesions   70–71
   kunkers, tissue grains or sulphur granules   62
   lymph node   71
   microorganisms   71–76
   microscope set-up   11
   needle cores   63–64
   neoplasia   59–60, 76–78
   otic *see* otic cytology
   staining methods   12–13
   techniques   60–64

dark field microscopy   11
deafness   255
Demodex   36, *40*
   cytology   62, *62–63*
   ear canal samples   25, *29*
   hair plucks   29, *30*, 50, *50*
   host faeces   34, *35*
   PCR test   36
   purulent material   33
   secondary infection   193, *194*
   skin scrapes   22, 32, *32*, *33*
   tape-strips   29
Dermacentor reticularis   *40*
dermal atrophy   113
dermatohistopathology *see* histopathology
dermatomyositis   **273, 274**

Dermatophagoides spp.   146, **147**
Dermatophilus   61
dermatophytes
   coat brushings   *87*, 87–88
   cultures   5, *6*, 99–101
   cytology   72–73, *73*
   dermoscopy   55, *56*, 99
   hair plucks   50–52, *52*, 88
   microscope set-up   11
   PCR diagnosis   210–211
   reclassification   101
   sampling methods   *87*, 87–88
   species identification   100–101,
      100–101, **102**
   transient   81
   Wood's lamp examination   97–98,
      98
dermatophyte test medium (DTM)   5, *6*,
   99–101
   identifying pathogens   100–101,
      100–101, **102**
   interpreting growth   99–100
   sample transfer   87, *88*
dermoscopes   53, *54*
dermoscopy   53–56
   dermatophytosis   55, *56*, 99
   uses   **55,** 55–56
dexamethasone suppression test
   cats   194
   high dose (HDDST)   192
   low dose (LDDST)   186–187, 189,
      189–191
   urinary cortisol:creatinine ratio
      (UCCR)   190–192, 195
dietary exclusion trials *see* food trials
dietary history   130
diet challenge   144
Diff-Quik® type stains   5, 12–13, **16**
diffuse dermatitis   121
discoid lupus erythematosus (DLE)   **168,**
   273, 274
dorsoventral (DV) view, tympanic
   bulla   217, **220,** *221*
doxycycline   **96**
dry eye and curly coat syndrome   **282**
dwarfism, pituitary   196, **283**
dyskeratosis   112

ear
   anatomy, dog   *242*
   examination   235–246
ear canal
   biopsy   255–256
   canalography   223, 246
   hairy   244, *244*
   normal appearance   *243*, 243–244
   radiographic changes   217, *218–219*,
      220, **220**
   sample collection   5, *5*, 25, 62–63, 89
   stenosis   *219*, 246
   visual inspection   238–240, *239*, *264*
   see also otic cytology; otoscopy
ear cleaners   240
ear cones, otoscopic   240, 241, 246
ear disease   235–256
   bacterial cultures   253
      see also antimicrobial sensitivity
        testing
   biopsy   255–256
   canalography   223, 246
   CT scanning   224–225, *226*, 247
   cytology *see* otic cytology
   imaging   215–225
   middle ear evaluation   254–255
   MRI   224, 247
   radiography   216–223
   ultrasonography   223–224
ear margin vasculitis   **273**
ear mites   22, *27*, 244
ectodermal dysplasia – skin fragility
   syndrome   **282**
ectoparasites *see* parasites
ectothrix spores   52, *52*, 72, **102**
Ehrlichia   210
electron microscopy (EM)   211
ELISA (enzyme-linked immunosorbent
   assay)   201, *201*
endocrine disease   173–197
   biochemical tests   179–180
   clinical signs   173–174
   haematology   177–179
   hair plucks   178
   imaging   226–229
   specific tests   181–197
   urine analysis   180–181

enrofloxacin   92–93, 95, **96**
enterococci   75
environmental allergens
  allergy testing   145–157
  extracts and mixes   146–148
  selection   146, **147–148**
  see also allergy testing
environmental parasites   35
eosinophilic granuloma   *59*
eosinophils   *68*, 68–69, 71
epidermal atrophy   113
epidermal hyperplasia   112
epidermal necrosis   114–115
epidermolysis bullosa
  acquisita (EBA)   **168, 273, 275**
  dystrophic   **282**
  junctional   **282**
epidermolytic hyperkeratosis
  (EHK)   **282**
epiluminescence microscopy *see*
  dermoscopy
epinephrine   107
epithelial cell tumours   76
epitheliotropic lymphoma   120
equipment   1–6
  essential   1–5
  optional   5–6
erosions   272–275, **273–275**
erythema chronica migrans   209
erythema multiforme (EM)   *116*, **168,**
  273, **276**
erythrocytes   64–65, *65*
erythromycin   **96**
erythropoietin   178
Escherichia coli   95, 253
Eutrombicula (chiggers)   22, 35
exclamation point hairs   45, *46*
exclusion diets
  commercial   131–141, **132–140**
  home-cooked   130–131, **131**
  hydrolysed foods   **132–140,**
    141
exocytosis   113, *113*
extended spectrum beta-lactamase
  (ESBL) producing organisms   95,
  96
external laboratories   15–17

faecal examination,
  ectoparasites   34–35, *35*
familial cutaneous vasculopathy   **273**
Felicola subrostraus   *39*
feline calicivirus (FCV)   212
feline hyperthyroidism *see*
  hyperthyroidism, feline
feline immunodeficiency virus
  (FIV)   *213*, 213–214
feline leukaemia virus (FeLV)   214
feline lung digit syndrome   231, *231*
feline paraneoplastic alopecia   231
feline thymoma-associated exfoliative
  dermatitis   *119*, 232
FIAD *see* food-induced atopic dermatitis
fibroblasts   67
fine-needle aspirates   5, *7*, 64
  see also cytology
Finn chamber   156
flea allergic dermatitis (FAD)   37–38,
  128–129, 259
flea comb   2, *2*, 23, 24
flea faeces
  coat brushings   24
  tape-strips   28
  visual inspection   22, *26*
  wet-paper test   24, *28*
fleas   22, 37–38, *39*
  allergens   37
  eggs   24, *28*
fluorescence-activated flow cytometry
  (FACS)   204, *204*
fluorescent antibodies   204
follicular casts   46, *47*
folliculitis   122–124, **168**
food allergens   126–129
  cross-reactions   143–144
  serology and patch tests   145
food-induced atopic dermatitis
  (FIAD)   125–145
  allergen testing   145
  food trials   125–144
food trials   125–144
  compliance   142–143
  dietary options   130–141
  diet challenge   144
  duration   141–142

managing animals during   143
see also exclusion diets
footpad hyperkeratosis   **282**
forceps, fine-tipped   *2*, 4, 41, *42*
formalin   5, 207
fractured hairs   46, *48*
fructosamine   179
fungal cultures   83–89, 99–101
    antifungal susceptibility testing   104
    identifying pathogens   100–101,
        100–101, **102**
    indications   83–85
    interpretation   99–100
    media   99
    sample collection   85–89
    see also dermatophytes
fungi
    commensal   81
    cytology   71–74
    detecting unusual   103–104
    identification   97–104
    mucosal reservoirs   83
    stains   14–15
    transient   81
    see also dermatophytes
furuncles, sampling from   33, 61, 89
furunculosis   122, 123

genetic conditions   **282–284**
genetics   277–287
genetic terms, glossary   **286**
genetic tests   280–287
    results   281–284
    submitting samples   280–281
    uses   284–285, **285**
gentamicin   **96**
German Shepherd dog pyoderma   **273**
giant cells, multinucleate   70, 71
Giemsa stain   14, **16**
glucagon assay   197
glucocorticoids   106, 143, **149,** 241,
        255
glucose   180
glutens   130
Gram staining   14, **16**
granulocytes   70
grey collie syndrome   **283**

Grocott–Gomori's methenamine
        silver   **16**
growth hormone (GH)   196

haematoxylin and eosin (H&E)   15, **16**
hair bulb abnormalities   45
hair follicle
    growth phase   42–44, *43*
    pathology   122–124
hair plucks   41–52
    endocrine and metabolic
        disease   175–176
    findings   42–52
    fungal cultures   88
    parasites   29–31, *30*, 50
    technique   41–42, *42*
hair removal
    biopsy site   106–107
    equipment   3–4
    intradermal allergy testing   150, *150*
hairs
    dermoscopy   55–56, *56*, 99
    normal   46, *47*
    pigmentation   48–50, *49*
    Wood's lamp examination   97–98, *98*
hair shaft
    abnormalities   48
    defects   46–48
hand lens   2, 21
harvest mites *(Trombicula)*   22, *26*, 35
head shape, ear imaging and   217, 220,
        221, 223
heat fixation   13
Henry's pocket   21
hepatocutaneous syndrome   196–197,
        196–197, 230, *230*
hereditary equine regional dermal
        asthenia (HERDA)   **282**
hereditary nasal parakeratosis   **282,** 285
Herlitz junctional epidermolysis
        bullosa   **282**
herpesvirus, feline   212
hidradenitis   122
high-dose dexamethasone/ACTH test,
        feline combined   194
high-dose dexamethasone suppression
        test (HDDST)   192

histiocytes 69, *69*
histiocytic sarcoma 77
histiocytoma, benign cutaneous 77
histopathology 17, 105–124
    hair follicle pathology 122–124
    immune-mediated skin
        diseases 160–164
    indications 105
    non-specific/misleading results 110
    pattern analysis 116–122, **117**
    report interpretation 110–124
    terminology 111–115
Histoplasma 73
honeycomb pattern, liver 230, *230*
house dust mites 146, **147**
hydrolysed diets **132–140,** 141
    see also food trials
hydropic degeneration of cells 113–114
Hydrotaea 35
17-hydroxyprogesterone (17OHP) 187,
        189–190, 195
hyperadrenocorticism (HAC) (Cushing's)
    adrenal dependent (ADH) 187–188,
        189, 192
    biochemical tests 179–180
    cats 174, *178*, 193–195, *194*
    clinical signs 173–174, *177, 177–178*
    confirmatory tests 185–195
    dynamic testing 186–192
    ferrets 186
    haematology tests 178
    iatrogenic 188, *188*
    imaging 195, 226–229, *227, 228*
    pituitary dependent (PDH) 189, *189,*
        191, 192
    urine analysis 19, 180, 186
hyperandrogenism 195
hypercholesterolaemia 179
hyperkeratosis 112, **168**
hyperoestrogenism 195
hyperpigmentation **117,** 269–271
hyperthyroidism, feline
    biochemical tests 180, 184–185
    clinical signs 173
    haematology tests 178, 179
    imaging 229
    urine tests 181

hyphae, fungal 72, 73, *73*
hypopigmentation **117,** 271
hypopituitarism 196
hypothyroidism, canine
    biochemical tests 179, 181–184
    clinical signs 173, *174–176*
    congenital **283**
    haematology tests 178
    imaging 229
    therapeutic trial 184
    trichograms 173, *176*

ichthyosis 269, *271,* **282,** 287
IGRA *see* interferon gamma release assay
imaging, diagnostic 215–234
    ear disease 215–225
    endocrine disease 226–229
    paraneoplastic syndromes 229–233
immersion oil 3, *4*
immune-mediated haemolytic anaemia
        (IHA) 169–170
immune-mediated skin
        diseases 159–171
    biopsy and histopathology 160–164,
        168
    cytology 159–160, **160,** *160–161*
    immunostaining 164–169
    other tests 171
    routine tests 159–160
    serology 169–171
    urinary protein 171
immune-mediated thrombocytopenia
        (ITP) 170
immunostaining 164–169
impression smears 60–61
    direct 60–61
    examination 64–78
    indirect 61
    wet-prep 61
indirect fluorescent antibody (IFA or
        IFAT) 204
infectious diseases 199–214
    diagnosis 205–211
    laboratory techniques 199–204
    virology techniques 211–214
inflammatory cells 67–70
inflammatory lesions 70–71, 106

inflammatory polyps,
    nasopharyngeal   215, **220**
inheritance   277–279
injection site vasculitis   **273**
insects   *39*
insulin-like growth factor-1 (IGF-1),
    plasma   196
interface dermatitis   117–120, *119*, **168**
interferon gamma release assay
    (IGRA)   **103,** 103–104
internal (in-house) laboratory   15–17
International Committee on Allergic
    Diseases in Animals
    (ICADA)   125, 148
International Society of Veterinary
    Dermatopathology (ISVD)   105
intradermal allergen tests
    (IDTs)   146–155
  consensus guidelines   149, **150**
  drug withdrawal   148–149, **149**
  equipment   6, *8*
  evaluation   153–155, *154–155*
  flea allergic dermatitis   37–38
  procedure   149–153, *151–153*
  see also allergy testing
intra-epidermal bullous or pustular
    dermatitis   121
ivermectin sensitivity   **283**
Ixodes ticks   *40*

karyorrhexis   67
keratinocytes   65, *66*, 248, *248*
keratohyalin   76
Kirby-Bauer disc diffusion test   90–92,
    91
Koehler (Köhler) illumination   10, *10*
KOH *see* potassium hydroxide
kunkers   62

laboratories, internal and
    external   15–17
lactate dehydrogenase (LDH)   180
lactophenol cotton blue   5, 14–15
Lagendium   73–74
lamellar hyperkeratosis   112
lateral oblique (LO) view, tympanic
    bulla   217–220, **220,** *221*

lateral view, tympanic bulla   **220,** 223
lavender foal syndrome   **284**
Leishmania   205–209
  bone marrow samples   206–209
  cytology   76, 205, *205*
Leishman's stain   14, **16**
lentigo   269
leptocytes   178
lethal acrodermatitis   **282**
lethal white foal syndrome   **284**
leucocyte adhesion deficiency type III
    (LAD III)   **283**
lice   22, *39*
lichenification   112, **274**
lichenoid band   **168**
lighting   1
ligneous membranitis   **284**
linear IgA dermatosis   **275**
Linognathus setosus   *39*
lipids, serum   179, 180
lipomas   76
liquid paraffin   2, 4, *5*
  coat brushings   24
  ear canal samples   25
  hair plucks   29, 41
  purulent material   33
  skin scrapes   31, 32
  vs. potassium hydroxide   34
liver enzymes   179, 180
long coat mutation   **282**
louse eggs (nits)   *39, 50, 51*
low-dose dexamethasone suppression test
    (LDDST)   186–187, 189,
    189–191
luminal folliculitis   122
lung digit syndrome, feline   231, *231*
lupus vasculitis   **168**
Lyme disease (borreliosis)   209
lymph node cytology   71
lymphoblasts   70, 71
lymphocytes   70, 71
lymphoid cells   70
lymphoma   77, *77*, 120

Mackenzie brush technique   87, 87–88
  see also dermatophytes; fungal cultures
macroconidia   72–73, *73, 74,* **102**

macromelanosomes   48–50, *49*
macrophages   *69*, 69–70
macular melanosis   269
macules   271, 272
magnetic resonance imaging (MRI)   247
  ear disease   224, *225*, 247
  hyperadrenocorticism   192, 228
  other uses   234
magnifying glass   2
magnifying lenses   2, *2*
Maillard reaction   129
Malassezia
  allergy testing   156
  cytology   71–72, *72*
  lesion distribution   **128, 129**
  otic cytology   248, *249–250*, 253
  otic discharge   240
  video-otoscopy   *245*
male feminisation syndrome   195
malignancy, cytological features   78
marbofloxacin   92–93, **96**
marking, skin   5
  biopsy site   107
  intradermal allergy testing   150, *151*
mast cells   70
mast cell tumours, cytology   *59*, 59–60,
  77
May–Grünwald stain   14
melanin   48–50, *49*, 75
melanoma   78
melanosis, macular   269
mesenchymal cells   67, 76
metabolic epidermal necrosis *see*
  hepatocutaneous syndrome
metabolic skin diseases   173–197
methylene blue   15
meticillin-resistant *Staphylococcus aureus*
  (MRSA)   95, **96**
meticillin-resistant *Staphylococcus*
  pseudintermedius (MRSP)   95, **96**
microbiome, skin   81, *82*
micrococci   75
microconidia   72, *73*, **102**
micromelanosomes   48, *49*, 75
microorganisms
  commensal   81, *82*
  culture and identification   83–104

cytology   71–76
  extracellular   71, 74–75
  intracellular   71
  mucosal reservoirs   83
  transient   81
microscope   2, *3*, 7–12
  buying guidelines   7–8
  cleaning   3, 12
  dark field microscopy   11
  essential equipment   3, *4*
  eye-pieces and illumination   9–11,
    10
  location   9
  scanning the field   11–12
  set-up   9–11
Microsporum audouinii   98
Microsporum canis   97–98, *100, 101*,
  102
Microsporum distortum   98
Microsporum gypseum   **102**
Microsporum nanum   **102**
middle ear
  evaluation   254–255
  radiographic changes   **220**
  sample collection   63, 89, 254
  ultrasonography   223–224
minimum inhibitory concentration
    (MIC)   90–95, *91*
  breakpoints   92, 93
  calculating drug doses   93, 94
  intermediate results   94
  predicting treatment response   92–94,
    93
  topical therapy and   94–95
  vs. Kirby-Bauer disc diffusion   90–92
  see also antimicrobial sensitivity testing
mites   *39, 40*
monocytes   69–70
MRI *see* magnetic resonance imaging
mucocutaneous lupus erythematosus
    (MCLE)   **168, 273**
mucosal reservoirs   83
mucous membrane pemphigoid
    (MMP)   **168, 273, 274, 275**
multinucleate giant cells   70, 71
mural folliculitis   122, **168**
mural isthmic folliculitis   **273**

mutant prevention concentration (MPC)   97, *97*
mycobacteria
  cytology   71, 75
  identification   **103,** 103–104
  staining   15
mycosis fungoides   120
myringotomy   63, 254–255

nail loss   **274**
necrolysis   115
necrolytic migratory erythema *see* hepatocutaneous syndrome
necrosis   114–115, **168**
needle cores   63–64
negative predictive value (NPV)   18–19
neoplasia
  cell types   76
  cytology   59–60, 76–78
  malignancy   78
Neospora   76
Neotrombicula see harvest mites
neutrophils   67, *68*
  degenerate (toxic)   67, *68*, 70
  non-degenerate   67
Nikolskiy's sign   273, **275**
nitrofurantoin   **96**
nits (louse eggs)   *39*, 50, *51*
Nivea Clear-Up Strips   29
nodular dermatitis   120, **168**
nodular dermatofibrosis   232–233, *232–233*, **284**
nodules   **117**
non-thyroidal illness (NTI)   179, 181, 183, 185
  see also hypothyroidism; thyroid function tests
Northern blot   199, *200*
Notoedres   *40*
nuclear streaming   67, *68*

oclacitinib   143
oedema, intracellular   *113*, 113–114
oestrogen   195
one-stain method   13
orthokeratotic hyperkeratosis   112, 269

otic cytology   *62*, 62–63, 247–253
  interpretation   248–253
  parasites   25
  sample collection   62–63, 247–248
  sample fixation   63, 240, 247
  see also ear disease
otic discharge   240, 244
  cultures   86, *86*
otic neoplasia   224, *225*, 253
otitis externa   215, 263–265
  antimicrobial sensitivity testing   92–93, *93*, 253
  clinical signs   215, 216, *264*
  cytology   247, 248–253, *249–252*
  minimum database   265
  otic discharge   240
  otoscopy   244–246, *245*
  radiography   *218–219*, **220**
otitis interna   215
otitis media   215
  clinical signs   215, 216
  imaging   **220,** 223–225, *225*, *226*
  sample collection   254–255
Otobius   22, 244
Otodectes   36, *40*
  cytology   25, 62–63
  otic discharge   240
  visual inspection   22, *27*, 244
otological examination   235–246
otoscopes   3, *4*, 240, *241*
  cleaning   246
  types   243
otoscopy   240–246
  abnormal findings   *244–245*, 244–246
  detection of parasites   21–22
  normal findings   *243*, 243–244
  procedure   241–243, *242*

panniculitis   122
papillated/papillomatous acanthosis   112
papillomaviruses   212
papules   271, 272
parakeratotic hyperkeratosis   112, 269
paraneoplastic associated skin disease   229–233
paraneoplastic pemphigus   162, 165

parasites   21–38, 257
  coat brushings   24–25
  common mistakes and pitfalls   38
  environmental   35
  faecal examination   34–35
  hair plucks   29–31, *30*, 50
  identification guide   38, *39–40*
  KOH vs. liquid paraffin   34
  management during diet trials   143
  microscope set-up   11
  purulent material   33
  skin scrapes   31–33
  tape-strips   26–29
  test specificity and sensitivity   35–38
  vacuuming   34
  visual inspection   21–23
patch testing   156–157
  food allergens   145
  open   157, *157*
PCR *see* polymerase chain reaction
pemphigoid of gestation   **275**
pemphigus erythematosus   162, 164,
    165, **168**
pemphigus foliaceus (PF)   **273**
  cytology   *66*, 67, 159, **160**, *160*, *161*
  histopathology   *113–115*, 114, *120*,
    163, *164*, **168**
  immunostaining   167
  lesions to biopsy   162, *162*, *163*
  otic cytology   253
  pinnal   238, *239*
  serology   169
  vs. pyoderma   67, **160**, **272**
pemphigus vegetans (Pveg)   **168**
pemphigus vulgaris (PV)   **168**, **275**
  histopathology   162, 165, *166*
  serology   169
perifolliculitis   122
periodic acid-Schiff (PAS)   15, **16**
peripheral neuropathy   **128**, 259
perivascular dermatitis   116–117, *118*
petrous temporal bone, sclerosis   220,
    220
pigmentary changes   269–271
pigmentary incontinence   115, *116*
pigmentation, hair   48–50, *49*
pinged hairs   45

pinnae
  alopecia   *237*, 238
  curling, in cats   238, *239*
  erythema   *237*, 238, *238*
  examination   235–238, *236–238*
  pemphigus foliaceus   238, *239*
pinnal–pedal scratch reflex   37, 235–238
piperacillin   93, *93*
pituitary dwarfism   196, **283**
pituitary tumours   192, 228, *228*
plasma cells   70
plasmacytoma   77–78
platelet factor 3 test   170
pollen grains, faecal   34, 35
pollens, allergy testing   **147–148**
polymerase chain reaction (PCR)   103,
    199–200, *200*, 210–211
polyomavirus, avian   214
positive predictive value (PPV)   18–19
potassium hydroxide (KOH)   4
  coat brushings   24
  ear canal samples   25
  hair plucks   29, 41
  skin scrapes   31, 32
  vs. liquid paraffin   34
poxvirus   212
precipitation test   202, *203*
prednisolone   106, 143
primary skin lesions
  ectoparasites   31, *31*
  fungal and bacterial cultures   86
  histopathology   106, **106**
processed foods   129–130
proteinuria   171, 180, 181
Proteus   75, 253
Prototheca   74
protozoa   76
pruritus   257–263, 276
  allergy testing   125–126, 146
  diagnostic algorithm   *127*
  differential diagnosis in cats   261–262,
    263
  differential diagnosis in
    dogs   **128–129**, *258–259*,
    258–260
  histopathology   **117**
  management during diet trials   143

minimum database in dogs   260–261, *261*, 262–263
pseudocarcinomatous acanthosis   112
Pseudomonas   75
    antimicrobial sensitivity
        testing   92–93, *93*, 94–95, 253
    otic cytology   *68*, *252*, 253
    otic discharge   240
pseudopelade   **168, 274**
psittacine beak and feather disease
        (PBFD)   214
psoriasiform acanthosis   112
Psoroptes   23, 24, 34
punch biopsy   107–108
purulent material
    impression smears   61
    kunkers, tissue grains or sulphur
        granules   62
    sampling   33, *58*, 86, *86*, 89
pustular dermatitis
    intra-epidermal   121
    subepidermal   121
pustules   271, 272
    histopathology   **117,** 121
    immune-mediated diseases   **168**
    pemphigus foliaceus   162, *162*
    sample collection   33, *58*, 61, *86*, 89
pycnosis, nuclear   67
pyoderma (staphylococcal)
    bacterial cultures   *84*
    canine hypothyroidism   173, *175*
    cytology   67, *85*, 159, **160,** *161*
    sample collection   *58*, 86
    serology tests   169
    vs. pemphigus foliaceus   67, **160, 272**
pyogranulomatous inflammation   70
Pythium   73–74

radiography
    ear disease   216–223
    hyperadrenocorticism   229
    other uses   231, 232, 234
radio-immunoassay (RIA)   201–202
Rapi-Diff® stains   **16**
'rat tail'
    canine hyperadrenocorticism   174, *177*

canine hypothyroidism   173, *176*
raw foods   129–130
red blood cells   64–65, *65*
referral, specialist   276
renal cystadenocarcinoma   232, **284**
resident bacteria and fungi   81
rheumatoid factor (RF)   170–171
Rhipicephalus   40
rod-shaped bacteria (bacilli)   75, 83, *83*
Romanowsky-type stains, modified   4, 12–14, **16**
rostrocaudal open-mouth (ROM) view, tympanic bulla   **220,** 220–222, *222*
round cell tumours   76, 77–78

Sabouraud agar   87, *88*, 99
sample collection
    bacterial and fungal cultures   85–89
    cytology   60–64
    equipment   2, *2*, 4, 5, *5*
    hair plucks and trichograms   41–42, *42*
    parasites   24–35
sample containers   5, 6, 109–110
sample submission, to external
        laboratory   17, 109–110
Sarcoptes mites   36–37, *40*
    serology   18–19, 37
sarcoptiform mites   *40*
satellitosis   115
scaling   21, 23, 269, *271*, **274**
    differential diagnosis   **270**
    histopathological patterns   **117**
    minimum database   269
scalpel blades   2, 5, 32
scintigraphy, thyroid   229
scissors, curved   4
sebaceous adenitis (SA)   122, **168**
sebaceous hyperplasia, ear
        canal   245–246
secondary skin lesions   106, **106**
self-trauma, trichograms   46, *48*
sensitivity, test   18–19
serology   200–204
    allergen-specific *see* allergen-specific
        (IgE) serology

serology (*Continued*)
  ectoparasites   37–38
  immune-mediated diseases   169–171
Sertoli cell tumours   174, 195
severe combined immunodeficiency
    (SCID)   **283**
sex hormone assays   195
sex-linked dominant disorders   279, *280*,
    281
sex-linked recessive disorders   277–279,
    279, **280**
Simonsiella   75, *75*
sinus tracts, draining   33, 61, 89, **274**
skin prick testing (SPT)   156
skin scrapes   *24*, 31–33
  common mistakes   38
  lesions to target   31, *31*
  technique   31–33, *32*, *33*
slides, microscope   *2*, 3, *4*, 11–12
smooth straight coat mutation   **282**
Southern blot   199
specialist referral   276
specific gravity (SG), urine   180, 181
specificity, test   18–19
specimen *see* sample
spindle cells   76
spongiosis   113, *113*
Sporothrix   73
spur cells   67
stains   5–6, 12–15, **16**
  cytology   12–13
  specialized   14–15
  tape-strips   13, 14–15, 60
staphylococci   75, 156, 253
  see also pyoderma
Staphylococcus aureus   90
  meticillin-resistant (MRSA)   95, **96**
Staphylococcus pseudintermedius   90,
    90, 248
  meticillin-resistant (MRSP)   95, **96**
steroid hepatopathy   179, 229
Stevens–Johnson syndrome (SJS)   **168,**
    273, **276**
sticky tape *see* adhesive tape
storage mites   **147**
streptococci   75
stress leucogram   178, 179

subepidermal bullous or pustular
    dermatitis   121
Sudan stains   15, **16**
sulphamethoxazole   **96**
sulphur granules   62
surgical kit, basic   5
swabs, bacteriology   5, *5*, 88–89
  external ear   89
  middle ear   63, 89
  skin sampling   88–89
symmetric lupoid onychodystrophy
    (SLO)   **168, 274**
syringes   5, *7*
syringohydromelia   **128,** 257, 259
systemic lupus erythematosus
    (SLE)   **168, 273**
  bullous   **168, 275**
  serology   169–170, 171

T3 (triiodothyronine)
  autoantibodies (T3AAs)   181–182
  free (fT3)   *181*
  suppression test   185
  total (TT3)   *181*, 183, 185
T4 (thyroxine)
  autoantibodies (T4AAs)   181–182
  free (fT4)   *181*, 182–183
  free, by equilibrium dialysis
      (fT4ed)   182–183, 185
  total (TT4)   *181*, 182, 185
tape-strips   *2*, 5
  common mistakes   38
  cytology   60
  ectoparasites   *23*, 26–29
  staining   13, 14–15, 60
telogen effluvium   44
telogen hairs   42–44, *43*, 44
tests, choosing appropriate   257–276
tetracycline   **96**
third phalanx (P3) amputation   108
thymoma-associated exfoliative
    dermatitis, feline   *119*, 232
thyroglobulin autoantibodies
    (TgAAs)   183
thyroid function tests
  canine hypothyroidism   181–184
  drugs influencing   181

dynamic   184, 185
  feline hyperthyroidism   184–185
thyroid hormones   *181*, 181–183
thyroiditis, autoimmune
      (lymphocytic)   182, 183
thyroid-releasing hormone (TRH)
      response test   184, 185
thyroid scintigraphy   229
thyroid-stimulating hormone (TSH)
  canine (cTSH)   183
  feline   185
  response test   184, 185
thyroid tumours   229
ticarcillin   93, *93*
ticks   22, *39, 40*
tissue grains   62
tobramycin   93, *93*
toluidine blue   **16**
toothbrushes   5, *6*, 87, *87*
topical antibiotic therapy   94–95
toxic epidermal necrolysis (TEN)   **168,**
      273, **276**
Toxoplasma   76
'tragic' facial expression   173, *175*
transient microorganisms   81
transmissible venereal tumour   78
trapped neutrophil syndrome   **283**
treats, food   143
Treponema paraluiscuniculi   210
Trichodectes canis   *39*
trichograms   29, 41–52
  canine hypothyroidism   173, *176*
  follicular casts   46, *47*
  hair bulb abnormalities   45
  hair follicle growth phase   42–44, *43*
  hair shaft defects   46–48
  normal   46, *47*
  pigmentation   48–50, *49*
  pruritic cats   261, *262*
  technique   41–42
Trichophyton equinum   99, **102**
Trichophyton mentagrophytes   *100, 101,*
      102
Trichophyton schoenleinii   98
Trichophyton terrestre   *73*
Trichophyton verrucosum   **102**
trichorrhexis nodosa   46–48

triglycerides, serum   179, 180
Trixacarus caviae   *40*
Trombicula see harvest mites
two-stain method   12–13
tympanic bulla radiographic
      series   217–223
  changes detected   217, *218–219,*
      220
  patient positioning   217, 220,
      221–222, 223
tympanic membrane (TM)
  assessing integrity   246–247
  deliberate rupture *see* myringotomy
  otoscopic appearance   *243*, 243–244
  ruptured   63, 245, *245*, 246–247
tympanometry   247
Tzanck test, positive   253

ulcers   272–275, **273–275**
  cytology   58, *59*
ultrasonography
  hepatocutaneous syndrome   230, *230*
  hyperadrenocorticism   195, 226–228,
      227
  middle ear   223–224
  nodular dermatofibrosis   233, *233*
urea nitrogen, blood (BUN)   180
urinary cortisol:creatinine ratio
      (UCCR)   19, 186
  dexamethasone suppression
      test   190–192, 195
  feline   195
urinary tract infections   180
urine analysis   171, 180–181
uveodermatological syndrome   **273, 274**

vacuuming, skin   34
vasculitis   121, **168, 273, 274**
vasculopathy   **168**
venereal tumour, transmissible   78
ventrodorsal view, tympanic bulla   223
video-otoscope   *6, 9*, 63, 243
virology   211–214
virus isolation   211

Warmblood fragile foal syndrome   **282**
wedge excision biopsy   108

wet-paper test, flea faeces   24, *28*
wet-prep impression smears   61
Wood's lamp   *2*, 3
    examination   97–98, *98*
Wright's (Wright–Giemsa) stains,
        modified   12–14, **16**
Wright stain   14, **16**

X-linked severe combined
    immunodeficiency
    (X-SCID)   **284**

Ziehl–Nielsen (ZN) stain   15, **16**
zone of inhibition (ZI)   90, 92
    see also antimicrobial sensitivity testing

Printed and bound by CPI Group (UK) Ltd, Croydon, CR0 4YY
25/05/2022
03125735-0001